The Weight of Grace

The Weight of Grace

EXPERIENCE THE FREEDOM FROM OVEREATING
THAT YOU ALREADY HAVE

PAULA NEALL COLEMAN

In Collaboration with
Scope Ministries International, Inc.

Weight of Grace Ministries, Inc., Gladstone, MO 64118
© 2008 by Weight of Grace Ministries, Inc.
Printed in the United State of America
ISBN 978-0-9798487-0-4

All Scripture quotations, unless otherwise indicated, are taken from the *Holy Bible, New International Version*®. NIV®. Copyright © 1973, 1978, 1984 by International Bible Society. Used by permission of Zondervan Publishing House. All rights reserved.

Scripture quotations marked "KJV" are from the King James Version.

Scripture quotations marked "NASB" are taken from the *New American Standard Bible*®, © Copyright The Lockman Foundation 1960, 1962, 1963, 1968, 1971, 1972, 1973, 1975, 1977, 1995. Used by permission.

Scripture quotations marked "AMP" are taken from the *Amplified Bible*, Copyright © 1954, 1958, 1962, 1964, 1965, 1987 by The Lockman Foundation. Used by permission.

Scripture quotations marked "NKJV™" are taken from the New King James Version®. Copyright © 1982 by Thomas Nelson, Inc. Used by permission. All rights reserved.

Scripture quotations marked "GNT" are taken from the *Good News Translation - Second Edition* © 1992 by American Bible Society. Used by permission.

Cover design by Reagan Coyle.
Cover concept suggested by Tena Ford.

For the grace of God that brings salvation has appeared to all men. It teaches us to say "No" to ungodliness and worldly passions, and to live self-controlled, upright and godly lives in this present age…

Titus 2:11-12

CONTENTS

DIAGRAMS

ACKNOWLEDGEMENTS

In the 1960's, Jim Craddock, an area director for Campus Crusade for Christ, was challenged by Christian psychologist Henry Brandt to explore the Scriptures for answers to the many problems Jim was observing in the family lives of fellow believers. Jim's dedicated and intense study of the Bible eventually led him to establish Scope Ministries International, which has offered to countless people insights and discipleship leading to Christ-centered emotional healing.

I was one of the broken people who sought counsel at Scope Ministries International, and my experience there resulted in such transformation that I decided to join Scope's staff so that I could participate in extending to others the freedom I had found in Christ. Many of the concepts presented in this book are inspired by and adapted from the writings and teaching of Jim Craddock and others on Scope's staff, such as Terry Coy, Steve Johnson, Judi Boyer, Donna Edwards, Richard Patzke, and Dub Rogers. This book exists because they were faithful in diligent Christian service and because Scope offered an environment in which I could minister to women in the context of small groups.

Going from leading small groups to writing a book was a long journey, which started with a challenge from Scope contributor Jody Humber in early 1998. He asked me if I was ready to turn my small group materials into a book and video series, and I surprised myself by answering, "Yes, and its title will be *The Weight of Grace*." Shortly after Jody threw down the gauntlet, Mike Coleman asked me to marry him. Mike has been my greatest supporter and biggest fan ever since. A few months after our wedding, I started working on the first draft of this book. I cannot thank Mike enough for his unwavering encouragement and unconditional love.

I would like to sincerely thank my partners in Weight of Grace Ministries, Inc., Lydia Rose, Harry Rose, and Francie Martin. They have generously given of themselves to join me in fulfilling the vision of making this book a reality. Others who have given advice, assistance, and encouragement are Robin and Karen Noad, Marci Maddux, Kathy Young, Ethylen Wilson, Renee Ridgeway, editor Sharon Smith, and every generous donor to Weight of Grace Ministries.

I would also like to express my deep appreciation to all the women who so honestly and bravely shared their struggles and victories with one another and with me in Weight of Grace small groups over the past 16 years. These women never cease to amaze me with their fervor to live their lives in submission to God's will.

Of course, my greatest thanks goes to the Lord Jesus Christ, who has extended to me the grace and mercy that not only allowed me to overcome many years of torment obsessing over eating and weight, but also continually provided inspiration and affirmations that kept me on track through the long process of writing this book. And I know that it will only be through Christ's ministry in each reader's life that any of the information in this book will have a meaningful effect.

The Weight of Grace

EXPERIENCE THE FREEDOM FROM OVEREATING
THAT YOU ALREADY HAVE

WILL *YOU* BENEFIT FROM READING THIS BOOK?

The women who are helped most by the information presented in this book have certain experiences and behaviors in common. *See if you identify with most of the following*:

- ✓ You have tried several different diets only to regain the weight you lost – or you can't — seem to stick with a diet for long. You are sick of dieting and have given up on it.
- You feel God is disgusted with you for having so little self-discipline and for being so ~no~ fat.
- ✓ You eat when you're bored, angry, depressed, and/or lonely. *transitions, reward* — *transition*
- You feel you always have to eat a snack right at bedtime (or right before or after some other routine event) or you get up in the middle of the night to have a few cookies.
- ✓ You find yourself constantly thinking about food – especially about what you should *yes* and shouldn't eat – and about your weight. You want to stop obsessing about eating, dieting, your weight, and your appearance.
- ✓ You have told yourself to be obedient to God in this area and berated yourself for your — *no* disobedience, but you just don't ever change.

Even more important than these points is whether you are open to considering a whole new way of thinking about yourself, your eating, your body, and how God fits into these areas of your life. If that is true, you are certainly going to find a lot of freedom as a result of applying the concepts presented in this book.

This Is Not a Weight-Loss Program

Even though, over the past decade or so, there has been an increasing number of books and articles about the negative aspects of dieting, there seems to be little decrease in the number of women who address their overeating unsuccessfully through dieting. Many women still desperately hope to find that miracle diet that will finally work for them. Therefore, I want to make it clear at the outset that this book does *not* provide a weight-loss plan or a diet program. Instead, this approach is aimed at *revealing the underlying issues that motivate overeating and gaining a proper understanding of the work God has done and is doing in your life in order to set you free from overeating.* For some women – and this was the case for me – weight loss may be a byproduct of putting into practice the principles presented within this book, but that may not be the case for all women. This book will teach you how to appropriate the grace and truth of God in order to live your life without being obsessed with food, eating, dieting, your weight, and/or your appearance. It's likely that, up until now, you've considered "success" to be reaching a particular (very low) weight goal. Usually, that kind of "success" is hard to attain and even harder to maintain. If, however, you are more interested in living by God's truth and in the freedom of his grace than you are in rapid weight loss, you will find true success when you start applying the concepts presented in this book.

This approach is aimed at revealing the underlying issues that motivate overeating.

Dive on In!

Two of my closest friends – I'll call them Jane and Jodi – started on the "journey" toward freedom from overeating about the same time I did. A few years after we had "set out," we were comparing notes about our differing levels of success. Jodi noted that, even though we were exposed to the same biblical concepts and literature, the three of us had taken three different approaches as we tackled our struggle with overeating and "fat." She likened each approach to a recreational activity. Jane was compared to a person taking a tour in a helicopter, looking down at the scenery as it whizzed past below. She had scanned several of the books each of us purchased, but she hadn't actually read any of them! She listened to what we said about what we'd read and what we'd heard from God, but she hadn't read or heard any of it on her own. She just flew by and observed with interest what was going on with us "down on the ground." It was about two and half years after we'd started down this road when we had this little discussion about our progress, and Jane, the "helicopter rider," had almost no freedom from fairly extreme compulsive eating and purging behaviors.

Jodi likened herself to a water skier. She had skimmed over the surface of the materials and the issues they raised. She felt frightened about going very slowly because she might fall into the water and not be able to swim to the shore. She kept on moving, reading all the books, but never really thinking through what was presented. Some of the books we were reading had exercises in each chapter. She skipped the exercises to move quickly through each book. She covered a lot of territory but never got very wet. As a result, Jodi's overeating wasn't as intense at it had been before, but she was still obsessing about food and about wanting to lose weight.

I found total freedom from overeating, dieting, obsessing about my weight and appearance, and 24 years of binge eating.

Finally, Jodi compared me to a deep-sea diver. I'd plunged into the books, exercises, articles, and the Bible, and looked at everything there was "down there." I'd soaked myself in prayerfully considering the underlying issues. I'd gone very slowly, exploring and pondering each new concept I encountered. I'd stayed in the water until I looked like a prune! And, I'd found total freedom from overeating, dieting, obsessing about my weight and appearance, and 24 years of binge eating.

If you're reading this introductory section, there's hope for you. You've already taken a dip into the water. People who skip the introduction of a book are probably going to fly or water ski over the rest of it. So, be encouraged, you're already a likely candidate for getting a great deal of benefit from this book!

Two Are Better than One

Each chapter in this book is based on a weekly session of the 14-week Weight of Grace small groups I have led for the past 16 years. For at least two-thirds of each 100-minute session, group participants engage in discussion about a lesson that's been presented. During this discussion – and when women do the "homework" that is assigned every week – a lot of "light bulbs" go on for group members. The benefit these women receive from interacting with each other is reminiscent of Ephesians 4:15-16:

...speaking the truth in love, we will in all things grow up into him who is the Head, that is, Christ. From him the whole body, joined and held together by every supporting ligament, grows and builds itself up in love, as each part does its work.

When we share truth, in love, with one another – when we contribute to one another's lives – we do grow spiritually. You'll get the most from this book if you go through it with at least one other person and discuss with one another the questions and "homework" provided in each chapter. (There is more information about the book's format in the following brief section, "How to Effectively Use this Book's Format.")

An Open Bible Really Helps

God's Word has more effect on us than any other written document. Therefore, I hope you take the time to carefully read referenced Scripture passages. Take advantage of the Scripture's power to transform (Isaiah 55:11; John 17:17; Hebrews 4:12). It was in understanding Scripture that I realized and experienced the freedom I already had from overeating. My prayer is that you, too, will experience this same freedom.

Do You Know Your ABC's?

This book is directed to women who have faith in Jesus Christ. If you haven't yet put your faith and trust in Christ, let me encourage you that it is as simple as "**ABC**" – not necessarily easy, but simple.[1]

Acknowledge that you have sinned.
The word "sin" actually means "missing the mark" God has set for you. We all have missed the mark at some time or another! This sin separates us from God, and it's why we need to accept his forgiveness to spend eternity with him.
Romans 3:23: For all have sinned and fall short of the glory of God.

Believe in Jesus.
Belief is more than "head knowledge" of Jesus. It's a belief that leads to an action – placing your total trust and faith in Jesus for forgiveness of your sins.
Acts 16:31: Believe in the Lord Jesus, and you will be saved.

Commit your life to Jesus and follow him.
When you place your full trust in Jesus, you are surrendering control of your life to him, so it's only natural that you will want to live in a way that glorifies him. His Word in the Bible and the Holy Spirit who will live within you will guide you in living that life day-by-day.
Luke 9:23-24: Then he said to them all: "If anyone would come after me, he must deny himself and take up his cross daily and follow me. For whoever wants to save his life will lose it, but whoever loses his life for me will save it."

Then *pray...*
Placing your trust in Jesus begins with a simple prayer telling God that you cannot live up to his holy standards and need him to guide your life. You can receive Christ right now by simply talking with God, who is not as concerned with your words as he is with the attitude of your heart. Here is a suggested prayer:

> *Lord Jesus, I want to know you personally. Thank you for dying on the cross for my sins. I surrender my life to you and confess that you are my Savior and Lord. Thank you for forgiving me for my sins and giving me eternal life. Take control of my life. Make me the kind of person you want me to be.*

Does that prayer express what you desire in your heart? If it does, pray a prayer like this right now, and Christ will come into your life as he promised!

HOW TO EFFECTIVELY USE THIS BOOK'S FORMAT

The information in this book is most effective when two or more women go through it together. Each chapter is structured to facilitate group interaction and is divided into the following sections: (*See the Facilitator's Guide, provided on pages 271-274.*)

- *Presentation of Information*: The "lesson" portion for the chapter.
- *Reflection*: These are questions that are intended to help you apply the information presented in each chapter. Write your answers and discuss them with others who are reading the book also. Whether you're working through this book on your own or with friends, writing your answers to questions will be helpful. When you commit answers to writing, you have to face exactly what you're thinking rather than having some vague idea rolling around in your head. You'll get the most out of the reflection questions if you do not proceed to the next section of the chapter until you've discussed and/or written your answers.
- *What Others Have Experienced:* Once you've responded to the reflection questions, this section provides some food for thought that is based on my own experiences or on how women in Weight of Grace small groups have answered the questions. No fair reading ahead into this section, though, until you've already answered the reflection questions for yourself!
- *Homework:* These are exercises for you to do on your own. Sometimes the homework consists of simply reading an article that is provided, or you may be asked to write down your thoughts or fill in short answers. Usually, the homework takes between one and two hours to complete and is best done in one or two sittings. A few of the homework assignments involve an activity you'll need to repeat several times over the course of a few days. Completing homework is a vital part of making the kind of personal application necessary for you to experience change.

  Completing homework is a vital part of making the kind of personal application necessary for you to experience change.

- *Homework Follow-up:* These questions will enable you to meaningfully reflect on your homework and how it has affected your perspective. You'll benefit most from these questions if you write your answers and/or discuss them with others who are also going through the book *before* moving on to the last section of the chapter. If you're meeting weekly with others, it is probably best to save these questions for the opening of your next meeting.
- *Comments on the Homework:* This section discusses how other women have responded to the homework and/or provides additional pertinent information.

Over and over again, I have seen this format really flow, and I trust it will work for you and your group as well as it has for participants in previous Weight of Grace small groups.

Small Group Dynamics and Guidelines

You're probably familiar with the common wisdom that a small group is best kept to 12 members or fewer. (Jesus knew this way before the psychologists figured it out.) A group size limit certainly holds true for this material. I've conducted a Weight of Grace group in which 16 women regularly attended, and I was amazed at how everyone managed to participate to some degree in discussion. However, these women were all well acquainted with one another and encouraged each other to speak up. But, we rarely got to thoroughly discuss truly personal application for more than one or two participants during any one session. The best interaction I've seen has been in groups with four to six participants. We were able to get on a more intimate level, and each week each participant was able to discuss her personal application of the concepts. Also, there were just enough of us to have a variety of experiences to discuss and compare. As an aid for small groups making use of this book, on page 7 are the small group guidelines I use for Weight of Grace groups.

Even If It's Just You, Don't Go It Alone

Ask God to show you how the information being presented applies to you personally.

Whether you are going through this book with a friend, in a small group, or on your own, the most important person to invite into the process with you is God. Before you read each chapter, ask God to show you how the information being presented applies to you *personally*. Ask him to help you be honest with yourself. Ask him to help you through any shame that may be keeping you from facing some of the circumstances and thinking that have contributed to your overeating. Remember to apply the forgiveness of the Cross to areas where you have fallen short.

Invite God to help you do your homework. Ask him to bring to your mind the real answers to the questions rather than just the answers you think you *should* give. He knows much more about you than you do, and he remembers your life perfectly. He knows what's in the back of your mind that you don't admit to even yourself. This is where God helped me the most as I studied the Bible and read books – including doing the exercises in those books – regarding overeating and weight. There were a number of thoughts, beliefs, and feelings I hadn't admitted to myself and certainly to no one else. Once these came to light through prayer and what I call "prayerful pondering," I was able to change my mind about them. Also, once I started discussing with others some of my faulty thinking and the issues with which I struggled, I found that no one was repulsed or offended. Usually, others were relieved to know they weren't the only ones who had had thoughts and beliefs similar to mine. This type of sharing was enormously helpful in reinforcing the concepts I was learning and starting to apply.

As I write this, I am praying for you, each and every person who will read this book, and asking God to make this a journey that is not just a road to freedom from overeating, but also a path to greater intimacy with him.

WEIGHT OF GRACE
SMALL GROUP GUIDELINES

1. Every effort will be made to start and end on time.

2. Confidentiality:

   Nothing personal said in the group goes out of the group. When you go home and discuss your group experience with a friend or husband, share only what **you** gained or learned. Share no one else's experiences but your own. Do not share any names, descriptions of group members, occupations of members, etc., with people outside the group. During the week, do not discuss among yourselves any other group members. We all need to feel free to express ourselves openly without the fear of being discussed later, even by other group members.

3. Communication with each other:

   - Don't try to "fix" anyone else. That's God's job.

   - Use "I" statements, not "you" statements. An example would be, "I feel you may have misunderstood me," instead of, "You got that wrong!"

   - Keep Ephesians 4:15 and Ephesians 4:29 in mind as you interact with one another: (bold print indicates my emphasis)

     *...speaking the truth **in love**, we will in all things grow up into him who is the Head...*

     *Do not let any unwholesome talk come out of your mouths, but only what is **helpful for building others up according to their needs**, that it may benefit those who listen.*

   - You will get more out of the group if you participate by sharing your thoughts, experiences, and feelings. All the group participants will benefit from one another, so don't deprive others of your input. Your transparency will help you. Go ahead and risk judgment; it's better to be transparent and risk disapproval than to keep your thoughts to yourself. Trust that each member of the group wants the best for the other members.

1   HERE'S MY STORY – WHAT'S YOURS?

It was embarrassing! No, it was humiliating and I felt terribly ashamed. I was standing in my own kitchen, staring at a cabinet that was locked shut with a bicycle lock! While I was at work, my roommate had moved all of her groceries into one cabinet, placed the lock on it, and hidden the key. It seemed so extreme, but I knew it was her only way of making sure she'd have something to eat for breakfast in the morning. Almost every night, I raided the fridge and the cabinets, eating "everything that wasn't nailed down." Actually, I left most of the canned vegetables, but Karen really didn't enjoy green beans with her coffee!

How did it get this bad?! I had been a Christian for 12 years. I was in full-time Christian work, at a biblical counseling ministry no less. I was the assistant to the president and edited all of the counselor training materials, which meant I was very familiar with how Scripture applied to the struggles of life. Why then did I constantly fight – without ever winning for any length of time – the "battle of the bulge"? How many times had I pleaded with God to help me stick to a diet? How many times had I lost and regained the same 30 to 60 pounds?

Overeating and weight gain had plagued me since childhood. I started binge eating on candy and was considered a "chubby" girl when I was eight years old. I even stole change from my mother's purse in order to go to the local drugstore and tank up on Pixie Stix® and banana taffy. At ten, after a long bout with the flu, I was briefly very slender and started noticing that being thin garnered attention. The attention I especially liked was from the teenage boys who saw me walking home from school as they drove by and, assuming I was older than I was, gave me wolf whistles and asked me if I wanted a ride. It wasn't long, however, before I became chubby again. So, starting at the age of 11, deeply longing to regain the attention I'd had while slim, I was either on a diet or breaking a diet until shortly after I turned 31.

Overeating and weight gain had plagued me since childhood.

Through the years, my weight constantly yo-yoed, usually taking big swings every six to ten months. I could stay on a diet for several weeks, but I'd always reach a point at which I felt I had to either binge or die! When I wasn't dieting, I "grazed," continually nibbling and snacking on whatever food was available. Each day, I'd postpone taking my first bite, knowing that once I started eating, there was no end until bedtime. When I was 24, I stayed on a diet program for exactly one year without "cheating." The weeklong binge that followed was of such proportions that my friends still tell stories about it. By the time I was 30, I was regularly sticking to a strict diet for three days and then binge eating on the fourth.

The contradictions I saw in my life were extremely painful and bewildering. On the one hand, I appeared to others to epitomize the "committed Christian" who "had it all together" spiritually. But, on the inside, I felt like a failure. Far from living in Christian victory, I was expending a tremendous amount of emotional energy on obsessing over my weight, begging God to help me get thin, and worrying about every bite of food I ate. Even today, over 20 years later, I cringe when I remember the depression and self-loathing I felt during my late twenties when my overeating and weight were rapidly escalating.

The contradictions I saw in my life were extremely painful and bewildering.

In the fall of 1984, the locked cabinet was only one alarming sign that my life was becoming increasingly out of control. I had discovered a doctor's scale stashed away in one of the storage closets at work, and I was sneaking in there to weigh myself four or five times a day. I was constantly checking to make sure I didn't weigh as much as I thought or to beat myself up for the previous night's binge. Even worse, I was occasionally using laxatives to expel large meals and binges, thinking I would prevent the calories from getting a chance to "stick."

It was the potential of seriously abusing laxatives that scared me enough to venture into a new way of thinking about my eating and weight. A friend was hospitalized for bulimia and complications from laxative abuse. Witnessing her struggles caused me to become terrified of the intestinal problems that might result from my purging through laxatives. I felt I had to take action before I ended up in a hospital bed too. Thinking I could forego hospitalization if I did the "treatment" on my own, I bought all the books my friend's doctors recommended. Starting with the first book, even though it was secular, I felt as though I had been hit with a bolt of lightening. Because the author was describing how women's beliefs motivate their overeating, it suddenly dawned on me how the biblical counseling concepts to which I'd been exposed for years applied to my battle with overeating. This was the beginning of the end – the end of all the diets, binge eating, obsessions with food, and multiple wardrobes. But the end came through a process, a process I want to lead you through in the course of reading this book.

The title of the first book I read can sound offensive to some evangelical Christians because of negative associations with modern "feminism," but what this book said made a lot of sense. *Fat Is a Feminist Issue* by Susie Orbach pointed out various reasons why women, more than men, struggle with overeating, obesity, and obsessing over their body size and appearance. Ms. Orbach also saw dieting as part of the problem, not the solution.

I thought dealing with my weight and overeating was all up to me and that God was so disgusted with my failures that he was not interested in helping me.

After reading Ms. Orbach's book, I started reading other books along the same lines. (I've listed them in Chapter 14.) All of them emphasized the thoughts and beliefs that motivate overeating and weight gain. Here were secular authors unwittingly making use of biblical principles. For other areas of emotional struggle I had learned to identify underlying beliefs and then "renew my mind" in light of God's truth. Empowered by the Holy Spirit, I had exchanged erroneous beliefs for the truth found in Scripture and had experienced a great deal of freedom from a sharp tongue, panic attacks, and destructive religious legalism. But when it came to my overeating, I had believed it to be strictly a matter of my own self-discipline. I thought dealing with it was all up to me and that God was so disgusted with my failures that he was not interested in helping me. Seeing secular authors examining underlying motivations and erroneous beliefs, changing their thinking and, thus, finding freedom from overeating and related obsessions, I thought, *How much more should I, in whom the Comforter dwells and who relies on the authority of Scripture, be able to change my thinking and find freedom in the truth?*

And that was exactly what happened. Over the course of about 19 months, I slowly reexamined basic biblical counseling principles and applied them to my overeating, dieting, and obsessions with my appearance and weight. The Weight of Grace small groups I lead and this book are my attempts to help others through a process such as the one I experienced. I've found that very few Christians have been exposed to the biblical counseling principles – which amount to basic discipleship principles – that I learned at Scope Ministries International, where I worked for 16 years. Not only are very few Christians exposed to these principles and concepts, but almost none would think of applying them to overeating and overweight.

When it comes to addressing overeating, the thinking among many Christians tends to fall into only a few categories. Some Christians think as I did – that overeating is completely due to a lack of self-discipline and that the cure is to crack down harder on themselves. They think, *If I'd just get my act together and keep a tighter rein on myself, I'd lick this thing.* Some Christians feel the cure is to "guilt" themselves into "behaving" (i.e., sticking to a diet) by pronouncing themselves "gluttons." They believe that naming their sin will bring them out of denial and motivate them to avoid continued sinning. A related line of thinking is the "obedience" approach in which eating when not hungry or eating foods not on your diet is seen as disobedience to God and a sign of not trusting him to take care of your needs. The solution, then, is to confess this sin and repent by returning to right behavior. All of these approaches leave out addressing underlying beliefs and motivations, something the Bible does not leave out in its understanding of how people are transformed!

The following points give an overview of my understanding of overeating, being overweight, and experiencing true freedom in these areas. I will elaborate on each of these points in later chapters.

- Overcoming overeating is *not* simply a matter of having self-discipline. I had a lot of discipline in nearly every other area of my life. Why did I lack it in this area alone? Not only is overeating not a matter of lacking self-discipline, but also trying to *control* eating results in having *less* control, less discipline. Later in the book we will examine Scripture passages such as Romans 7:7-8 and Colossians 2:20-23 in regard to this point.

  Overcoming overeating is not simply a matter of having self-discipline.

- There are reasons why women feel a need to be large or to consider themselves "fat," despite cultural and social pressures to be "thin." Being overweight serves purposes in women's lives. Women's beliefs about what it means to be "fat" or "thin" can lead to their being more emotionally comfortable when they're "fat" than they are when they're "thin," even though they feel a great deal of pain about being "fat." Throughout the New Testament, the authors of the Epistles addressed erroneous beliefs that resulted in negative behavior and asked their readers to believe in God's truth, expecting this would change their behavior. Until beliefs about "fat" and "thin" and what these concepts mean to the individual are revealed and changed, the behaviors that result from these beliefs (overeating and remaining overweight) will not change.

  Being overweight serves purposes in women's lives.

- Eating is often a way women try to meet their emotional needs or suppress painful emotions. When women understand the provisions God has made for meeting their needs and expressing negative feelings, the desire to overeat in the face of uncomfortable emotions diminishes.

- Our culture puts way too much emphasis on women's appearance and on being "thin." The "world system" (Romans 12:2) tries to get our focus away from God's values and onto assessing our worth on the basis of our weight or appearance. Seeing yourself as God sees you relieves the pressure to be an unrealistically thin size.

- We were not designed to mentally control our food intake. Our bodies are designed with an excellent signaling system that tells us when we need to eat, how much we need to eat, and even what we need to eat. This system is called physical hunger, but most women are convinced that they cannot trust their bodies to tell them what they need to eat and when. It is clear in Ephesians 5:29 that we naturally do what is good for our bodies. Also, as Christians, by virtue of our rebirth in Christ, we have a new nature, and one of the attributes of that new nature is *self-control* (Galatians 5:23). Self-control is not the same as the "discipline" that's involved in dieting, because that kind of discipline is imposed through rules and regulations from outside ourselves. A Christian's self-control is the natural outgrowth of the inward presence of the Holy Spirit. When we act in ways that are not good for our bodies or are not self-controlled, we are not "being ourselves." We can learn to be our true selves in regard to eating.

We have a new nature, and one of the attributes of that new nature is self-control.

My experience is that knowing the truth in these areas has set me free (John 8:32). I don't diet. I don't weigh myself. I don't worry about what I can and cannot eat. I don't panic or celebrate if I get a little bigger or smaller now and then. I almost never feel overly full. I almost always like my body and appearance. I have stayed pretty much the same size for over 20 years. Many of you who are reading this book will understand the significance of the fact that I am still wearing some clothes that I wore in 1986 (trust me, they're classics), and many of my clothes have been discarded, not because I got too fat or too thin for them, but because they wore out!

Reflection: What about You?

You'll get the most from the following questions if you discuss them with one or more women who are going through this book too. If you don't have someone with whom to discuss these questions, write your answers (and don't worry about grammar or spelling). Only after you have talked over these questions with others or written your answers, move on to the next section of this chapter, "What Others Have Experienced."

1. When did you first start thinking of yourself as "fat" and what were some circumstances surrounding your starting to eat more than what seemed appropriate? In other words, when did you start having a "negative relationship" with food?

2. What were the attitudes about body size, eating, and dieting in your home when you were growing up?

3. What are your feelings about the idea of working on underlying issues as opposed to going on a diet? Do you see any possible emotional issues that might underlie your overeating or a "need" to be "fat"?

What Others Have Experienced

- When did you start having a "negative relationship" with food?

There is not always a "traumatic event" that marks the beginning of having a struggle with overeating and weight gain, but sometimes there is. In looking back at when I started to overeat, I can see that it started at the same time my stepfather started sexually molesting me. Hopefully, what was going on in your life wasn't that difficult, but maybe it was worse. Even if I wasn't familiar with the statistics that are often quoted about the number of girls who experience sexual abuse, I couldn't help but notice that at least a third of the participants in Weight of Grace small groups report having had some form of negative sexual experience during childhood and seeing this as contributing to their overeating. Other factors, such as a mother who is diet conscious or an alcoholic family member, also can trigger a pattern of overeating and weight gain. Or, you may have started turning to food for comfort or to escape painful emotions because you were teased by kids at school or when your parents divorced or when a loved one died. Almost always there are several contributing factors and a progression in eating behaviors.

Women tell of starting to have a "weight problem" beginning with puberty or after having their first child or at the onset of perimenopause. These may sound strictly

At least a third of the participants in Weight of Grace small groups report having had some form of negative sexual experience during childhood.

physiological due to hormonal changes. However, many women go through these same life changes and do not start "fighting fat." Were you already someone who got a few "strokes" from being slender and then a life-passage weight gain threatened that? Because our culture does not allow for the natural ups and downs of women's weight, as soon as a woman gains a little weight for any reason, even pregnancy, there is a great deal of pressure to get it off as soon as possible. Many women who would naturally, gradually lose weight following pregnancy jump into dieting, not realizing they are setting themselves up for a lifetime of yo-yo weight gains and losses. (In Chapter 10, we will look at why dieting backfires in this way.)

As you progress through this book, keep in mind when your struggles with overeating began. Several chapters will provide ways for you to uncover why you turned to food at that particular time and in that particular context. These insights can enable you to think and act in news ways and break out of the patterns in which you've been trapped ever since.

- What were the attitudes about body size, eating, and dieting in your home?

Attitudes among family members, especially parents, have a tremendous influence on what we believe about our appearance and weight and how we behave toward food. There seem to be a lot of mixed messages regarding food and appearance directed at girls, particularly for those growing up in Christian homes. On the one hand, many are told to "clean their plates," which requires girls to eat more than they physically need. At the same time, being thin is often touted as a Christian virtue, seen as evidence of self-discipline or taking care of one's "temple." Attractiveness is rewarded but working too hard at being attractive garners disapproval. After all, one ought not take pride in one's appearance. These conflicting values can result in young women just giving up and giving in to being "fat."

"For as he thinks in his heart, so is he." (NKJV™)

One translation of Proverbs 23:7a is: "For as he thinks in his heart, so is he" (NKJV™). Often, what our parents tell us about ourselves is what we believe and then what we become. Many women in Weight of Grace groups tell how a parent called them "fat" or a "cow" even though, in looking back at old photos, they were within a normal weight range. However, the message was taken to heart and resulted in their living up to those descriptions.

Any time there is a great deal of emphasis put on outward appearance, it seems there is a greater chance for eating problems. In some cases, being overweight is a form of rebellion, a means by which a child can demonstrate to her parents that they cannot control her. For others, the pressure to be a certain size forces a child to start dieting at a very young age, and the dieting backfires for them at a young age too. One woman who came to me for counsel – I'll call her Meg – was so obese she could only weigh herself on a cattle scale. Because Meg was a large baby, her mother was afraid Meg would be a "fat" child and adult. Therefore, her mother started restricting Meg's food from the moment she was born. Some of Meg's earliest memories are of sneaking food because she always felt hungry. The ultimate result of her mother's efforts to keep Meg thin was that Meg became exactly what her mother dreaded.

• What are your feelings about working on underlying issues instead of dieting?

Many women have said to me in a panicky tone something along these lines: "If I were to give up dieting, I'd just get fatter and fatter until I was a blimp." Because of feelings such as these expressed by many Weight of Grace participants, I don't really expect anyone to give up dieting at the onset of their small group experience. My hope (and this hope has often been realized) is that once women are introduced to biblical principles that ring true for them, they will be excited about stepping out in faith and pursuing a new direction in regard to their overeating. Act upon the faith that you have in this area. If you currently believe that dieting is not helping you, you will probably find it relatively easy to do all the exercises in this book. If, however, you do not feel you can just give up dieting – for fear that your weight will go beyond what you can emotionally handle – don't worry about it right now. Read the book, do the exercises as well as you can, and ask God to show you whether this approach is right for you. God is more interested in you having freedom in this area than you are. If not right now, you will eventually find freedom, because that is the way of the Holy Spirit and God's work of sanctification.

Ask God to show you whether this approach is right for you.

Homework

The information in this book won't be of value to you unless you take the time to personally apply and prayerfully think through the concepts presented. One way to do that is by answering the reflection questions. Another way is by completing the homework assignments. Most of the assignments are designed to be completed in about one to two hours. Hopefully, you are working your way through the book along with one or more friends. If so, complete the homework on your own before comparing notes about it with others. Following the homework, there are follow-up questions and comments on the homework in the "Before You Go on to the Next Chapter" section of each chapter.

1. Read the following excerpts from *Tufts University Diet & Nutrition Letter* "Special Report"[1] that Is reprinted here with permission. Underline the portions of the article that stand out to you. Write how these portions relate to you personally (in the past or currently).

SPECIAL REPORT

At what price the quest for thinness?

"I was bad today" has become the confession of a large group of self-professed sinners, a particularly recalcitrant bunch whose offenses do not include the ordinary coveting of a neighbor's goods or lying or stealing but rather transgressions like eating something sweet or rich, getting up from the table feeling full, and perhaps worst of all in their minds, enjoying more food than they intended to at the start of the day.

Eating, in other words, or at least deriving pleasure from eating, has become somewhat of a moral lapse. The reason? It has largely to do with the incessant demand made of Americans to diet—to remain or become thin no matter what.

A historical perspective

To avoid fatness at all costs wasn't always part of the American prescription for good, clean living. As late as the end of the 1800s, amply fleshed people were viewed as cheerful, well adjusted, productive, and prosperous, explains historian Roberta Pollack Seid, PhD, in her excellent book *Never Too Thin: Why Women Are at War with Their Bodies* (New York: Prentice Hall Press). Today, however, a large body is regarded as the sign of a piggish slob who has no control over himself.

Body shape's relatively new role as an indicator of moral character comes from a variety of developments in the fields of medicine, psychology, culture, and fashion that all converged to bring about an urgency to diet in the 1940s and '50s. A belief began to take hold in the health care community, for example, that biologic or genetic differences were not sufficient for explaining why certain individuals maintain a high weight. It was felt that all people are meant to be slim, and that all fat people *could* slim down if they just made more of an effort to stop eating too much.

In effect, obesity had largely been reduced to an equation of too many calories going in for the number of calories going out, with the blame for the imbalance placed invariably on the overweight person's lack of willpower. ... That shift in attitude did not result from a mean-spirited callousness on the part of medical professionals. They were merely responding to the latest "evidence" that excess weight is bad for health and can lead to an early death. ...

Psychology, the newest health field "on the block" in the mid-twentieth century, fueled the fear of fat—along with the prejudice against fat people. Obesity, psychological theories suggested, may not be a physiological problem at all but rather one caused by emotional tension, insecurity, oral fixations, unresolved infantile neuroses, sexual repression, or lack of love. In other words, fat people were coming to be thought of as necessarily mentally handicapped, not worthy or capable of self-esteem—in short, damaged goods.

The cultural factor

America's fear of "going soft" in the post-World War II era of plenty probably also contributed to the view of a fat person as less than emotionally whole or "correct," or at least as someone who lacked character. ... When the abundance of ease of the 1950s brought more of the "good life" to the middle class, there was concern that the very backbone of the nation, the so-called common man, would be corrupted by money and leisure time and even less able ... to exercise the self-control and moral restraint needed to keep the country—and himself—in good shape. ...

The media fueled the notion that lean was desirable with unremitting intensity. Models in fashion magazines became thinner and thinner. And their influence grew as more and more people acquired the money and the time to buy and study them to see how they themselves should strive to look. Likewise, television, which brought fashion and fashionable bodies into people's living rooms with an immediacy never experienced before, drove home the thinner-is-better theme all the more. Momentum for thinness in the media kept building into the youth- and youthful-body-loving 1960s, when an emaciated Twiggy appeared on the scene. At five feet seven and a half inches and 91 pounds, that one-time paradigm of the fashionable body was clearly skinny enough to meet the clinical criteria for anorexia. Small wonder that eating came to be referred to as bad, that those with big bodies came to be seen—and often saw themselves—as misfits, sloppy, weak-willed sorts who couldn't get hold of themselves.

To diet or not to diet?

Beyond a shadow of a doubt, morbid, or extreme, obesity raises the risk for such ills as heart disease and hypertension. And many people who are just slightly overweight but have problems like high blood cholesterol or diabetes are also in greater jeopardy of compromised health than others. That is, there are millions upon millions of Americans who would reduce their health risks if they lost some weight.

But whether it is possible for all of them to lose weight and keep it off is another matter entirely. In the last decade, more and more evidence has come to light that some people simply are predestined to weigh more than the medical and fashion communities say they should. For instance, University of Pennsylvania obesity researcher Albert Strunkard, MD, has found that identical twins separated early in life and raised in different environments by different sets of parents are just about as likely to end up being overweight to the same degree as identical twins raised in the same household. …

What it all comes down to is that some people are more prone than others to becoming—and remaining—overweight. That's not to say environment and lifestyle have no influence on how much a person will weigh. But it does seem that to at least some degree, biology is destiny. And for individuals whose destiny may be to stabilize at relatively high weight, repeated failed attempts to lose weight and keep it off may do more harm than good, not just emotionally but also physically. Research suggests that each time a person sheds pounds and then puts them back on, he ends up with more body fat and less lean muscle mass at the higher weight than he had previously. And the more fat someone has, the more disposed he may be to developing such ills as heart disease.

The emotional toll dieting takes

"Typical diets, by prohibiting certain foods, reinforce the fear that those foods are inherently dangerous, thereby intensifying a profound sense of helplessness in handling them. In addition, by characterizing certain foods as illicit, diet regimens make them all the more desirable and harder to eat in moderate amounts." So says Emily Fox Kales, PhD, a psychologist on the attending staff of McLean Hospital in Belmont, Massachusetts, who coordinates outpatient groups for eating disorders and obesity.

It's as if a weight-loss plan's failure is built right into it, a fact borne out by recidivism rates as high as 98 percent for most diets. Unfortunately, however, unsuccessful dieters usually think the failure is theirs rather than the reducing regimen's and end up with eroded self-esteem. Going off a diet has come to signify a fall from grace, Dr. Kales says. And it not only adversely affects how someone feels about himself but also may literally obstruct a person's going forward in life.

"I've seen women with lots of intelligence and creativity divert all their energy into an obsession with food and weight," she explains. "At times many of my patients, ordinarily hard-driving and ambitious, will stay home from work and miss a crucial meeting because they binged the night before or gained five pounds or are afraid they look fat. They feel powerless in the grip of these 'secrets,' which handicaps their careers and personal relationships. Some women organize their lives specifically around their eating problems. One of my clients, an executive in a large corporation, passes up opportunities to take business trips that would advance her career because she's afraid to eat in restaurants; she's afraid of the mini bars in hotel rooms. In other words, she limits her professional success because of her concerns about going off her

diet. Despite all she's achieved, her self-esteem is still tied up in her body weight and shape. It has reached the point," Dr. Kales adds, "where women do not even know when they're hungry anymore. Years of cycling on and off diets has the unfortunate effect of making a person very insensitive, almost numb, to his own bodily signals. What many people don't realize is that we're born with a wonderful apparatus that lets us know when we're physiologically hungry. There are all kinds of cues of nutritional status depletion that under normal circumstances lead a person to correctly identify hunger. The stomach rumbles, you feel a little weak and headachy, maybe even somewhat tired. But people who diet continuously are more responsive to external cues, such as foods' caloric content, and lose touch with the internal signals. Or at least they override them."

Indeed, hunger has become a frightening sensation for many, women in particular. A woman is often panic stricken when she feels hungry…because she fears losing control once she begins to eat. …

Getting in touch with hunger

With the anxiety felt by people preoccupied with their weight and, at the same time, faced with the abundance of foods that is available to most Americans, it is not hard to understand how the instinct of hunger has become submerged beneath the uncomfortable feelings of confusion and guilt. Another problem for many overeaters is that emotional stress from other sources often replaces physical hunger as a reason to eat.

"People often use food to medicate anxiety," Dr. Kales says. "That is the most common thing I see in my practice—food used as anesthesia for anxiety and depression." …

Dr. Kales recommends that people start to become aware of the *absence* of physical hunger, to ask themselves what they are really feeling when they're anxious. For instance, a person's throat and stomach might be clenched, but that could be muscle tension arising from the desire to scream at her mother-in-law, not a need for food. In other words, it is important to become more aware about the true source of any anxiety or stress…and then to find ways to tolerate your feelings, to express them rather than to "swallow" them by eating.

Of course, getting in touch with the internal, physiological signals of hunger doesn't guarantee thinness. Some people are going to be fatter than others no matter how much they eat… [L]earning to handle food without tension, to find out for yourself how much food feels right for you, can at least help redirect the enormous amount of energy so many people waste trying to eat and look the way society's rigid and largely unfounded standard has come to say they should.[1]

2. Spend time in prayer, asking God to show you whether you should commit to completing this book, especially in light of the fact that it will not involve a weight-loss program. If you do not already have a partner or others with whom to go through this book, ask God to show you if there is someone who would be a good partner for you. Write what you believe God is telling you in answer to these prayers.

God is telling me to rely on Him. Trust Him. My needs will be met. He will tell me when I need to stop eating — what I should eat.

BEFORE YOU GO ON TO THE NEXT CHAPTER

Before beginning Chapter 2, discuss the following questions with one or more women who are also reading through this book and/or write your answers.

Homework Follow-up

1. Is it "okay" for you to spend the time it may take to start "listening" to your body/hunger as was suggested near the end of the Tufts article? Compare the amount of time and energy you spend on dieting and being concerned about your weight with the amount of time you'd spend on becoming aware of your hunger.

2. Did reading the Tufts article excerpts result in your feeling discouraged or encouraged? Why?

3. What does it seem that God is telling you about what you've read in this book so far? How interested in and committed to proceeding through the rest of this material are you? Is it helpful to have a partner or others with whom to work through this book?

Comments on the Homework

- Is it okay to spend time listening to your body/hunger? How does this compare to the time and effort involved in dieting?

Many women have expressed feeling guilty over spending time learning to get in touch with their bodies' signals of hunger. They feel they're concentrating too much on themselves, which is not a "godly" thing to do. Two chapters of this book will address the topic of reconnecting with true physical hunger; but for now, consider whether an investment now in what you may feel is "self-centered" could result in your later being able to end your self-absorbed obsessions with fat, dieting, constantly paying attention to what you eat, and worrying about your appearance. Often, women feel much less guilty about staying on a diet than they do about taking the time to discover their hunger signals. This is despite the fact that dieting requires a great deal of self-centered activity and usually results in everyone around you having to make adjustments to accommodate your diet. I once joined a family's gathering where, because of one woman who was on a diet, all twelve of us went to a restaurant that only she preferred. And, had she not been dieting, I doubt she would have preferred it!

My experience is that dieting always costs more in time and money than not dieting. Aren't the extra expense and all the other special effort you have put forth to be on your diet pretty self-centered? However, because so many Christians believe dieting is a sign of godly self-discipline, it can feel more comfortable to spend time and energy dieting than to spend time and energy learning to listen to and respond to one's body's true physical hunger. Dieting and maintaining weight loss are exhausting work. Consider the possibility of being like the people you know who stay at a normal weight and don't worry about every bite they eat. How do they do that? They were born with hunger signals and, unlike dieters, never learned to ignore those signals. You can return to that natural way of relating to food, eventually not having to work at recognizing the signals you were created to respond to, but just responding automatically.

My experience is that dieting always costs more in time and money than not dieting.

- Did reading the Tufts article excerpts encourage or discourage you?

Most women who read the Tufts article excerpts say they really identify with a lot of what it says. Many, however, feel very discouraged by the possibility that they have a "large body type." Although this will be addressed at greater length in later chapters, for now, start asking yourself who told you that being larger than a certain size was bad, wrong, or ugly, and where did they get that information? Is it God who has set this standard? What makes you think so? It is encouraging to many who read this article that their experience of failure with dieting is validated. It may not be something horribly wrong with them, but with dieting as the means of addressing overeating. This opens the possibility that there may be a more effective alternative.

If by any chance you're thinking that the Tufts article is dated, a line from a recent movie encapsulates how our culture has become even more obsessed with thinness since that article was published. An actor portraying an associate editor at a New York-based fashion magazine told the female protagonist who wore size 6 clothes, "Size 6 is the new size 12." Then her boss referred to her as "the fat one" because the other female employees all wore size 0 or size 2!

- What does it seem God is telling you so far?

If the idea of not dieting and losing weight immediately is just more than you can bear right now, it's okay to set this book aside for a while. God does not work on every area of our lives at the same time. There may be many other issues in your life God feels are more important to address at this time. I've long ago stopped trying to figure out God's timing. I would have preferred that God free me from my struggle with overeating as soon as I accepted Christ. But, instead, he first enabled me to experience freedom from anxiety reactions, suppressing my emotions, and religious legalism. He knows in what order we can best handle changes that need to take place.

If it seems God is giving you a go-ahead with this book, go forth with gusto! Some indicators that God is leading you in the direction this book will take you are that you're excited about what you've read so far, you're curious to know what's next, and you feel hopeful that God is going to change you once and for all in this area of your life.

There is almost nothing that reinforces concepts more than discussing them with others.

It is my hope that you are not going through this book by yourself. Even if there is no obvious partner or small group available to you right now, keep praying that God will give you the opportunity to share what you're learning with others. There is almost nothing that reinforces concepts more than discussing them with others. An even greater reinforcement is teaching what you've learned to another. I've found that teaching is my best teacher. Many participants in Weight of Grace groups have started to tell their friends about what they've learned in their small group only to discover they were telling it more to themselves, as well as helping themselves understand and remember the concepts much better.

2   GOD WANTS YOU TO HAVE FREEDOM (AND HE'S NOT DISGUSTED WITH YOU)

To start this chapter, let's do a little experiment. Jot down five or six adjectives that describe who your father was to you as a person when you were growing up. Write down what immediately comes to your mind.[1]

_____

_____

_____

Believe it or not, many biblical counselors would tell you that those adjectives are indicative of how you subjectively feel about God as your heavenly Father. No matter how good a father your father was, no human being is perfect. And, for many of us, our fathers were very far from perfect. Without realizing it, we can impose on God whatever our understanding of a "father" is. In addition, there are usually several other authority figures, both male and female, who make an impression on us and, through their words, attitudes, and behavior, influence what we think about God. And what we think and how we feel about God have a very direct bearing on whether or not we will seek – and experience – God's intervention in the area of our overeating.

Without realizing it, we can impose on God whatever our understanding of a "father" is.

My parents divorced when I was five years old, and my mother had primary custody of my sister and me. My father was very faithful in sending child support checks twice a month and in taking us girls for the weekend every other week. When I was 11, the every-other-weekend pattern was broken by some events involving my mother's remarriage, and we started seeing Dad only on Thanksgiving and Christmas. He never called us and I believed at that time that he didn't want me to call him. The child support checks always arrived on time, but contact with Dad was rare. When we did see him, interaction was awkward and stilted.

My father seemed to me to be very hard to please. I made straight A's but he told me I was too bookish. When I made mistakes in doing chores around the house, he was quick to scold and often said, "You should have known better." When I did the exercise I've just asked you to do above, some of the adjectives I wrote about my father were "distant," "uninterested," and "demanding." Later in life, when I was confronted with the possibility that I was allowing my impressions of my father to influence my view of God's character and personality, this made sense. I had seen God as always faithfully providing my material needs but not at all interested in actually interacting with me or being emotionally involved with me. Also, I had felt God wanted me to figure out things for myself and not bother him. When it came to my problems and mistakes, I thought God was shaking his head and saying, "You should have known better."

This was especially true when it came to eating and being overweight. I just knew I should have gotten over this problem already and that God was terribly impatient with my failures in this area. It was such a simple issue – just have discipline. Discipline is easy, like sending the check twice a month. You just put your mind to it and you do it because it's the right thing to do. For years, I did not even question this view of God's attitude toward me. When I started being willing to see my eating in a new light, I also started to realize I needed to check out whether I'd made wrong assumptions about God and his desire to help me with my struggles with food and "fat."

Not only do we have a tendency to confuse our heavenly Father with our earthly fathers, but also there are a number of other factors that set us up for seeing God as less loving, trustworthy, and interested in our struggles than he truly is. First of all, as a result of our sinful nature, which we inherited from our distant ancestor Adam, we were born separated from God. In our most formative years, as any mother will tell you, we believed ourselves to be the center of the universe, and we did not have a close, dependent, personal relationship with God. For almost all of us, all we had to go on in regard to understanding what God is like were the models our authority figures set for us and the messages we got from our surroundings.

You probably drew many conclusions about God from the events in your life.

If you did not grow up in a Christian home, it is likely that one of the few facts you learned about God was that God is almost always referred to as "he." You put two and two together to come up with the belief that God is probably a lot like the significant man or men in your life. This would be even more the case if you were exposed to reference to God as "Father." Also, you probably drew many conclusions about God from the events in your life. When I was 16, after my stepmother attempted suicide, I wrote in my diary, "God, don't you see what a cruel game you're playing?" I interpreted the negative events I'd experienced as indicative of God being cruel. To this day, I struggle with that well-entrenched false belief about God.

If you grew up in a family that attended church, there are all sorts of inaccurate doctrines and ideas about the nature and character of God to which you may have been exposed. I have been a Christian for over 30 years and, as a result of working in interdenominational Christian organizations for 20 of those years, I've been exposed to dozens of Christian denominations and sects. Many denominations emphasize God's judgment over his mercy and his demand for holiness over his love and forgiveness. The greater part of preaching I've heard has in some way made use of guilt in order to motivate the believer to good works. The underlying message is that God is disapproving and expects much, much more than what we are giving to, or doing for, him. My own feeling that I could never do enough to please God led to tremendous emotional difficulties for several years during the early part of my Christian walk.

Almost all participants in Weight of Grace small groups admit that they have felt that God was very disapproving of them, not only for their difficulties with weight gain and overeating, but also because of many other real and perceived shortcomings. Those same women could recite a list of God's very positive attributes. But, when asked how God actually felt and acted toward *them*, those attributes did not seem to come into play.

But why do our perceptions about God matter when it comes to overcoming struggles with overeating and being overweight? Because without an accurate view of God and his role in every aspect of their lives, women do not access the only lasting solutions to their problems, which are all found in the context of a relationship with and reliance upon God. When women believe that God is disgusted with them and impatient with their failures to exercise self-discipline, they find it difficult to invite God to help them with their struggles. They do not *trust* that God will do anything even if they do invite him to help. Often, women have prayed and prayed for God's help to stay on diets or to lose weight and have seen no evidence that God has answered those prayers. This adds to their belief that God does not care about them in regard to their overeating. Because of their erroneous beliefs about God, women are either not asking for God's help at all or are asking him to help them in ways that do not provide permanent solutions to their underlying spiritual and emotional issues. Therefore, the starting point for experiencing real freedom from overeating must be to revamp the person's view of God and his desire to help her in this area of her life.

So, if we admit to the possibility that our view of God is less than accurate and needs to change, how do we become acquainted with him as he truly is? The best place to start is in God's Word, the Bible. However, many people, in reading the Bible, take it through their own mental filters that lead them to interpret Scripture in such a way that it reinforces their negative perceptions about God. At a turning point in my Christian walk, I was asked by a counselor to read the Gospels assuming that Christ was always using a pleasant tone of voice. It shocked me to realize that I'd previously "heard" Jesus speaking harshly to, or hollering at, most of the people to whom he spoke.

Instead of looking at Scripture using only our own mental lens, which may be colored by erroneous assumptions or vague notions about God, we can see his true nature through Scripture when we ask *him* to illuminate what we're reading and when we remember to interpret whatever we read in the Bible through the filter of the Cross. If God so loved us that he sacrificed to the extent of suffering death on a cross, if the Cross is indeed the focal point of all history, then all that we read in Scripture about him should be colored by that immeasurable love. So often, the harsh tones and impatience we imagine are God's are really the product of our imposing onto Scripture the preconceived notions we have because of our experiences in life and with others. Also, we need to remember that it is the work of the Holy Spirit, not our unaided intellect, that makes clear the truths of Scripture (John 16:13-15). When we are willing to set aside our prejudices, keep the Cross as our focal point, and ask God to show us himself as we read his Word, he will do exactly that.

So often, the harsh tones and impatience we imagine are God's are really the product of our imposing onto Scripture the preconceived notions we have because of our experiences in life and with others.

In looking to the Bible to understand God's attitude toward me and my struggles, one of the stories in the Gospels that helped me most to believe that God accepts me and has mercy on me even though I have sinned is that of the woman at the well (John 4:4-30). Jesus knew everything about her, right down to the number of men she'd lived with, but he didn't say a single harsh word to her. In fact, it appears that she was the very first person to whom he revealed that he was the Christ. Throughout his ministry, Jesus gently drew to himself those who were committing very obvious sins. Yes, he had some harsh words for a select few, but it is important that we realize who they were. Only the Pharisees, who were heaping regulations on top of the Mosaic Law and making it harder for people to be in relationship with God, were called "vipers" and "whitewashed tombs." These were stiff-necked, hypocritical leaders who needed to be called to task, not broken people who realized their shortcomings and their need for God's forgiveness and grace. (See Matthew 23:13-36.)

So, looking at Scripture through the lens of the Cross, let's consider some information God reveals in his Word about himself.

- God is our "Abba" or "Daddy." See Romans 8:15-17. Paul uses a term here that was used by small children, much as we might say *da da*. We can trust God as a small child unreservedly trusts his daddy. However, unlike some of our dads, God never changes or fails in his nurturing care for us.

- God loves us unconditionally (Romans 5:8; 1 John 4:19). God's love is not based upon how well we perform for him. His love predates any of our good deeds. His love is due to *his* character, not ours.

- God desires nothing but the best for us (Jeremiah 29:11; Romans 8:28). God does not want you to live in bondage to compulsions and obsessions of any sort. He is in the process of guiding you into being more and more like Jesus, and he's doing this because that is what will be most fulfilling for *you*.

- God *knows* you intimately (Psalm 139) and delights in you (Psalm 18:19). Delighting in someone is not just a "by the way" feeling. It is taking active pleasure in that person. When we feel disgusted with ourselves, it is very hard to accept that God is delighting in us, but God, more than anyone, knows who he created us to be. He knows how truly delightful we are and sees us that way when all we see are our faults.

- Because God is love (1 John 4:8, 16), we can view the "love passage" in 1 Corinthians 13 as a description of God. Read 1 Corinthians 13, replacing the word "love" (or "charity") with "God."

- God is not condemning of you (Romans 5:8 and 8:1). He does not condemn you for your weight or your eating behavior. He is at work in you to bring you into line with his purposes (Philippians 2:13). He knows he is able to do this (Philippians 1:6).

- God does not view you in the same way that most people view you (1 Samuel 16:7). He does not look at your outward appearance as a measurement of your worth. He is looking at your heart. And your heart desires to obey him, even if you have not found a way to do that fully yet.

It is likely that you don't yet *feel* all these facts about God's attitude toward you to be true. That is fine. What the Bible says about God is more true than what you feel or what you experience. And, the truth will win out if we keep it in mind. (See Philippians 4:8 and Colossians 3:2.) Here's where what I call "prayerful pondering" comes in. Over the next days and weeks, think about and pray about what God is really like. Ask God to reveal himself in special ways to you. My experience was that, when I prayerfully pondered God's character and love, I realized he had been revealing his personal love and care for me all along, but I didn't have the mindset to perceive it. When I started asking God for little reassurances that he really is as good and kind as the Scripture passages above would

What the Bible says about God is more true than what you feel or what you experience.

indicate, he did some pretty interesting things. The one I found most humorous was that every time I'd go for a walk, I'd run across at least one penny. At the time I started finding these pennies (without looking for them at all), my bright red hair had not yet faded with age, and the thought came to my mind that God was telling me, "You are my little copper penny." This was certainly a daddy-like expression of affection, and I secretly (because I felt too silly about it to tell anyone) cherished the childlike feeling I got each time I stumbled onto one of those pennies. Oh, by the way, I take walks several times a week and this penny-finding experience went on for about ten years!

Reflection

1. What people and events influenced your view of God and in what ways was that view affected?

2. To what degree do you "buy into" the fact that God unconditionally loves you? What are the barriers to you feeling that to be true? (For example, are you using your belief that he is condemning you as a means to keep yourself from sinning?)

3. How have you always thought God felt about your weight and eating? Where did you get this idea? What can you now start believing about God that you haven't believed before, and do you have a scriptural basis for your new beliefs?

What Others Have Experienced

- What people and events influenced your view of God?

For many women, their view of God is influenced by very overt messages from their parents. For example, one young woman told how her father once emphatically insisted she was a "pig." Without even questioning it, she had always assumed God thought this about her too. As I mentioned above, my own father often said, "You should have known better." It took me years to realize this was not God's attitude toward me. God does not ask me to know what I've never been told. Looking back, I realize God has many times intervened in my life so that I did not suffer the consequences of what I did out of ignorance. Later, he showed me the truth so that I would not continue to repeat my mistakes.

For other women, it wasn't so much what their parents did as what their parents didn't do that influenced their perceptions about God. Many women tell how their fathers just weren't really present all that much or that their fathers interacted with them very little. As a result, they believed God was indifferent toward them or that they had to "make a big splash" to get God's attention. Sometimes, only negative behavior got noticed. One woman told how she could see that being overweight was one of her ways of proving to God that she needed his attention.[2]

- Do you buy into the fact that God unconditionally loves you?

Some women hate themselves so much that they cannot imagine that God feels any affection for them.

Some women hate themselves so much that they cannot imagine that God feels any affection for them. They have the thought, *How can a* **holy** *God accept* **me***?* Here they are assuming that God's values are the same as their values or the same as the culture's. Our culture is obsessed with how terrible it is to be "fat" and how glorious it is to be "thin." Many of us accept these standards – assume that they are right and even godly – without even realizing it and certainly without analyzing these beliefs in light of Scripture. Also, Christian women who overeat often label themselves "gluttons" and assume God must despise them for this heinous sin. However, there is debate among Bible scholars over whether the word translated as "gluttony" really has as much to do with eating food as with participating in orgy-like banquets.[3] The word is usually used side by side with a reference to drunkenness, so the two terms probably go together as an idiom for a certain lifestyle or form of "partying." Christian women's struggles with overeating rarely take place in the context of riotous living. In fact, quite often overeating is done in secret – not at all as a form of rebellion against God or a desire to "live high."

Another reason women find it difficult to believe and accept God's love and forgiveness is because they fear they will have no reason to "do good" if God accepts them even when they are doing poorly. They are basically using their perception of God's disapproval – and their own guilt – as the means by which they motivate themselves to behave. A verse that contradicts this logic is Romans 2:4: "*...do you show contempt for the riches of his kindness, tolerance and patience, not realizing that* **God's kindness leads you toward repentance***?*" (emphasis mine). God has provided many ways in which to positively motivate us to obey him. We will not become "out of control" if we no longer use guilt to keep ourselves in line. In later chapters, the ways in which God motivates Christians will be addressed more fully.

• How have you always thought God felt about your weight and eating?

The word women use most to answer this question is "disgusted." As mentioned previously, women point to Scripture references about gluttony. They also cite 1 Corinthians 6:19, which refers to our bodies as temples of the Holy Spirit. In looking at such verses, they are not taking into account the context. Women use these verses as "proof texts" for what they already believe about themselves, and their beliefs did not originate with their study of the Bible. For the most part, women believe themselves to be disgusting because of the messages they have received from their families, peers, and the culture in which they live. But according to 1 Samuel 16:7, God does not judge us by our outward appearance in the way people tend to. Also, we know from King David's history, for example, that God does not cease to love us when we sin. (See Psalm 51, especially verse 1.) So, even if our overeating is indeed sin (which may be debatable in many cases), this does not cause God to love us less or care about us less. God knows our failings. That is why Christ died for us! (See Romans 5:8.) But, as long as we are convinced God is disgusted with us, we will not reach out to him for the kind of help that we need to overcome our struggles.

God does not judge us by our outward appearance in the way people tend to.

I hope that as a result of reading this chapter, and especially after doing the homework below, you will start considering how God is indeed "on your side" when it comes to your overeating and weight – because he's on your side in every area of your life. In fact, God knows that if you start trusting him to work in this painful, shame-ridden area of your life, you will then be better able to trust him in every other area. This has certainly been the case for me. There is nothing that reminds me more of how trustworthy God is than when I remember that I no longer have to fight a battle against overeating thanks to how God has worked in my life. There was a time when I was *sure* I would have to contend with overeating, dieting, and weight gain for the rest of my life. But now, at some point in nearly every day, I think about how grateful I am that I was mistaken! I am now convinced that freedom from this kind of bondage is the birthright of every Christian.

Homework

1. Read the following excerpt from "FatherCare," a booklet that is reprinted in its entirety, with permission, in Addendum One at the back of this book (beginning on page 207). If you have time, read the entire "FatherCare" manuscript, fill out the workbook section, take the "Relationship Test" on pages 239 through 241, and choose one of the "Characteristics of the Father" studies to complete (pages 243 through 252).

FatherCare

A Fresh Perspective on the Character of God

No relationship is more crucial to children than that of the parent/child relationship. In our culture, we sometimes forget how important the father/child relationship is. I have often stated that every daddy needs a little boy or little girl, and every little boy and little girl needs a daddy. What a loss when we realize that the average father spends approximately six minutes a day with his children. We live in a society that not only condones, but encourages, absentee fatherhood. What a refreshing and astounding difference it makes when we realize that God is our Father and is never absent, but always available to us every moment of every day.

Two passages of Scripture, among many others, confirm this fact of God's fatherhood to us:

> **A father of the fatherless, and a judge and protector of the widows, is God in His holy habitation.** Psalm 68:5 (Amplified)

> **"And I will be a Father to you, and you shall be sons and daughters to Me," says the Lord Almighty.** 2 Corinthians 6:18 (Amplified)

Allow me to digress here for a moment to demonstrate how easily we have been deceived into erroneous thinking about God. In this passage from the Psalms, you will note that God selects two segments of society to specifically mention, widows and orphans. It is interesting to note that at the time of this writing, both widows and orphans were considered a detriment to society, a non-productive drain upon the culture.

In this passage, God is called a "judge." Now what image comes to your mind when you think of a judge? Normally, we see in our mind's eye an image of a judge behind his bench, dispensing justice from his perspective – and we feel guilty. Place this mental image of a judge over onto God and we come up with the concept of a "cosmic policeman" just waiting for us to step out of line.

However, God is not a judge in that sense. First, all judgment has been placed in Christ (John 5:22). Second, there is no condemnation to those who are in Christ (Romans 8:1). Third, all of our punishment was placed on Christ (Isaiah 53:5). Fourth, God doesn't remember our sins and transgression (Hebrews 10:17). Fifth, our transgression is forgiven and our sins covered (Psalm 32:1). So, if God is not a judge in the way we conceive of a judge, then how are we to define the way "judge" is used in Psalm 68:5 (NASB)?

The way that the word "judge" is used here is "one who evaluates worth"!!! Get this, for it is important – God as Judge is not one who condemns, but one who evaluates what is of worth. In this passage, He is evaluating as worthy the two segments of society which were considered worthless. Therefore, God doesn't judge you in the sense of passing judgment unto condemnation, but He evaluates your absolute WORTHINESS!!!

Now, what is a father? William Barclay says this:

> There are two English words which are closely connected, but whose meanings are widely different. There is the word "paternity" and the word "fatherhood." "Paternity" describes a relationship in which a father is responsible for the physical existence of a son; but, as far as paternity goes, it can be, and it not infrequently happens, that the father has never even set eyes on the son, and would not even recognize him if in later years he met him. "Fatherhood" describes an intimate, loving, continuous relationship in which father and son grow closer to each other every day.[4]

It is this "fatherhood" that describes God's relationship to us. Thus, this is the greatest benefit of all in knowing God as Father – a continuing, growing intimacy with the Father.

However, this tends not to be our experience because on what basis do we build our concept of the Father? Humanly speaking, we establish father concepts through experiential relationships with our earthly fathers. Unfortunately, this produces erroneous concepts of a true father, because there is no absolutely perfect human father who can provide a role model for us.

Therefore, it is only through the Bible, our absolute standard of truth, that we can know what a father truly should be. It is the Bible that shows us, in the humanity of Jesus as He lived His life here on earth, the perfect role model as to what a true father is. It is there in the pages of Scripture that we see Jesus as the Father, a real Father in action.

What I am saying is that our normal father concepts tend to be erroneous, and it is only through the love and care of God, as we know Him as Father, that we can establish the proper concept of "father." It is in this biblical dimension that we discover what a father truly is, that is, by seeing, in the Person of Jesus Christ, the Father at work here in our lives on earth![5]

2. Write what you have assumed God thinks about you in the areas of your weight and eating. Write how you're willing to believe he totally accepts you whether or not you "shape up."

3. Make a decision to trust God with your overeating, overweight and related issues – write this out – even though your emotions may not necessarily line up right now. At least tell God you are willing to believe he is interested in giving you freedom in this area. (Remember "faith is not a feeling."[6])

BEFORE YOU GO ON TO THE NEXT CHAPTER

Homework Follow-up

1. What is new in your thinking about what God is like and how he feels about you, your eating, your weight, and your appearance?

2. What old beliefs about God have you now rejected?

Comments on the Homework

- What is new in your thinking about what God is like and how he feels about you?

What is important here is a willingness to believe differently about God. This involves a willingness to admit to having erroneous beliefs about God. Among Weight of Grace participants, many – especially women who are older in their faith – have a difficult time admitting to the possibility that they think anything at all negative about God. They feel this in some way insults God. However, it's really pretty silly to think that we could be born in sin, live in a sin-filled world, and have Satan constantly lying to us about God and still have a 100 percent accurate view of God. Also, God is aware of our doubts and erroneous beliefs, whether we admit them or not, so what's the harm in owning up?

Many have a difficult time admitting to the possibility that they think anything at all negative about God.

In addition to the fear of insulting God, there can be a fear of God's disapproval – even more disapproval than we already suspect God has for us – if we admit we doubt his character in any way. However, look at the numerous psalms in which people basically told God he was not doing a good job, he was forgetting them, he was being unfair, or he was failing to live up to his promises. Not only did God not strike these people down for writing such sentiments, he printed their criticisms in his Word! Also, we see in these psalms a pattern of people admitting to God exactly how they feel about him and then being willing to think through the truth of the matter. Psalm 73 is a good example of this. Here was a guy who was totally put out with God because the wicked had it "made in the shade" and he'd been keeping himself pure only to find his lot in life wasn't all that great. He even said that when he thought about all this, he became a "brute beast" before God. When I read this I picture an enraged Incredible Hulk-like person. Aaaarrrr! *But*, when this psalmist stopped to think about it – when he went into the house of the Lord and got perspective – he realized God was totally faithful and just. It's important to realize that if we don't admit we're wrong in our thinking about God, we won't ever turn to what's right.

- What old beliefs about God have you now rejected?

The hardest part about rejecting old beliefs is that we tend to make our emotions our final authority. My emotions constantly tell me that God is going to do something cruel and that it's just around the corner. This is an old emotional habit I developed as a result of some painful childhood experiences and an attempt to avoid devastating disappointment.

The hardest part about rejecting old beliefs is that we tend to make our emotions our final authority.

My reasoning is: *If I think bad things are just around the corner, I won't be surprised and dejected when they happen; I'll be emotionally prepared.* Even though experience tells me that thinking this way has never really prepared me well for unhappy events and losses, every time I'm especially happy, thoughts about impending God-wrought tragedy flood in like waves.

When I find myself having thoughts about God being mean to me, I have learned to reason in the following way: *Either God is good or he is not good. If he is not good, we are all doomed. If he is not good, why did Christ die on the cross? Okay, God is good and not cruel. So, even if something "bad" happens, God will give me the grace to handle it and it will work out for my ultimate good.* To some, this may seem to be "mental gymnastics," but I believe this is exactly what Paul was talking about when he said to "put off the old self" and "put on the new self" (Ephesians 4:22-24). And, I believe it is the Holy Spirit who reminds me to rethink my beliefs when my old emotional habit of doubting God's goodness and expecting the worst from him kicks in. Instead of going by how I *feel*, with the help of the Spirit, I turn to what is *true*, which ultimately changes how I feel.

It may be similar for you when it comes to how you *feel* about God. Just like the short suggested prayer from "FatherCare," below, you may need to repeatedly "put off" your wrong ideas about God and "put on" the truth according to Scripture. Ask God to help you in this and to bring the truth to your mind. He is, after all, more interested in you knowing the truth about him than you are!

> *Instead of going by how I feel, with the help of the Spirit, I turn to what is true, which ultimately changes how I feel.*

My Father, I always considered You an unloving God, but now I know that You are a *loving* Father to me. I choose now in faith to put off my false belief and I choose to believe that You are loving to me. I choose to believe what Your Word has to say about You rather than my feelings or reason or past experiences, and I know that Your Word says that You love me as a person and that your love is not based on my performance or on what I have or achieve. Thank You, my Father, for loving me unconditionally.[7]

3 IF I'M A "NEW CREATION IN CHRIST," WHY AM I STILL FAT?

According to 2 Corinthians 5:17, when we put our trust in Christ as our Savior – when we become Christians – a dramatic change takes place. We become "new creations." For many Christians, however, it is very hard to reconcile this verse with their day-to-day behavior. "Old things are passed away; behold, all things are become new" (2 Corinthians 5:17b, KJV). Well, one of my "old things," which was quite an issue before I was a Christian, did not appear to "pass away" at all after my conversion! In fact, after I became a Christian, my overeating became worse, not better. I gained about 25 pounds during the first three months after I, at the age of 19, put my faith in Christ.

It was not until I had some fairly extreme emotional problems during my midtwenties that I was exposed to an explanation of what it truly means to be a "new creation." Up to that point, I had worked very hard to make myself into what I believed a "new creation" should be. I actively participated in not one, but two, churches, as well as in two Bible studies. I was teaching at a Christian school and sponsored the junior and senior high pep clubs and cheerleading squads, as well as the ninth grade class. That wasn't enough; in the evenings I also provided homebound education to children with long-term illnesses. I faithfully kept many "rules" regarding daily Bible study and prayer. I appeared to be a really good Christian, but my many good works were largely powered by self-effort and it was extremely exhausting. Eventually I ran out of steam. At 25, I collapsed. I had what most people would call a "nervous breakdown." I cried constantly, couldn't cope with stress of any sort, and had to quit my job. In fact, I couldn't even drive a car for about six months.

I appeared to be a really good Christian, but my many good works were largely powered by self-effort and it was extremely exhausting.

Thankfully, God allowed me to collapse in the context of a circle of friends that included two biblical counselors who had seen similar crises in the lives of believers before. In this chapter, I'll share with you what I learned from them about what it means to be a "new creation in Christ." Understanding this not only enabled me to recover fully and fairly rapidly from my "breakdown," but also eventually contributed dramatically to resolving my struggles with overeating and overweight.

There is debate among evangelicals over the basic nature of human beings, especially regarding "dichotomy" and "trichotomy" and those who eschew both of these views. Each camp has biblical evidence for its stance. However, for our purposes here, and because this is my own leaning, in discussing what it means to be a "new creation in Christ" and how that impacts overeating, I am going to take a "trichotomous" view of human nature. In other words, we are going to view people as having three ("tri") basic aspects to their nature: body, soul, and spirit. First Thessalonians 5:23 and Hebrews 4:12 make mention of these three aspects. There are numerous definitions used for each of these three terms, and in the Bible, the terms "body," "soul," and "spirit" can have different meanings in different contexts. However, the definitions I'm going to use in order to sketch an understanding of our basic nature are, very simply, as follows: The body is the aspect of you that you or your surgeon can see, the soul is the aspect of you that you and your surgeon can't see and is in fairly constant flux, and the spirit is the aspect of you that connects with that which is spiritual – either with God (John 4:24) or with Satan and his minions, who are evil spiritual beings, although they are in no way on a par with God as omnipresent, omniscient, or omnipotent (Ephesians 6:12). These definitions do not cover all the ground that is actually encompassed by "body," "soul," and "spirit," but we are looking at a somewhat simplified outline of human nature in order to eventually better understand the concept of "new creation" and the bearing that being a "new creation" has on overeating.

The term "body" is not too difficult to grasp. "Soul" and "spirit" are trickier. In saying that the soul is the aspect of you that you can't see but is in constant flux, I mean that there is much that is intangible about us and changes from moment to moment, such as our personalities, emotions, and thoughts. Many authors define the soul as "mind, will, and emotions." But keep in mind that the mind is not the same as the brain. The brain can have physical maladies that affect the mind. The brain is physical, tangible, a part of the body. The mind refers to our thoughts, which are not visible and are intangible and therefore part of the soul.

Unlike the soul, which is constantly in flux, the human spirit does not change once we are indwelt by Christ. Just as the Old Testament temple of God in Jerusalem, our physical temple has at its center a "holy of holies" where God dwells. Personality, emotions, and thinking (all aspects of the soul) may all change from moment to moment, but because God does not change, our spirit does not change once God dwells there.

Let's look at two diagrams that might help in understanding these three aspects of who we are. The diagram on page 35 shows that our "outer layer" – or as speaker Bill Gillham calls it, our "earthsuit" – is the body. Within the body are the soul and spirit, with the spirit at our very core. Prior to becoming Christians, we are spiritually dead to God and alive to sin and Satan. (See Ephesians 2:1-3.) This permeates our entire lives and imprints our souls (mind, will, and emotions) and bodies with ungodly thoughts, beliefs, and habits.

Because of our identification with the death of Christ on the cross, at the core of our being, all the bondage to Satan is broken.

The diagram on page 36 shows these three aspects after we receive Christ. God takes up residence within us – in our spirit. We become spiritually 100 percent brand new. This is what 2 Corinthians 5:17 refers to. Because of our identification with the death of Christ on the cross, at the core of our being, all the bondage to Satan is broken. (See Romans 6:6-7.) Then, because of our identification with Christ's resurrection, we begin a new life with a transformed spirit, which has become a holy place where God actually dwells. (See Romans 8:9-11.) For the rest of our lives we are participants in a process of the indwelling Holy Spirit transforming the rest of us – transforming our souls and our bodies – changing our false beliefs, erroneous thinking, and negative habits. Theologians refer to this process as "sanctification." When we put our trust in Christ's death and resurrection as the means for our eternal salvation, we are instantly spiritually "reborn." (See John 3:7.) From then on, we gradually become more and more Christ-like as we cooperate with the work of the indwelling Holy Spirit.

WHAT YOU WERE LIKE BEFORE TRUSTING CHRIST

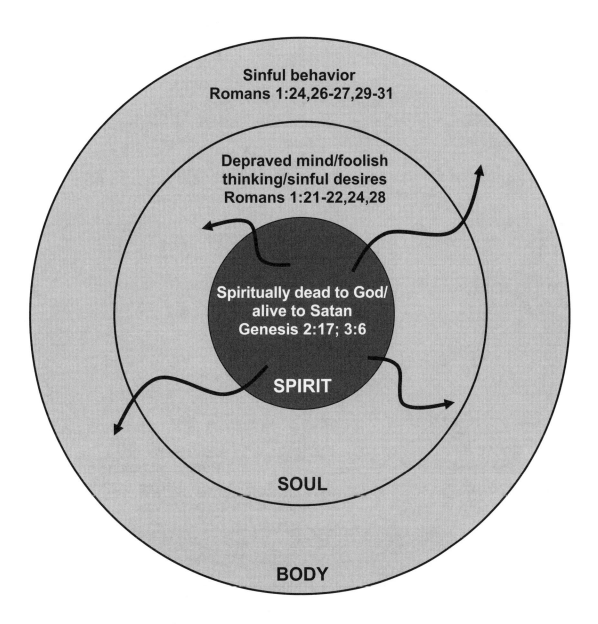

WHAT YOU ARE LIKE AFTER TRUSTING CHRIST
2 Corinthians 5:17

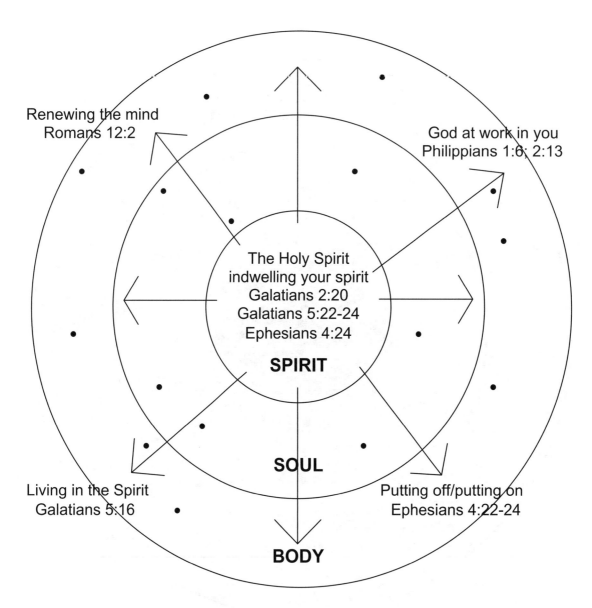

• Sin measles – Romans 7:21-23
   Examples: physical and emotional habits, wrong beliefs, and erroneous thinking

Throughout your life, the Holy Spirit is gradually curing you of the "sin measles," making you in your soul and body more and more like who you already are in your spirit.

This is not to say that our bodies won't continue to age and eventually die. Thank God that we will someday receive new, imperishable bodies (1 Corinthians 15:42). This does mean, however, that God helps us to overcome the physical dependencies – such as on drugs – that we developed while trying to maneuver through life without depending on him. It appears that some people are instantly delivered from dependencies at conversion and, for some, it is more gradual or comes later in their Christian experience. But, for every bondage, God is in the business of working it out of our lives and heading us toward freedom. (See John 8:36.)

In the diagram on page 36, I refer to our erroneous or sinful beliefs and thoughts and our negative emotional and physical habits as "sin measles." This is in order to address an unfortunate tendency people have to define themselves by their negative behaviors or by their sins. When someone has the measles, we do not say, "You are one big, red measle." In the same way, when a person becomes a "new creation in Christ," but continues to struggle with sin, we are mistaken when we say, "You are a dirty, rotten sinner." Rather, the person is a saint, a holy dwelling place of God, who still has sin in his or her soul and body. The Corinthians were engaging in sinful behaviors when Paul wrote to them and called them "sanctified in Christ Jesus" (1 Corinthians 1:2). They were spiritually totally "new creations," but they were still being influenced by the sin that remained within them and around them. Because we are "new creations," it is inappropriate for us to refer to ourselves with labels such as "compulsive eater" or "glutton." At worst, we are saints who still behave at times in ways that are not totally in line with who we are spiritually.

The Bible has a lot of amazing things to say about what we are like as "new creations" in Christ. We are holy (1 Peter 2:9), perfect (Hebrews 10:14), complete (Colossians 2:10), and adequate (2 Corinthians 3:5). We possess the "fruit" of the Spirit; therefore, we are loving, joyful, peaceful, patient, kind, good, faithful, gentle, and self-controlled (Galatians 5:22-23).

"Oh, right!" you might say. "I'm not like that!" When confronted with these "truths," the question immediately arises, "If I'm a new creation and all these things are supposed to be true of me, why don't I behave, think, and feel like it?!" The answer lies in those "sin measles." Although we have a 100 percent new spirit, the influence of having been born separated from God and having functioned under the influence of Satan remains with us. In Romans 7:21-25, this is referred to as "the principle of sin." Sin is at work within our "members" (Romans 7:23). There are a number of erroneous beliefs about which we became convinced as a result of sin's and Satan's influence. There are a number of negative emotional and physical habits that we developed apart from God's guidance. These do not totally vanish the moment we become Christians (although at least some of them do for most people). What totally vanishes is Satan's grip on our spirit. As Christians, because we are vitally linked with God – for he has taken up residence within us – we now have the freedom and power to choose whether we sin or not (although the ravages of our former bondage to Satan sometimes cloud our perceptions so that we don't always see our choices clearly). Despite all the negative influence of sin and Satan and the corrupted world in which we live, as new creations, we are on the mend! The indwelling Holy Spirit is guiding us into all truth (John 16:13), God is at work in us to enable us to obey him (Philippians

There are a number of erroneous beliefs about which we become convinced as a result of sin's and Satan's influence.

2:13), and we are being transformed into the likeness of Christ (2 Corinthians 3:18). The Spirit is gradually curing us of the "sin measles."

This is not to infer that we can just sit back and watch this take place. There are a number of imperatives in the New Testament that indicate we have a role to play in our own transformation. Romans 12:2 tells us to "be transformed by the renewing of your mind." Ephesians 4:22-24 tells us to "put off" the "old self" and "put on" the new. Galatians 5:16 tells us to "live by the Spirit." Colossians 3:15 says to "let the peace of Christ rule in your hearts." And, there are many, many more verses along these lines. These passages indicate that the process of becoming more and more on the "outside" (in our souls and bodies) like our "inside" (spirit) requires our participation. This process can be compared to a ballroom dance, where God and the believer are partners[1]. God leads and the believer follows. As a result of the death and resurrection of Christ, God has made you a new creation and given you the power through the indwelling Holy Spirit to live a godly life, but you won't live like a new creation until you respond by believing you are a new creation and acting in light of this truth.

A story which is a good illustration of how we can be "new creations" and yet not act or feel like we are may be "urban folklore," but useful nevertheless. The story is that there was a small boy who was left to be reared by his senile grandparents. The grandparents were so senile that they actually put the child in the backyard kennel with the dogs and left him there. The grandparents apparently fed the child and gave him water, but they rarely brought him into the house. By the time neighbors called in the authorities, the child had for all intents and purposes become one of the dogs. He ate from a dog dish, lapped water with his tongue, went around on all fours, and lifted his leg to relieve himself.

Now, what was this boy behaving like? A dog. What was he really? A boy. What do we sometimes see ourselves behaving like? A sinner. What are we really? A "new creation," a "saint" who has a new, pure spirit. In the same way as the little boy, we were conditioned to believe we were "dogs." Satan has us convinced – by our feelings, history, and circumstances – that we are "dirty rotten sinners," but God has recreated us into holy, pure saints. This is not just God looking at us through "rose-colored glasses" and seeing us as we someday will be in heaven because of the blood of Christ. This is an actual change that he has wrought in our natures. (See Hebrews 8:8b-12.) It is because of the sacrifice of Christ that we have changed so that the Spirit is able to take up residence within us. (See Galatians 2:20 and Colossians 1:21-22.)

When we behave in ways that are "out of control," we are not "being ourselves."

What this means for those of us who struggle with overeating is that, despite evidence in our behavior to the contrary, we can start believing that what God says about us is more true than what we feel and think about ourselves. If God says that he has given us "self-control" (Galatians 5:23), then we know when we behave in ways that are "out of control," we are not "being ourselves." The *real* you, even though none of us has fully experienced that yet, is a person who is free of compulsions and eats moderately. There are just a few "sin measles" (mostly well-suppressed false beliefs) getting in the way of you eating in moderation – and you'll likely recognize and address those "measles" in the course of reading this book. (Look at the title of the next chapter!)

Reflection

1. What are some of the negative things you have believed to be true about yourself, either because society or your parents – or even you – have convinced you of them?

2. Can you see specific ways in which what you've believed about yourself has affected your eating and weight?

What Others Have Experienced

- What are some of the negative things you have believed to be true about yourself?

The most typical, immediate answers to this question are: "I'm ugly and fat," "I'll be fat all my life," and "I just can't control myself." There are two aspects of our culture that feed into such beliefs. First, our culture equates beauty with thinness, thinness that is unrealistic for most women. Also, our culture accepts the idea that once a person displays a "compulsive behavior," this is evidence of a "disease" that can never be cured but only treated (usually through a "program") for the rest of one's life. A later chapter in this book will go into depth about the thinness-equals-beauty lie. But what this chapter discusses strikes directly at the "this-is-my-disease-that-I'll-always-struggle-with" lie.

I have referred to "sin measles," which are the thoughts, beliefs, and habits that were developed apart from God's influence and still affect us even though we are 100 percent spiritually regenerate. The Bible term for this is "the flesh." In *Lifetime Guarantee*, Bill Gillham provides an excellent discussion of the flesh – what it is and how it manifests itself in different people. The definition he uses for "the flesh" is "the old ways or patterns by which you have attempted to get all your needs supplied instead of seeking Christ first and trusting Him to meet your needs."[1] Before we were aware of the ways in which God has planned for our needs to be met, we worked out ways to meet them ourselves. Many times, compulsive behaviors are the ways we seek to meet our emotional needs. In my own case, I had a terrible inner conflict between 1) wanting to be attractive to men so I could get the male attention I craved, and 2) wanting to shun sexual advances because I was afraid I'd be unable to resist them. I developed two ways of coping with this conflict. I felt a little nauseated whenever I was alone with a man, and I compulsively ate so that I'd stay just "fat" enough to feel no one would "hit on" me. This was how my "flesh" dealt with my inner conflict. Once I realized that as a new creation in Christ, the Holy Spirit would empower me to say no to sexual advances, I stopped feeling nauseated while on dates and I started binge eating less and less. Instead of acting in accordance with my "flesh" – my old ways of dealing with life apart from the Holy Spirit – I started living in the power of the Spirit more and more.

I did not have an incurable, lifelong ailment; I had some erroneous beliefs and I was ignorant about how God works in people's lives. The "cure" to compulsion is found ultimately in a Spirit-led life. Ephesians 5:18 points to this, as does Galatians 5:16.

- Can you see specific ways in which what you've believed about yourself has affected your eating and weight?

Here are three comments that Weight of Grace small group participants made and some "new creation" thinking in response to each of them.

- *"If I were thin, I'd be proud and feel superior to others."* In this woman's family, pride was the ultimate no-no. As a young teen, she had gotten attention for her emerging, yet lithe, figure. She had also been elected cheerleader. She'd felt quite good about her looks and the popularity she believed resulted from them. Oops! That was pride! That wasn't right! She was a Christian. Christians are never supposed to be proud. In fact, didn't her pastor claim that pride sends some people to hell?! Knowing how proud she'd felt as a teen and remembering the resulting guilt over that pride, she now dreaded a repeat of that sinful attitude if she lost weight. As an alternative to her fears, the "new creation" thinking is, yes, in "the flesh," she might from time to time feel pride, but the indwelling Spirit will motivate her to have the humble attitude of Christ (Philippians 2:5-7). The Spirit will also remind her that God judges people, not by outward appearance, but by the attitude of the heart (1 Samuel 16:7). Knowing that God will guide her away from pride, she can give up being fat and risk having a figure for which people might pay her compliments. She'll know their attention is being directed to something of much less value than her right standing and intimate relationship with God. Her inner motivation, under the influence of the Holy Spirit, will lead her away from a prideful attitude.
- *"I really can't control myself when it comes to eating."* More than one small group participant has made this comment. Sometimes this belief comes from what parents, peers, or treatment programs have communicated, and sometimes it's just the result of experiencing over and over again that seeming inability to stop eating when one feels she really should be able to do so. But, despite all of your experience so far (and

perhaps for a while yet), as a "new creation," God has given you "self-control" (Galatians 5:23) and has designed you in such a way that you naturally take proper care of yourself (Ephesians 5:29). This means that, after some work on your particular "sin measles," you will actually be able to be just as God has created you – self-controlled – when it comes to eating.

- *"I don't deserve to be thin."* When a small group participant made this statement, I completely understood the pain she felt, but my knee-jerk, smart-alecky (totally silent) mental response was, *None of us deserves any good thing – and why do you think being "thin" is such a reward anyway?* The truth is that, as sinners, we didn't deserve anything from God. In his love for us, however, God bestowed upon us through Christ not only eternity with him in heaven, but also a transformed inner self. It doesn't depend on whether you deserve it or not; it depends on the love and character of God. But this woman wasn't making a theological statement about total depravity and grace. She was expressing her belief in her lack of worth as a person and her belief that being "thin" is a state only for those who are "worthy." The "new creation" truth, however, is that by dying on the cross for her, Christ has established just how worthy she truly is. She's worth his dying for. And by resurrecting her into a new life as a new creation, Christ affirms her as being worthy enough to be his dwelling place. She has tremendous worth because of who she is to Christ and in Christ. Also, a "new creation in Christ" has the mind and values of Christ, who does not evaluate people by their appearance. Therefore, she need no longer see being "thin" as a validation of worth. She can see that her relationship with Christ and resultant inner beauty are to be greatly prized more than achieving a lower weight.

Being transformed doesn't depend on whether you deserve it or not; it depends on the love and character of God.

Homework

1. Set aside at least an hour for this assignment. Ask the Holy Spirit to reveal to you events that took place in your life that resulted in you having beliefs about yourself that are not true. Then, using the "age span sheets" on the following pages, in the first column, write down how old you were (or approximately how old you were) and, very briefly, what the circumstances were. In the second column, write the false belief that resulted. If you know of one, in the third column, write a truth from Scripture that contradicts the false belief. (You don't have to know the chapter and verse; you can just write a general principle from Scripture. However, if you can make the time, look up Scripture passages that apply.) Be careful not to be overly introspective. Allow the Holy Spirit to bring to your mind the events and false beliefs that are important for you to consider right now. It is not necessary to put something on every sheet. Once you have completed the sheets, ask other members in your small group or ask a godly friend to help you with the "God's Promises" column for each "Lie Believed as Truth." Here is an example of an "age span sheet" entry:

Age and Circumstance	Lie Believed as Truth	God's Promises
12 – Boys made fun of me for being "fat."	I am "fat" and, therefore, ugly.	1 Peter 3:3-4 – God says I'm lovely because of my inner nature.

RENEWING THE MIND – AGE SPAN SHEETS – YEARS 0 THROUGH 10[2]

Age & Circumstance	Lie Believed as Truth	God's Promises

RENEWING THE MIND – AGE SPAN SHEETS – YEARS 11 THROUGH 20

Age & Circumstance	Lie Believed as Truth	God's Promises

RENEWING THE MIND – AGE SPAN SHEETS – YEARS 21 THROUGH 35

Age & Circumstance	Lie Believed as Truth	God's Promises

RENEWING THE MIND – AGE SPAN SHEETS – YEARS 36 AND OLDER

Age & Circumstance	Lie Believed as Truth	God's Promises

2. In the following "Becoming Who You Already Are" chart, find some statements in the first column with which you identify and put a checkmark by each of them. Read the contrasting statements in the second column and look up the Bible verses in the third column. Ask God to make these truths more and more real to you.

Becoming Who You Already Are[3]

What I Feel or Think About Myself	What Is True About Me According to Scripture	Scripture
I am unworthy/unacceptable.	I am accepted/worthy.	Ps. 139; Rom. 15:7
I am alone.	I am never alone.	Rom. 8:38-39; Heb. 13:5b
I feel like a failure/inadequate.	I am adequate.	2 Cor. 3:5-6; Phil. 4:13
I have no confidence.	I have all the confidence I need.	Prov. 3:26; 14:26; Eph. 3:12; Heb. 10:19
I feel responsible for my life.	God is responsible/faithful to me.	Ps. 138:8; Phil. 1:6; 2:13; 2 Thes. 3:3
I am confused/think I'm going crazy.	I have the mind of Christ.	1 Cor. 2:16; Eph. 1:17; 2 Tim. 1:7
I am depressed/hopeless.	I have all the hope I need.	Ps. 27:13; Rom. 5:5; 15:13; Heb. 6:19
I am not good enough/imperfect.	I am perfect in Christ.	Eph. 2:10; Col. 2:10; Heb. 10:14
There is nothing special about me.	I have been chose/set apart by God.	Ps. 139; 1 Cor. 1:30; 2 Thes. 2:13
I don't have enough.	I have no lack.	Phil. 4:19
I am a fearful/anxious person.	I am free from fear.	Ps. 34:4; 2 Tim. 1:7; 1 Pet. 5:7
I lack faith.	I have all the faith I need.	Rom. 10:17; 12:3; Heb. 12:2
I am a weak person.	I am strong in Christ.	Is. 58:11; Dan. 11:32; Phil 4:13
I am defeated.	I am victorious.	Rom. 8:37; 2 Cor. 2:14; 1 Jn. 5:4
I am not very smart.	I have God's wisdom.	Prov. 2:6-7; 1 Cor. 1:30; Eph. 1:17
I am in bondage.	I am free in Christ.	Ps. 32:7; Jn. 8:36; 2 Cor. 3:17
I am miserable.	I have God's comfort.	Jn. 16:7; 2 Cor. 1:3-4
I have no one to take care of me.	I am protected/safe.	Ps. 32:7; Ps. 91
I am unloved.	I am very loved.	Jn. 15:9; Rom. 8:38-39; Eph. 2:4; 5:1
I am unwanted/don't belong to anyone.	I have been adopted by God. I am His child.	Rom. 8:16-17; Gal. 4:5; Eph. 1:5; 1 Jn. 3:1-2
I feel guilty.	I am totally forgiven/redeemed.	Ps. 103:12; Eph. 1:7; Col. 1:14,20
I am a sinner.	I have been declared holy, righteous and justified.	Rom. 3:24; 1 Cor. 1:30; 6:11; 2 Cor. 5:21
I have no strength.	I have God's power. I am indwelt by the Holy Spirit.	Acts 1:8; Rom. 8:9-11; Eph. 1:19; 3:16
I can't reach God.	As a believer-priest, I have direct access to God.	Eph. 2:6; Heb. 10:19-20; 1 Pet. 2:5,9
I feel condemned.	I am not condemned/am blameless.	Jn. 3:18; Rom. 8:1; Col. 1:22
There is no direction/plan.	God directs me/has a plan for me.	Ps. 37:23; 138:8; Jer. 29:11; Eph. 2:10
Nothing will ever change.	I've been given a brand new life.	2 Cor. 5:17; Eph. 4:22-24
I am afraid of Satan.	I have authority over Satan.	Col. 1:13; 1 Jn. 4:4; Rev. 12:11
Sin overpowers me.	I am dead to sin.	Rom. 6:6, 11, 17-18

BEFORE YOU GO ON TO THE NEXT CHAPTER

Homework Follow-up

1. What was a striking lie that the Holy Spirit revealed you have believed about yourself? Where did it come from? What is the truth?

2. For the statements in the first column of the "Becoming Who You Already Are" chart that stood out to you, do you believe the contrasting truths? Why or why not?

Comments on the Homework

- What is a striking lie you've believed about yourself?

The following are some examples of "lies believed as truth" women have reported (and I've paraphrased):

- *My grandmother always told me, "You can't do anything right," and "You'll never amount to anything."* This group member realized that she had believed her grandmother's pronouncements to be true and that she had done a great deal to either fulfill them or overcompensate for them. In light of Scripture, she chose to start believing that God does indeed adequately equip her for any circumstance to which he calls her (Philippians 2:13; 4:13). She started to expect to succeed or, if her efforts did not turn out as she hoped, she chose to believe that God had a purpose in that also.

- *Throughout my adulthood, I married mainly because I was tired of supporting myself. I couldn't seem to stop myself from marrying the wrong kinds of men. So, I started believing that the only way to keep from marrying again was to stay so fat that no one would come around and tempt me to marry him.* This woman had had four unhappy marriages and had started to truly trust in Christ after her fourth husband died. Ironically, shortly after she realized she held this false belief and even though she was quite large, a man she was seeing and who appeared to her to be a "nice man" (but apparently not a vital Christian) asked her to move in with him. Being "fat" hadn't succeeded in fending off opportunities to be supported by a man! However, as a result of believing God would direct her to do what was right and what was best for her, even though the man presented her with a more convenient financial circumstance, she turned him down. She credited this to the work of the Holy Spirit in her life.

- *In reaction to my father molesting me, I tried to be perfect so no one would know how weird I really was. When the truth came out about Dad, I gave up on being perfect because everyone knew I wasn't. Now I stay fat so I won't have to be "perfect."* It's a horrible strain to be perfect. And in our culture, for women, being thin equals being perfect. Many women equate staying thin with having to engage in a constant effort to remain at an ideal weight or size. Rather than working so hard at what they feel will eventually result in failure anyway, they just give up and get "fat." In light of her new understanding about her nature as a new creation in Christ, this woman stopped viewing herself as "weird" because she'd been molested. She also saw that there had never really been a need to be perfect, because God does not insist on our perfection in order for us to be acceptable to him. Therefore, she no longer had to do anything (such as stay fat) to combat the pressure to be "perfect."

- For the statements that stood out to you in the chart, do you believe the contrasting truths?

In the back of Campus Crusade's evangelistic booklets, there's a diagram of a little train. The engine is "Fact." The first car behind the engine is "Faith," and the caboose is "Feeling."[4] This illustration is a reminder that the *feeling* that we are "created to be like God in true righteousness and holiness" (Ephesians 4:24) and in possession of all the fruit of the Spirit may not come right away. What's important is to be willing to "be transformed by the renewing of your mind" (Romans 12:2). When I do what I call "prayerful pondering," I ask God to help me think through his truth and how it applies to my life. I often do this while I'm on a walk or driving to work. I think through the scriptural principles that tell me what I'm really like, pondering how they are true even though my behavior doesn't always line up. I remind myself – and I believe the Holy Spirit prompts me to do this – that at the very core of my being, in my true nature, I am a person who wants to live according to truth, who loves unconditionally, who is patient toward people, and who deeply desires to be in total dependence upon God and to live a holy life. I ask God to do whatever it takes to eliminate whatever is in me that results in my behaving in ways contrary to my true nature. While pondering, I sometimes realize I'm trying to meet a need through a "fleshly" behavior. Then Scripture passages come to mind that show how *God* meets that need. This thinking is evidence of God at work in me. This is part and parcel of having an intimate relationship with God – thinking his truth through, talking it over with him, and allowing him to bring issues and pertinent Scripture to light. Ultimately, this leads to my *feeling* that what God says about me as a "new creation in Christ" is really the truth. Sometimes my

Many women equate staying thin with having to engage in a constant effort to remain at an ideal weight or size.

At the very core of my being, in my true nature, I am a person who wants to live according to truth.

feelings change in just a moment and sometimes it has taken several years. What's important is to realize that the truth doesn't always *feel* like the truth to us, but that doesn't change how true it really is!

4 IDENTIFYING UNDERLYING BELIEFS: WHAT MOTIVATES OVEREATING AND OVERWEIGHT?

There is a way that seems right to a man... Proverbs 14:12a

The "ways" that seem right to us are our beliefs.[1] And, our beliefs influence absolutely everything we do. For example, when you sit down on a chair, you do so because you believe it is sturdy enough to support your weight. You don't think through this basic belief. You just make an assumption (an assumption is a type of belief) based on experience. From repeatedly sitting on chairs and having your weight supported, you formed a belief that most chairs, which have certain recognizable characteristics, are sturdy enough to hold you.

Christians may have many beliefs that are accurate, but because we still suffer from the "sin measles" and because we are influenced by our "flesh," by ungodly aspects of our culture, and even directly by Satan, we also have a number of inaccurate beliefs. These are the "ways" that seem right to us – but lead to our destruction. (Look at what the second half of Proverbs 14:12 says.) When it comes to continuous overeating and struggles with overweight, the beliefs that we hold – the ways that seem right to us – are what keep us in defeat no matter how many diets and programs we try. As long as certain beliefs are present, they will affect how we behave. As long as I believed that I would automatically succumb to the temptation to engage in sex outside of marriage, I also believed I needed to stay "fat" in order to ward off being faced with that temptation. No diet could change that basic belief. Being "thin" just didn't feel right to me, and I repeatedly sabotaged my efforts to lose weight. Also, as long as I believed that overeating was a lifelong addiction, I saw myself as someone who was either "on the wagon" or who had totally fallen off of it. I didn't believe I was capable of moderation. I either rigidly dieted or ate like a fiend. My beliefs seemed right to me. They were totally wrong. But, they totally influenced my behavior.

We have formed beliefs about every aspect of life, and they are the basis upon which we make decisions and take action (or take no action). Also, our beliefs are the grid through which we perceive everything. For example, if you hold the belief that you are not really good at public speaking, when you are put in the position to give a public address, and then receive a compliment for it, you will very likely say to yourself, *Oh, he just said that to be nice.* It wouldn't matter if the compliment was truly deserved; your belief would lead you to interpret the compliment as insincere (albeit "nice").

Time and time again, I have heard husbands complain about how their wives do not accept their compliments, especially in regard to their appearance. This is particularly true for women who believe themselves to be "fat" and therefore ugly. I recently saw a greeting card on which a woman is depicted asking her husband about ten times, "Am I fat?" and he answers "No" each time. The punch line inside the card is: "Happy anniversary to the man

When it comes to continuous overeating and struggles with overweight, the beliefs that we hold – the ways that seem right to us – are what keep us in defeat no matter how many diets and programs we try.

who has all the right answers." So many women have a basic belief that they are "fat" and that being "fat" is totally unacceptable to anyone – no matter how much affirmation they receive to the contrary.

We were not born with the beliefs we have. They were formed as a result of our experiences. Some of our beliefs were taught to us, directly or indirectly, by family, teachers, and churches. Some of what we were taught was positive and based upon biblical truth, but if you're like just about every Weight of Grace small group participant, most wasn't. We also pick up beliefs from our peers, the media, literature, and our culture. And so much of our media, literature, and culture is not influenced by God and is, in fact, antagonistic toward God and his Word. Many Christian women have a belief that "if I love this man, then God must have put him in my life and it's okay that I'm living with/sleeping with him." This is not based upon Scripture. It opposes many verses about avoiding sexual immorality and reserving sexual intimacy for marriage. This belief, however, does jibe with a pervasive cultural standard that it is acceptable to live with or have sex with someone as long as you love him or her.

Most of the time the errors in our beliefs are not obvious. An example of a subtle erroneous belief is the person who, when he was a small child, was told by his parents that he was clumsy. The parents did not realize that what they called clumsy was really a display of normal motor skills for a toddler. To them, how clumsy "Junior" was, was their little family joke. However, Junior formed the belief that he really was clumsy. He then went through life perceiving all of his behaviors as either evidence of his clumsiness (when he'd knock something over as most of us do from time to time) or as an amazing departure from his "norm" of clumsiness (when he didn't bump into anything or drop anything as the opportunities arose). A person having a belief such as this will either actually act clumsily because he believes that he is clumsy or become overly careful in order to avoid acting as clumsy as he fears himself to be. Remember, the "clumsy" person was never actually clumsy in the first place! And, he's probably totally unaware of the erroneous belief that's motivating his behaviors.

Most of the time the errors in our beliefs are not obvious.

The belief that was a big motivator for my remaining "fat" is one common to many victims of incest. My stepfather made comments and behaved toward me in ways that inferred I had brought his advances upon myself. Also, since this was the only male attention available to me, I had on occasion actually put myself in his way with the hope he would molest me. These factors led me to believe that I was the type of person who, given half a chance, would behave in sexually inappropriate ways and that the resulting guilt would be unbearable. Because of this belief, I developed a "flesh pattern," a way of coping using my own devices. (Remember, "the flesh" is our attempt to get needs met in our own way instead of allowing God to meet our needs his way.) I kept myself just "fat" enough to feel sure that no one would be attracted enough to me to make any advances and, therefore, tempt me to become sexually involved. My reaction to the belief that I was a "slut," as I used to hear myself say in my head, was to be overly careful not to act like the slut I knew myself to be.

I know a woman whose childhood experiences were very similar to mine. She, too, had the belief that she was a "slut." But, she reacted in a very different way as a result of that belief. Her thinking was, *Since I am this way, there's no use in fighting it.* So, she became sexually active at an early age and "slept around." What was sad about both of us was that, especially as Christians, neither of us was a slut! I was overcompensating for how promiscuous I believed myself to be on the inside, and she was living out what she believed herself to be.

It really should be no surprise to us that we hold inaccurate, twisted beliefs. Romans 1:21-22 tells us that our "thinking became futile" and we became "fools" as a result of our separation from God. Also, Romans 12:2 refers to how the "world" – our culture, media, and institutions – tries to "conform" us, tries to "press us into its mold."[2] Jesus told us that, for now, Satan is the prince of this world (John 12:31). Satan uses the world to pressure us into thinking we should all look and act as he desires. So, movies, advertisements, magazines, and television shows lead women to believe they should be "thin" and that "thin" equals success and happiness while "fat" equals failure and misery. (And often their version of "thin" is not normal for anyone and "fat" is what is perfectly normal for most!) But those same movies, ads, TV shows, and magazines also tell us that chocolate is an emotional cure-all and that "fat" people are humorous and loveable. Satan loves the confusion and inner conflict that result from these contradictory beliefs.

What is really scary about our inaccurate beliefs is that they control us. Proverbs 23:7a says, "For as he thinketh in his heart, so is he" (KJV). What we hold to be true controls who we are and how we behave. Most people around my age (I was born in 1953) remember the singer Karen Carpenter. She got the idea that she was "chubby." She spent most of her adult life overcompensating for her chubbiness by starving herself – until she died as a result. That appears to be an obvious and easily identified false belief. But, it wasn't obvious to her, just as the beliefs that control us aren't obvious to us.

What is really scary about our inaccurate beliefs is that they control us.

So, if our beliefs are oftentimes erroneous and they also control us, is there any hope for us? Read Romans 12:2 and Ephesians 4:22-23. Now that we are new creations in Christ and are no longer controlled by sin, we have the power to change our beliefs. Because of the indwelling Holy Spirit and the inspired Word of God, we have the ability to identify false beliefs, turn from them, and start accepting beliefs that are based upon God's truth. In Romans 12:2, this is called "renewing the mind." In Ephesians 4:23, it's called being "made new in the attitude your minds." Second Corinthians 10:4-5 refers to "strongholds," "arguments," and "pretensions" that try to block our knowing the truth. In response to them, we are directed to enter into the process of "taking every thought captive to the obedience of Christ" (NASB). When we become aware that a belief is erroneous, we can exchange it for the truth. But, *how* do we do this? How do we renew our minds?

Now that we are new creations in Christ, we have the power to change our beliefs.

To begin with, we must realize that the Holy Spirit is our guide. As the one who leads us into all truth (John 16:13), he will show us what specifically needs to be renewed, when it needs to be renewed, and then will provide us with the power to do so. This is an integral part of our relationship with God. We are not engaged in a "religion" of only rituals and dogma, but in a vital *relationship* with the living God, who desires to interact with us, to

To begin with, we must realize that the Holy Spirit is our guide.

personally communicate with us, and to transform us. This means we can expect to "hear" from the Holy Spirit.

Hearing the Spirit can happen in a number of ways. It is said that the Scripture is the vocabulary of the Holy Spirit. When we read Scripture, no matter what passage we may be reading at the time, God speaks to us through his Word. According to Hebrews 4:12, Scripture judges our thoughts and attitudes. Just the other day, as part of preparation for our church Bible study, I was reading the passages in Luke about the trials of Jesus. When I read how Pilate, against his better judgment, succumbed to the loud, insistent, demanding shouts of the people to crucify an innocent Jesus, it popped into my head that I, too, was allowing "insistent shouts" to influence me. The shouts were from my culture, trying to tempt me to consider myself ugly and unworthy because I don't fit into a size 9 skirt. I was a little shocked by what seemed to be a trivial application of so grave an event in the life of Christ. Nevertheless, I believe the Holy Spirit was willing to use the passage I was reading to speak to me about my lapsing into old, false beliefs.

Not only does the Holy Spirit speak to us through the Scripture we're reading, but also he brings passages of Scripture to our minds at appropriate times. My feelings toward God have not always been of the warm, fuzzy, affectionate variety. As a result, I used to berate myself for not loving God. Believing myself to be a second-class Christian, I would use Deuteronomy 6:5 (and those passages in which Jesus quoted that verse) as the club with which I beat myself up because I didn't *feel* affectionate toward God. However, an experience when a verse popped into my head at just the right moment cured me of the false belief that I was a disappointment to God because of my lack of affectionate feelings for him. I was very much in love with the man I was dating, and although we were not having sex, I believed we were too physically involved. (This was after I got over my "be nauseated around men to stay away from sex" flesh pattern.) The morning after an evening of particularly heavy "necking," I called my boyfriend and told him I could not date him any longer. Given how much I craved affection, I could hardly believe I was doing this. This was the first man I had dated in quite a long while and I greatly feared it would be the last. Nevertheless, I truly felt giving the relationship up was what God was asking me to do in order to be obedient to him. After I hung up the phone, I heard a verse in my head: "This is love for God: to obey his commands" (1 John 5:3). Then I also heard, "And you say you don't love me." I realized that my love for God did not have to be a "mushy" feeling. As the old chorus goes, "Love is something you do, not something that you feel, but it's real." I changed my belief about myself and God's acceptance of me. God used bringing his Word to my mind to very personally communicate to me about a false belief I had.

Although the Holy Spirit would never contradict Scripture, the Spirit is not limited to only Scripture in speaking to us. Nearly every day I hear the "still, small voice" of God. (See 1 Kings 19:12 in the King James Version.) I hear that voice in thoughts such as, *It's all okay; things will work out for the best,* or *Just do the best you can; I'll take care of your reputation,* or *No, you're not an irritating person; that's an old belief that's untrue.* Yes, these could just be my own thoughts, but I believe if you're seeking to be in humble submission to God, he puts thoughts into your mind to encourage and direct you. (See Daniel 10:12.) You know a

God used bringing his Word to my mind to very personally communicate to me about a false belief I had.

thought is really from Satan or from one of your false beliefs if it's contrary to Scripture or evokes condemnation (Romans 8:1).

Other ways in which the Spirit speaks to us about our false beliefs are through fellow believers (Ephesians 4:15 and Colossians 3:16), Christian music (Ephesians 5:19), and even in dreams and visions (Acts 2:17-18). Of course, you can't base important life decisions on impressions or dreams. It is necessary to carefully test them against Scripture and to seek the affirmation of mature Christians with whom you're in fellowship (1 Thessalonians 5:21). However, even though it is possible to be led astray by Satan or by our own desires, this does not discount how God can and does communicate to us in unusual ways. I have many times been greatly encouraged by visions I have had or by those that others have had about me. Still, our most reliable source for direction is in the Scriptures with the Holy Spirit as our guide and interpreter.

Let's go through an example to better understand how beliefs can influence overeating and can be changed by the renewing of the mind. As I mentioned in Chapter 1, I struggled for years with going on horrendous eating binges. I always considered them to be caused by a profound lack of self-discipline. However, when I started considering that my eating was motivated by beliefs rather than the result of a lack of self-discipline, I began to ask God to show me the thinking behind these wild binges. Initially God used my roommate, Karen, to show me the main issue. She noticed that I would frantically eat and eat but seemed to feel no emotions. When I was binge eating, she would ask, "Are you upset about something? Do you feel stressed?" I'd always say, "No, I just want to eat the world. I don't feel anything." But Karen noticed on several occasions that when I'd gotten to the point of having eaten so much I felt ill, I'd start crying and telling her about some incident in which I'd had a negative interaction with a friend or co-worker.

When I started considering that my eating was motivated by beliefs rather than the result of a lack of self-discipline, I began to ask God to show me the thinking behind my wild binges.

After we realized the pattern, the next time I started to binge, Karen asked me, "What happened today?" She didn't ask me how I felt because she knew I didn't *feel* anything. She just asked me to tell her the events of my day. When I did, she said in regard to an exchange I'd had with a co-worker, "If he had talked to me like that, I would have felt really mad!" I said, "No, I don't feel angry about it at all," and continued on my binge. As usual, though, when I could eat no more and felt terribly ill, I started to cry and realized how hurt I felt because of the incident that day with my co-worker, who was also a friend. Later, I mentioned this pattern to a trusted counselor, who said that it seemed pretty obvious to him that I was suppressing anger by eating. Once I ate as much as I possibly could, I wasn't able to hold down the anger and hurt any longer. He also suggested that I was punishing myself for feeling angry toward someone I believed I should never feel anger toward.

I started praying about what Karen and my counselor friend were seeing as one of the underlying beliefs motivating my binge eating. Then I heard that "still, small voice" saying, "You believe anger is so horribly threatening that you are trying to punish yourself enough that you will avoid ever being angry again. You think that, if you get angry with someone, you will lose your relationship with that person." Then I remembered a lesson I'd heard on Ephesians 4:26 and how anger, in and of itself, is not necessarily sin. I realized that I could feel the anger but didn't have to express it inappropriately; therefore, I need not alienate a dear friend just because I felt anger toward him or her. God used two friends, prayer, a Bible lesson I'd heard, and his Word to change my wrong belief of "If I get angry at someone, I'm a horrible person and I'll lose that friendship." As a result, the painful, bulimic-like binges tapered off. However, anger was not the only motivator for my binge eating. Other beliefs needed to be addressed before the binge eating stopped altogether.

Hopefully, you noticed there was no formula involved in how God revealed to me my erroneous belief about anger. Formulas are not the same as relationship. God desires a relationship with us. Each of my false beliefs that have been changed to align with the truth have been changed through a different means, but each time God's Spirit and God's Word have been at the core of the process. My role was a willingness to enter into and participate in the process.

Reflection

1. Briefly, what do you believe to be bad about being "fat"?

2. What is good about being "fat"? What does being "fat" do *for* you? What about being "fat" are you afraid to lose?

3. Briefly, what are the good things you associate with being "thin"?

4. What is bad about being "thin"? What do you fear about being "thin"?

A Note about the Use of the Word "Fat"

In this book, the reason "fat" usually appears in quotes is because I don't believe that anyone *is* fat. All of us *have* varying degrees of fat cells on our bodies. However, for most people who struggle with the issues addressed in this book, *being* "fat" is a way they've come to describe themselves, and by describing themselves in that way, they mean "larger than I believe to be acceptable," even if no one else would think that. It's very subjective, but always extremely negative and reflects a belief to some degree in one's unworthiness as a person. Even for the woman whose weight is unusually high, *she* is not "fat" even though she has a large number of fat cells on her body. Who she is should not be defined by her physical characteristics alone and certainly not by only one physical characteristic. On the other hand, being "thin" is just as subjective as being "fat" and is considered every bit as positive as being "fat" is considered negative. "Thin" is the usually unobtainable ideal that we assume will, once reached, make life absolutely blissful. It is a totally unrealistic belief and no real woman experiences it.

What Others Have Experienced

- What do you believe to be bad about being "fat"?

Of course, it's pretty easy for most group participants to list the many ways in which being "fat" is bad: People think you're ugly. You are ugly. It's hard to find clothes that fit and look okay. You can't wear a swimsuit in public. Your husband or boyfriend doesn't like your looks. No man will ever like your looks. Every time you eat anything you really like, you feel guilty. You look silly in sexy lingerie. You aren't sexy. Your feet get tired faster. You don't fit into small places well, like between rows of desks or chairs. You are often short of breath. And so on. We all know – and are told constantly by the culture, friends, and relatives – how very bad it is to be "fat."

- What is good about being "fat"?

It's a little hard at first for most Weight of Grace participants to figure out what's good about being "fat." But, usually it takes just one or two examples to jump-start a stream of responses. You don't have to worry about men making unwanted advances. If people like you, it's for you and not for your looks. You don't have to worry that you'll get too proud about your appearance. Women aren't threatened by you. Men feel comfortable having you as a friend. You feel less likely to be attacked or assaulted. You don't have to constantly work at staying thin. You feel more nurturing. People expect less of you. You feel you're taken more seriously when you give your opinion. In some cases, husbands actually prefer "more to love" or that you're "out of the running" with other men. There is a great deal about being "fat" that is actually difficult to give up! Unless we acknowledge this, we will never be able to undo the thinking that is motivating us to stay "fat."

There is a great deal about being "fat" that is actually difficult to give up!

- What is good about being "thin"?

Again, it's usually very easy for group participants to identify the positives of being "thin." You can wear just about any clothes that you want. You can wear a bathing suit.

You can move about more easily. Your husband or boyfriend is proud to be seen with you. You're more likely to be or feel sexy. You like yourself more. People don't pity you. You feel better physically. Many of these aren't really true, but they're what we believe to be true for "thin" women.

- What is bad about being "thin"?

As much as women deeply long to be "thin," there are compelling reasons why being "thin" is repugnant.

By the time we get to this question, most group participants have picked up on the drift and can pretty easily come up with answers. My favorite is: "I'd have to be perfect and stay that way." That's the deal with being "thin"; it's "perfection" and that's quite a responsibility and burden. Once you're there, you have to maintain it or hate yourself. And maintaining it requires tremendous, exhausting effort. Other bad or scary aspects of being "thin" that group participants have mentioned are: You are more likely to be "hit on" by men. You're more tempted to flirt or engage in sexual sin. You feel small and more vulnerable. You don't feel you "carry as much weight" with people and aren't taken as seriously. You're tempted to feel prideful about your looks. People, especially men, like you primarily for your looks. Women are jealous of you and threatened by you. Men feel you're too attractive to be "just friends." And so on. As much as women deeply long to be "thin" and feel being "thin" is essential to their happiness, they also believe there are compelling reasons why being "thin" is repugnant. Overeating can often be motivated by a desire to avoid the perceived pitfalls of being "thin."

Homework

The following exercise is taken from *Breaking Free from Compulsive Eating* by Geneen Roth. (This book was recently reissued with the title *Breaking Free from Emotional Eating*.) Through this exercise God revealed to me beliefs that were greatly influencing me to overeat so that I would stay "fat." It strikes many people as a strange exercise, but I hope you make an attempt to complete it. Ask the Holy Spirit to guide your thoughts as you do. Scripture refers to a war that wages between our flesh and our true desires to obey God (Romans 7:21-23). This exercise helps those two aspects of ourselves come into the open and engage in a discussion. Remember, "the flesh" is our way of meeting our needs rather than allowing God to meet those needs. The flesh is really our way of trying to help ourselves, although misdirected and ultimately ineffective.

> Give the fat you a name and write a dialogue between…her…and you. (Give yourself at least two hours to complete this because it usually takes longer than you'd expect to quiet yourself enough to distinguish your voice from the voice of the fat you.) Speak to this part [of you], ask it what it wants, what it needs, how it is taking care of you.
>
> Tell it how you feel about it. Let yourself speak from your heart. If you are angry, be angry. If you are sad, be sad. But begin to make contact with what you have shunned and disliked for so long: the part of you that eats and eats and eats.[3]

BEFORE YOU GO ON TO THE NEXT CHAPTER

Homework Follow-up

1. What did your dialogue between you and your "fat self" reveal to you about the purposes being "fat" serves in your life?

2. What did the dialogue reveal about what you fear would happen if you were "thin"?

Comments on the Homework

Many Weight of Grace participants have felt so uncomfortable with the fat self/real you dialogue that they did not do this homework assignment. However, almost every woman who has done it has had a revelation about beliefs that motivate her to stay "fat." By far the most common theme is the avoidance of inappropriate behavior with men or the fear of having to contend with unwanted advances from men. The concerns range from anticipating a feeling of guilt about flirting to a terror of rape. Often the underlying false belief reflects 1) a lack of faith in what it means to be a "new creation" and in the power of the indwelling Holy Spirit, and/or 2) a lack of faith in God's willingness to protect.

Let's look at the "new creation" belief first. It's especially difficult to believe you'll behave appropriately when you've failed to do so in the past. One woman – I'll call her Lois – told of having been promiscuous during her teens. Even after becoming engaged, she had sex with men other than her fiancé. In doing the dialog exercise, Lois realized that she feared she would cheat on her husband and that staying "fat" was a way to ward off that temptation. She felt such temptation would be especially irresistible because her husband was having personal struggles that resulted in his being relatively inattentive to her. Lois's "fat self" reasoned with her about how she was a Christian when she slept around. What assurance did she have that she wouldn't do so again now? Lois needed the "fat self" to protect her from sinning. The "real Lois" piped up, however, with some additional information. Lois was reared in a denomination that emphasized rule keeping but taught little about God empowering the believer to engage in good works. During her teen years, Lois became aware of leaders in her church excusing themselves from obeying the rules they told others to keep. Her promiscuity was one of the ways in which she rebelled against the rules she saw others breaking while still requiring her to adhere to them. Since that time, she had come to understand the pitfalls of attempting to live the Christian life through her own efforts and was learning about the power to live a holy life that is available only from the indwelling Spirit of God. Before, she was living in "the flesh," working out her emotional turmoil (resentment toward overly rigid restrictions) her own way. Now, she was seeking to "walk in the Spirit." Lois made a decision to trust that, thanks to her new nature in Christ and her reliance upon the Spirit, engaging in sexual sin, even when sorely tempted to do so, would no longer be her means of meeting her emotional needs. She renewed her mind in regard to herself and God's role in her life, and as a result, she stopped constantly overeating.

In looking at beliefs about God's protection, I relate all too well to the fear of rape and having a lack of faith in God's willingness to keep me safe. I can't honestly say that this issue is totally resolved for me. Many people have told me that, when called upon, God protects his children from rape, but I know of several God-fearing women for whom this was not true. I've come to believe that God never allows anything in our lives for which he doesn't also give us sufficient grace to find victory in it. But, that's not wildly reassuring to me. When I did the dialog exercise several years ago, one role my "fat self" was playing became clear to me. She was allowing me to feel that a would-be attacker would take one look at me and think, *There's a big one!* and pass by me. My "real self" pointed out that I was

She renewed her mind in regard to herself and God's role in her life, and as a result, she stopped constantly overeating.

trying to protect myself in my own power through overeating and staying large. In light of this, I made a decision to put faith in God's sovereignty and not in my "fat."

The point here is not to completely resolve every issue you may have. It is, rather, that you become aware of what your erroneous beliefs are and how they may be motivating you to overeat and stay "fat." You can change your mind about your beliefs and turn to God to help you with your struggles rather than "taking care of yourself" through food and overweight.

5   ARE YOU REALLY GETTING IT SO FAR?

It is no trouble for me to write the same things to you again, and it is a safeguard for you. Philippians 3:1b

The concepts presented in the first four weekly sessions of each Weight of Grace small group are for many women very new ideas and not always easy to personally apply or even accept. They may at times even fly in the face of teachings or theology women have up to this point believed to be sacrosanct. Because this material can meet with surprise, uncertainty, or resistance, and because subsequent sessions hinge on group members really "getting it" when it comes to the foundational principles presented so far, during the fifth weekly session, we spend some time going back over what has been covered and seeing how much of it is really making sense to, and being personally experienced by, group members. As Paul notes in Philippians 3:1, reiteration of important principles is a safeguard. So, in this chapter, we will go back over the following concepts that are key to experiencing the freedom God has already given you from overeating, taking care to make very *personal* application: 1) being confident in God's personal concern for you, 2) understanding your nature as a "new creation in Christ," and 3) realizing the ability you have as a Christian to exchange erroneous beliefs for God's truth.

As you read this chapter, ask yourself the following questions – and ask the Holy Spirit to help you answer them:

- **Do I really comprehend what is being said here?**
- **Do I "buy it" – do I believe this is the truth?**
- **Do I believe this is really true *for me*?**

God's Character and Concern for You

Before you will experience true freedom from overeating and overweight, the most important question for you to answer is: Do you believe that God is interested in setting you free from overeating? There is a lot of "programming" that can influence even Christians to have erroneous beliefs about God (2 Corinthians 10:5), to see him in a negative light. The tendency among most women who struggle with overeating is to believe that God is critical of them, disgusted and impatient with them, and pretty much fed up. However, this is not the God that Jesus came to earth to reveal! These beliefs about God are usually based upon how *people* have behaved and especially upon the actions and attitudes of one's *earthly father*. But, the incarnation and death of Christ prove that God wants us to experience a loving and intimate relationship with him. He *is* concerned about the very painful areas of our lives, even if we think of them as unimportant or trivial (Psalm 139:1-4). We are in no way the objects of his condemnation (Romans 8:1).

Do you believe that God is interested in setting you free from overeating?

When it comes to our view of God, we need to ask the Holy Spirit to "test our thoughts" (Psalm 139:23), to show us where our thinking is off, and to show us the real truth. Without at least a willingness to believe that God is "in there with you," true freedom from overeating isn't possible for the Christian. If the truth about God's loving and intimate care for you does not seem to be sinking in for you personally, prayerfully return to the Bible studies at the end of "FatherCare" (Addendum One). Look up the Scripture passages in those studies and ask God to call to your attention examples in your daily life that show he is truly as loving and involved as he says he is. Also, you might read one of the excellent books that reinforce an accurate view of God, such as *Our Heavenly Father* by Robert Frost or *The Father Heart of God* by Floyd McClung.

Remember my friend's analogy in the first few pages of this book? Some of us tend to skim the surface of information, but there is no more important area in which to go "deep sea diving" than in one's understanding of what God is really like. Yes, no one this side of heaven has a 100 percent accurate view of God. As I mentioned before, I still struggle with thinking God is "mean." But, having it all figured out is not the prerequisite to experiencing freedom from overeating. Rather, a willingness to believe God is interested in your struggles and in helping you overcome them is what's vital to finding that freedom.

Okay, ask yourself those three questions on page 63. Decide whether you need to do more "work" on this issue before you move on – Bible study, meditation (prolonged, prayerful pondering, not the Eastern religion type of meditation – no lotus positions necessary), review of materials/homework, further reading, and/or discussion with fellow believers or with fellow small group members if you're studying this book with others.

Who You Are as a "New Creation in Christ"

There is a tendency in our culture for people to define themselves by their behaviors and/or appearance.

When it comes to what's important for finding freedom from overeating, second only to having an accurate understanding about God is having an accurate understanding about you. There is a tendency in our culture for people to define themselves by their behaviors and/or appearance. This is not only inaccurate, but also disastrous. Scripture tells us that we live out what we believe ourselves to be (Proverbs 23:7 – see KJV). If you think of yourself as a "big, fat slob," you will either actually live like one or expend massive amounts of energy fighting against looking on the outside like what you believe yourself to really be on the inside.

In many self-help groups, participants are asked to make statements such as: "Hi, I'm Paula, and I'm a compulsive eater." This type of "confession" is used to discourage denial. However, it also inaccurately brands the individual, locking her into a behavior that need not be a permanent part of her life. A better, more biblically accurate confession would be: "Hi, I'm Paula, and I'm a new creation in Christ who sometimes engages in overeating but is seeking God's power to transform me in that area." (This, however, is probably not succinct enough to recite when introducing yourself at a meeting without irritating others in attendance!)

As a Christian, your identity is spelled out for you in Scripture. God does not define you by your behaviors but by whom he created you to be. When you trusted in Christ for salvation, God made you into a "new creation" (2 Corinthians 5:17), empowered and motivated from within by the Holy Spirit. God has given you a new, pure heart that desires to be in total obedience to him (Hebrews 10:16). He has even given you "self-control" (Galatians 5:23). You may not have experienced this to any great extent yet, but this is because you were ignorant of the truth. And, remember, it is the truth that sets you free! (John 8:32)

What keeps us from wholeheartedly believing that we are "new creations" with self-control as part of our nature is our behavior, which seems to make the "fruit of the Spirit" Scripture passage look like a lie. If we're such wonderful "new creations," why do we engage in behaviors such as overeating, yelling at our kids, telling "white lies," gossiping, etc.? The answer is that, even though our spirits (our innermost selves where God has taken up residence) are totally new, pure, and holy, we are still affected in our souls (thoughts, personalities, emotions, will) and bodies by the experiences of having been born "in sin" (spiritually separated from God) and of living in this sinful world. Paul refers to this as "sin at work within my members" (Romans 7:23), and I've called it the "sin measles." It's a wretched state! (Romans 7:24). But, God is at work in us to deliver us from this condition (Philippians 1:6, 2:13). The indwelling Holy Spirit points out to us when we are acting out of "the flesh" (our attempts to meet our needs in our own way) or out of our erroneous beliefs (e.g., *I'm a failure*, or *I have no control*). He then points us to the truth and empowers us to live according to that truth. The Spirit knows what we can handle and when, so he does not hit us over the head all at once with every area in our lives that needs correction. This is a process, not only for "sanctifying" us, but also for teaching us to intimately relate to and depend on God. Through this process, little by little, we are becoming outwardly – in personality, emotions, thoughts, and choices – what we already are inwardly in our spirits (2 Corinthians 3:18).

Go back to the three questions on page 63. Ask God to show you what is standing in the way of your believing "new creation" truths about yourself.

Among Weight of Grace group participants, there are some reasons that come up again and again for why women find it difficult to accept that they are "new creations." The most common one is guilt. It usually manifests itself in one of two ways. One way is when a woman just cannot forgive herself for her behavior or perceived lack of character and, therefore, cannot allow herself to believe she possesses all the positive attributes of a "new creation." The thinking often runs along these lines: *If I believe all this good stuff about myself, I'm just getting off "scot-free" for all the rotten things I've done (or for being such a horrible person).* This is common among incest victims, because they often blame themselves for whatever was perpetrated upon them and they think of themselves as worthless and shameful. This is also common thinking for people who binge-eat. They see the binge eating as so repulsive that there has to be big-time punishment in store for them. And usually they mete out the punishment themselves in the form of self-loathing, rigid dieting and exercise, avoidance of friendships, and other "being hard on yourself" behaviors.

The other way guilt gets in the way of accepting "new creation" truths is when a woman feels she needs her guilt in order to keep herself in line when it comes to eating and other actual or potential "out of control" behaviors (such as promiscuity or misspending money). The thinking is: *If I really believe I'm forgiven and accepted, I'll just go hog-wild and misbehave horribly. If there's no guilt, what's to hold me back?*

Guilt gets in the way of accepting "new creation" truths when a woman feels she needs her guilt in order to keep herself in line when it comes to eating.

The answer to guilt is in focusing on the Cross. Accepting forgiveness is not "giving yourself a break." It's realizing that Christ took all our punishment on himself – there was no break involved. And the Cross is not just about punishment. It's about death to sin. Our identification with Christ's death means sin's grip on us is broken. Therefore, believing that you're forgiven and accepted doesn't mean you're giving yourself license to go "hog wild." It's realizing God has empowered you to behave in a godly manner, which brings us right back to the new person God has made you to be – someone who truly desires to do his will (Philippians 2:13) and to live a holy, righteous life (Ephesians 4:24).

Do you believe that you are a new creation in Christ, motivated at your core to live a godly life? If guilt is not what's standing in the way of your accepting that you are a "new creation," what is? Discuss this with God and prayerfully look back over the "Becoming Who You Already Are" chart on page 46. Look up the Scripture verses in the chart and ask God to reveal the truth to you about what you are really like. For further study, an excellent book that goes into depth about what it means to be a new creation in Christ is *Handbook to Happiness* by Charles R. Solomon.

Identifying Beliefs and Renewing the Mind

Another core concept that's important to "get" before moving on in this book is that of beliefs and how we operate out of the set of beliefs that we hold. The problem is that not all of our beliefs line up with God's perspective. We have been "programmed" by friends, family, denominations, and the "world system" to have beliefs that are the opposite of God's truth. For example, our culture influences us to believe that being "fat" means the same as "ugly" and indicates a lack of self-discipline. However, God does not evaluate us according to our appearance. He looks at our hearts to see what kind of people we are (1 Samuel 16:7). Also, cultures are fickle. What one culture calls ugly, another calls attractive. Many people in developing countries consider being what Westerners call "fat" a sign of affluence and success. This is not necessarily any more accurate than seeing "fat" as ugly and a sign of sloth. The world is not a good source for truth. Only Christ and his Word are. (However, we can sometimes impose our preconceived notions onto the Bible. This is why it is so important to look to God's Spirit to help us in our understanding of Scripture.)

Women hold many beliefs that override the desire to be "thin."

Most women in our culture have a belief that "thin" is always and only desirable. However, women also hold many beliefs that override the desire to be "thin." Some examples are:

- *"If I'm thin, I'll be perfect."* (And there's way too much responsibility, effort, and fear of failure associated with maintaining that perfection.)
- *"I'll feel small and vulnerable, easier to attack."*
- *"People will discount what I have to say and won't take me seriously."*
- *"I'll be much more sexually attractive."* (This can produce fear if sex is unappealing, scary, or "dirty" to you – or if you fear you'll give in to the temptation of sexual sin.)
- *"People will expect me to have it all together."*
- *"I'll be prideful about my appearance and pride is a sin."*
- *"People will like me primarily for my appearance."*

As you can see, not all beliefs about being "thin" would motivate someone to become and stay "thin." In fact, a number of beliefs about being "thin" motivate many to either stay "fat" or to regain lost weight. For them, it's just too uncomfortable to stay "thin." For years, this was certainly the case for me.

So, what do we do once we realize we have beliefs that are not in line with God's truth or that hold us back from change? This is one of the ways in which the "rubber meets the road" in our relationship with God. Go to God and ask him to reveal to you what you believe. Ask him for insight into why you hold the beliefs you do. For example, by believing it's safer to stay "fat," you may be trying to protect yourself from behaving inappropriately. Through various means – prayer, Scripture reading, friends, Christian music – God will reveal to you what your false beliefs are and what the truth is. When he shows you the ways in which you've been trying to meet your needs your own way, ask *him* to meet those needs in your life in *his* way. This process is what Paul calls "renewing of your mind" in Romans 12:2 – and it *is* transforming!

Ask yourself the questions on page 63 in regard to beliefs and renewing the mind. Do you accept that your beliefs – rather than just a lack of self-discipline – are in some ways motivating your overeating? Do you believe that God can and will reveal your wrong thinking to you? Will he also lead you into the truth? Perhaps you need to pause at this point and study what the Bible has to say about the work of the Holy Spirit in the believer's life. (A good place to start is John 14:15-26.) Or perhaps it would help to read a book that goes into depth about how beliefs affect our lives and how they can be changed through renewing the mind. Excellent works on this subject are *Be Transformed*, a workbook by Scope Ministries International; *Lifetime Guarantee* by Bill Gillham (as well as his tape series, "Victorious Christian Living"); and *Classic Christianity* by Bob George.

Do you accept that your beliefs – rather than just a lack of self-discipline – are in some ways motivating your overeating?

The participants in Weight of Grace groups who have the most success in experiencing freedom from overeating are those who either were already familiar with the core concepts presented so far in this book (but hadn't seen their relevance to overeating yet) or became more familiar with these concepts through further study (e.g., reading books and/or attending courses such as those offered at Scope Ministries International, Christian Life Ministries, or Exchanged Life Ministries — Internet links to each provided at www.weightofgrace.org). I had been immersed in these concepts for four years before the light went on and I realized how they applied to my overeating and staying "fat." It doesn't have to take four years of exposure to these principals for you to find freedom from over-eating, but the more you consider and live the truths of who God is, who you are, and allow the Holy Spirit to change your beliefs, the more likely it is you will experience that freedom.

Reflection

1. What beliefs about God are you now more aware of, and what bearing do you see these issues have on your eating and/or being "overweight"?

2. In what areas are you still unconvinced about being a new creation in Christ and how might these areas influence you staying "fat"?

3. What do you suspect (or even know) are some of the underlying beliefs you have about "fat" and "thin" that may be motivating you to overeat and/or stay large? What do you plan to do about these beliefs?

4. If you are going through this book in the context of a small group, are there any underlying issues someone else in the group has that seem pretty evident to you? If others in your group are open to input, based upon what you know about them, humbly share what you suspect some of their underlying beliefs might be. Notes:

What Others Have Experienced

It is at this point in the 14-week Weight of Grace small group experience that I am most grateful for the small group format. Christ does use his Body as a means of communicating his truth to believers. As women talk with one another, "speaking the truth in love," the result is growth (Ephesians 4:15-16). First, when women tell about their own struggles and what they are discovering to be their underlying faulty beliefs, others relate and start to see areas in their lives to pray about. Also, when the context is love and understanding, women can and do share what they suspect are underlying issues for their fellow group members. Because all the group members are "in the same boat," there is less defensiveness. Group participants are encouraged to couch their comments with phrases such as, "When I hear you say you were criticized by your mother, it makes me wonder if you think God is just as critical." No accusations, just humble guesses being offered to "try on for size" to see if they fit.

Hopefully, you have found others with whom to discuss what you have been learning so far in this book. Even if you know of no one else who is struggling with overeating, you no doubt do know of others who have emotional struggles of one sort or another. Getting to know God better, coming to an understanding of what it means to be a new creation in Christ who is motivated by the indwelling Holy Spirit, and looking to God to uncover erroneous beliefs so that they can be exchanged for the truth are the basics for overcoming most of the spiritual and emotional difficulties all of us face. Discussing with others, and praying with others, about these concepts and how they apply in your lives provide a tremendous means of reinforcing them, as well as "building up" fellow believers into greater maturity.

- What do you suspect are some of the underlying beliefs you have that are motivating you to overeat? What do you plan to do about these beliefs?

The best thing to *do* about underlying beliefs is to discuss them with God and ask him to reveal to you what's "off" in your thinking and what the truth is according to his Word. It is tempting for us to try to "get busy" and change ourselves. So many women try to psychoanalyze themselves and then use self-talk to change their thinking. This is ultimately ineffective because God wants us to experience what Jesus meant when he said, "Apart from me you can do nothing" (John 15:5). Self-sufficiency – being able to handle our lives ourselves – is not a virtue. In fact, it is "the flesh," which wars against the Spirit (Galatians 5:17, NASB). We are created for a dependent existence, dependent upon God. Struggles such as overeating can open a door to engaging in a more intimate and dependent relationship with God. So, if you *do* anything about your belief system, do prayer and prayerful Bible study, expecting God to speak to you and to transform you.

The best thing to do about underlying beliefs is to discuss them with God and ask him to reveal to you what's "off" in your thinking.

Homework

Spend at least one hour talking with God (or writing to God) about your beliefs concerning him, your identity as a new creation in Christ, being "fat," and being "thin." Ask him to reveal to you some of the beliefs that may be motivating your overeating and/or staying "fat." Conclude your time by entrusting him with these beliefs and writing the new beliefs you either already have or desire to have (space provided on next page).

BEFORE YOU GO ON TO THE NEXT CHAPTER

Homework Follow-up

What are some of the truths you are convinced of now that you weren't sure of before you started reading this book?

Comments on the Homework

At this point in Weight of Grace small groups, there are usually a few group members who make statements such as, "God's not telling me anything about what my false beliefs are." As group leader, my temptation is to make very pointed suggestions about what *I* suspect are the underlying beliefs operating within these women. However, as much as I believe Christ uses fellow members of his Body as a means of communicating with his people (exhortation, admonishing, teaching, preaching, etc.), I also believe it's very important for Christians to take care that they don't try to do the Holy Spirit's job for him, so I don't always offer my opinions. God is working in different areas of people's lives at different times. If now is not the time for a "word" from God about the beliefs that underlie a woman's overeating, you can bet now *is* the time that God is at work in some other area within that person. Forcing the issue may actually be opposing God.

That said, here are a few suggestions if you feel you're not getting anywhere with hearing from God about erroneous beliefs. First, honestly assess whether you are truly in submission to God. This does not mean that you absolutely never sin. This means that your desire is for God to have his way in your life.

Surrender to God is scary for many – it is for me. But we must give God the benefit of the doubt – accept that he wants what is best for us – and give him the access to our souls that he needs in order to change us. You may have to pray a prayer similar to the one I often pray: "Lord, you know I'm afraid of what you may do to me, but I'm totally at your disposal. I'm yours and want you to work in me and through me in whatever ways you see fit." God is still working on some of my erroneous beliefs about him. He can do that because I'm letting him. I am acknowledging that he is the Potter and I am the clay. Just as the old hymn says, my prayer is, "Have thine own way, Lord."

Another barrier to hearing from God about the beliefs that are motivating your overeating is engaging in blatant sin. There are some activities in which we can be involved that result in our getting so spiritually out of whack that we cannot hear from God. Or, we can be under God's discipline, which may include his not speaking to us about those areas where we most want to hear from him until we accept what he is already telling us about the areas in which we have refused to obey. (For an example, see 1 Samuel 28:6-18.) But, hyper-conscientious people, beware! Do not think you have to quit overeating before you can hear from God because you're a blatant "glutton." As discussed previously, most overeating is not done out of rebellion against God, nor is it biblical "gluttony." The types of activities that disrupt our hearing from God are sins such as sexual immorality, involvement in the occult, or stealing. My experience tells me that God tends to deal with such "biggies" before working on struggles that have to do mainly with false beliefs and emotions, as overeating does.

So, before moving on to Chapter 6, make sure you've made a way for God to speak to you by surrendering to him, listening to what he's already said, and acting on what he has already told you to do. Then, see if you hear from him about your overeating and "fat."

A barrier to hearing from God about the beliefs that are motivating your overeating is engaging in blatant sin.

6   EMOTIONS AND OVEREATING

What do you do when you get angry? When you're lonely? When you're bored? What do you do when you feel sad or anxious or stressed out? If you're like I was for many years, whenever you have any uncomfortable emotion, you either eat or think about eating. So far, we've looked at how our beliefs – about God, ourselves, and being "fat" or "thin" – influence overeating. Now, we'll turn to another big contributor to overeating – how we respond to our emotions.

Women have quite a few feelings about their feelings. They range from total denial that they feel anything at all to "letting it all hang out." Most Christian women have some degree of guilt over their emotions and perceived inability to control them as they feel they "ought." Because of this, many women see their emotions as their enemy. They try to eliminate them and suppress them, often through eating.

There are many emotions worth welcoming – joy, love, contentment – and even some that don't feel good but help us out, such as the fear that causes our adrenaline to pump when we see a big black bear approaching and we need to run, fast! However, emotions can be very unwelcome, not only because they feel bad, but also because of how we respond to them. Although they don't realize it, many people make their emotions the authority by which they decide what they do and don't do. So, often, rather than make choices based upon the truth of God's Word, people make choices based upon the emotions that are screaming within them, drowning out the truth, if they know the truth at all. [1]

An example of making emotions the authority in one's life is when a person is sure he has lost his salvation because he *feels* guilty and doesn't *feel* forgiven. This usually leads to a great deal of repeat professions of faith in Christ and "walking down the aisle" to pray the "sinner's prayer." It is the *feeling* of guilt, rather than the truth about the atoning death of Christ, that motivates this behavior.

Even when people deny their emotions, they still make them their authority, dictating their behavior. When I binged, it was because I *felt* as if I *had* to eat. I didn't realize I was suppressing anger. It was my fear of feeling angry that was controlling my decision to binge-eat.

Not only are people unaware that they're letting emotions run their lives, but also their beliefs about their emotions create even more emotional havoc. Many people believe that there are emotions that are, in and of themselves, sinful. This is especially true regarding anger. As a result, women experience constant guilt over every angry feeling and/or they suppress their anger through unhealthy behaviors, such as compulsive shopping, excessive TV watching – or overeating.

Given all of the negatives about our emotions, how is it possible to gain a positive perspective on them, even the ones that feel really horrible?

First, it is important to recognize that emotions are a God-given part of our nature. There are numerous references in Scripture to God's emotions, such as grieving, joy, affection, anger, and indignation. Since we are created in God's image, it is natural that we also have a full array of emotions.

Although they don't realize it, many people make their emotions the authority by which they decide what they do and don't do.

Emotions are serving as messengers, telling us to check out what is going on in our thinking and beliefs.

It's hard to accept all of our emotions, however, when we find them to be very painful and more in control of us than we are of them. It's certainly understandable that many women try to suppress their emotions through eating. However, when they do that, they are squelching what has the potential of being one of their best friends. You've heard the expression, "Don't shoot the messenger." Well, that's exactly what women do when they deny, suppress, and despise their emotions. What they don't realize is that their emotions are serving as messengers, telling them to check out what is going on inside of them. When we have painful emotions, *they* are not the "problem." They can be likened to a red light that shows up on a car's dashboard when the oil level is low. The light isn't what needs fixing. It's telling you there's an unseen problem that needs attention. In a similar manner, our emotions can and do tell us that something needs attention "under the hood," in our thinking and beliefs.

An example of emotions as messengers in my life is the anxiety I used to feel at my workplace when I was a legal secretary. When work stacked up on my desk, I got worried that my boss would disapprove of me for not working quickly enough. I knew I was working as quickly and efficiently as I was able, but I still feared that I was failing to meet my boss's expectations. Then my anxiety made it even more difficult for me to concentrate and get my work finished. This made me even more anxious, creating a vicious cycle. Before I realized that emotions are messengers, I used to address the anxiety itself and browbeat myself with thoughts such as, *Stop worrying! You know worry is a sin. After all, we are to 'be anxious for nothing.'* And, following through on the rest of Philippians 4:6, I would "pray about everything," but the prayers were all the same: "God, help me get this all done really fast!"

More recently, when this kind of anxiety hits me, now that I know it is a messenger telling me something is wrong "under the hood," I catch myself and turn to God, asking him to show me what I'm thinking that is resulting in anxiety. When I got really anxious at work the other day, God brought to my mind that I was returning to an old belief about needing constant approval from people in order to feel I'm okay. This time, instead of asking God to help me work more quickly, my form of "praying about everything" was more along these lines: "God, I know you are really the one I'm working for and you know I'm trying my hardest, so help me relax and accept that you will protect my reputation with my boss if it needs protecting." I also had the thought, *If my boss really does disapprove, that is his problem, not mine. If he fires me because I can't do this volume of work, God will provide me with a more suitable job.* The anxiety itself was not my problem. The problem was with my belief that I would be a worthless person if my boss disapproved of me or fired me. Once I prayerfully thought through the belief underlying my anxiety (which only took a minute or so), I no longer felt anxious.

But what about the big one, anger? Is it also a messenger, not a sin? People who believe feeling anger is a sin usually point to the Sermon on the Mount, where being angry is equated with murder (Matthew 5:21-22). However, by contrast, Ephesians 4:26 can be paraphrased: "You may be angry, only do not sin."[2] The inference here is that you can feel anger and yet not commit any sin. The dividing line has to do with allowing anger to be harbored and to turn into bitterness or acting on anger by verbally or physically lashing out or taking revenge. What is done with anger is what Jesus was condemning. It has been said that anger is not a sin until it travels to the end of your fist and punches someone in the nose. The *feeling* is not the sin; it's what you do with it that may be sin.

Even if you are not persuaded by this line of thinking and are convinced that anger is almost always a sin (of course, God's anger never is), sin or not, it still serves as a messenger. Just because it's a sin doesn't mean you'll never feel it. We are not, after all, fully regenerate. We still suffer from the "sin measles." Simply calling sin "sin" will not cure us of it. When we are willing to see anger as a "red light," we are then able to ask God to show us what needs addressing "under the hood" and thereby address the beliefs and thinking underlying the anger. We will look much more thoroughly at anger and a few other specific emotions in the next chapter.

Recognizing that our emotions are messengers can free us to accept and feel our emotions rather than "stuff" them or distract ourselves from them by eating. But, simply recognizing them as messengers is really just the first step in experiencing them in a healthy way. And, as with everything that has to do with "life and godliness" (2 Peter 1:3-4), the Bible is what gives us the best pattern for how we are to respond to our emotions. In looking at the Psalms, we certainly see a lot of emotions being expressed, many of them negative. Psalms 55 and 73 provide very clear examples of how godly people expressed and resolved their emotions in a godly way. For ease in remembering this pattern, I'll use an acronym, "REED." But, please note that this is *not* a formula by which *you* can take "four easy steps" to overcoming your every emotional difficulty. Rather, it is an aid for remembering to include God in your emotional struggles, to help you enter more fully into an intimate relationship with him that will transform you and your emotions.

Recognizing that our emotions are messengers can free us to accept and feel our emotions rather than "stuff" them or distract ourselves from them by eating.

The "R" in "REED" stands for "recognize." Before you can respond appropriately to an emotion, you have to acknowledge that you're feeling it. This isn't always easy if we've developed the habit of automatically suppressing our "unacceptable" feelings, such as depression, anger, and anxiety. Rather than actually feel an emotion, we just feel that we need to eat or shop or watch TV or play a video game. This is what I did when I got angry with close friends. I didn't *feel* angry; I just felt ravenous!

If you're eating when there's no real physical hunger, this is very likely a sign that there's an emotion you're trying to avoid feeling. When this happens, you can turn to God and ask him to help you recognize what you're feeling. Prayerfully look back over what has happened recently and ask yourself, *If this had happened to someone else, what would I assume she would feel in the same situation?* You may also want to try talking with a friend about your day to see what she thinks is likely bothering you. Remember that God uses fellow believers as one means by which he communicates with us. Read through some psalms and see if you find yourself identifying with any of them. Ask yourself, *What was this person feeling when he wrote this psalm?* You might want to prayerfully "test out" a list of emotions to see if one or more fit.[3]

What is most important about the "R" in "REED" is to realize that you can call upon the Holy Spirit to enable you to recognize what exactly it is that you're feeling.

Once you've recognized that you're feeling something – and even if you can't quite put a name to it yet – the next part of "REED" is "E" for "express to God." Time and time again, we see in the Psalms how the writers openly expressed to God exactly what they were feeling. Here are a few examples:

- Psalm 10:1: Questioning God about whether he really cares
- Psalm 22:1-2: Expressing doubts to God about his goodness
- Psalm 38:1, 4: Guilt and fear of reprisals
- Psalm 51:1-3: Remorse and confession of sin
- Psalm 64:1a, 3-6: Complaining and whining about others
- Psalm 70:1: Fear
- Psalm 74:9, 11: Anger at God

Not only was God willing to listen to these expressions of peoples' emotions, but also he recorded them in his Book. (This is a list of "negative" emotions. There were also a great number of "positive" emotions people expressed to God, such as praising him, joy, zeal, and affection.)

When you really think about it, who is best equipped to handle what you're feeling? There is nothing you can say to God that threatens him (unlike how many people might respond). Many women are terrified of offending God. This is certainly understandable, but not really very logical. God already knows what we're thinking. He understands our thoughts and feelings better than we do (Psalm 139:4). Whether or not we talk with him about our feelings, he is fully aware of them. We might as well go ahead and be honest with him, keeping in mind verses such as Romans 8:1, 31-39 and Hebrews 4:15-16, which assure us that, thanks to Christ, it's okay to boldly approach God and that we are secure in his love.

There are many people with emotional and relationship problems because they do not know they are supposed to turn to God with their emotions. Typically people respond to their emotions in one of two ways: 1) lashing out and dumping their emotions on others, which burdens or breaks their relationships, or 2) stuffing and suppressing their emotions, which lead to their emotions "coming out sideways" through ulcers, nervous breakdowns, high blood pressure, chronic depression, self-loathing, and what are commonly called "compulsive behaviors," including overeating.

God has demonstrated throughout Scripture that he is willing and able to listen to us when we need to express how we're feeling.

God has demonstrated throughout Scripture that he is willing and able to listen to us when we need to express how we're feeling. So, once we've recognized we are feeling something ("R"), we need to express what we're feeling to God ("E").

The next "E" in "REED" stands for "evaluate." Look at Psalm 73. Here was a man who nearly "lost it" with God. He said that when his "heart was grieved" and his "spirit embittered," he was a "brute beast" before God (vv. 21-22). He did the "R" and knew he was grieved and angry, and he did the first "E" and "let it all hang out" before God. *Then* he came to a turning point and did an about-face when he "entered the sanctuary of God" (v. 17). This psalmist was willing to listen to God, willing to check out what he had believed against what God had to say. And God revealed to this man where his thinking was off and gave him an accurate perspective of the situation. He had envied others who, for a time only, appeared better off than he, but God showed him how all would be fair in eternity.

Similarly, we too can invite God to show us what's going on "under the hood," what we're thinking and believing that is resulting in our feeling so upset. An example of an underlying issue would be if you flare and feel automatically defensive when criticized. This may be a sign that you are not secure in your beliefs about God's unconditional approval for you regardless of your performance. Or, if you're anxious, is this revealing that you're not all that sure God will come through for you in your situation? God has demonstrated in Scripture that he is interested in pointing out to us our "heart issues," the beliefs that underlie our emotions and behaviors. (See Psalm 25:9, 32:8 and 139:23-24.)

The "E" for "evaluate" is not intended to encourage you to psychoanalyze yourself! Allow the Holy Spirit to be who he is – the Counselor. If you're willing to hear it, he will reveal to you what underlies the emotions you're feeling. He will enable you to evaluate, in light of the truth of Scripture, the thoughts and beliefs you hold that result in the troubling emotions you feel.

Finally, the "D" in "REED" stands for "decide." It's not enough to give intellectual assent to the fact that what you've been thinking and believing is in error; you must decide to replace those thoughts and beliefs with God's truth. This is probably the most difficult part of responding to our "messenger" emotions. Many people are convinced they cannot believe in something until they *feel* that it's really true for them. But those feelings can be liars, programmed by years of erroneous messages from others or oneself. The fact of the matter is that, whether you feel it's true or not, what's true is true! Whether you feel God's Word is true or not, it's true! So, how do you make the decision to replace your wrong thinking and beliefs with God's truth?

As with everything we are called upon by God to do in life, the Holy Spirit is our power source. Ask him to help you take the steps necessary to believe in the truth and act upon it. Then be willing to thoroughly and prayerfully think through the truth and how that should affect you. For example, here's a "decide" line of thinking: *Even though I feel like a failure and feel I should conform to society's standard of thinness, I am not going to keep dwelling on these "things of the earth." I am going to continue to believe I'm a new creation in Christ, acceptable by God's standards, and that my spiritual fruit of self-control will guide my eating habits more and more.* The result should be less panic over being "overweight" and, therefore, no longer engaging in such behaviors as rigid dieting, compulsive exercise, abusing laxatives and diuretics, or throwing up to purge meals.

"REED" is not a four-step process that we follow and then feel we've "handled" our emotions. That would be responding to our emotions in "the flesh." Instead, "REED" is a reminder of how we need to turn to God with our emotions and allow him to lead us in working out the messages they're sending, as well as guiding us into his truth.

Let's look at an experience I had in applying the "REED" pattern. I used to have a habit of taking food to bed with me to eat right before I started to read and then fall asleep. It felt as though I just couldn't go to bed unless I had that snack to take to bed with me. Typical of my "stuff 'em before you feel 'em" pattern, I didn't feel any emotions at bedtime; I just felt I

We can invite God to show us what's going on "under the hood," what we're thinking and believing that is resulting in our feeling so upset.

It's not enough to give intellectual assent to the fact that what you've been thinking and believing is in error; you must decide to replace those thoughts and beliefs with God's truth.

really had to have that snack. Once I became alerted to how overeating behaviors likely point to suppressed emotions, I prayerfully thought through what emotions I was trying to avoid by eating those bedtime snacks. It came to me in that "still, small voice" that I was avoiding feeling lonely and depressed. I realized that, at bedtime, I was most aware of being single, and this was very painful to me. God helped me recognize ("R" of "REED") that I was feeling lonely, depressed, and discouraged about being single.

But recognizing what I was feeling wasn't enough. Once I knew what I was feeling, I needed to express (the first "E" in "REED") those feelings to God – to be honest about my emotions, getting them out instead of stuffing them down with food. It was at this time that I started writing a series of journal entries, passionately expressing the pain I felt over being single during my thirties and forties. (I married a couple of months before I turned 45.) Such feelings aren't necessarily resolved by thinking them through just once. They recur at different times and for different reasons. Each time is an opportunity to turn to God with our pain and invite him into our struggles. I poured out my heart to God in my journal.

Once I was perfectly honest with God about how I felt, I then gave him a chance to provide me with his input.

Once I was perfectly honest with God about how I felt, I then gave him a chance to provide me with his input. This is the next "E" of "REED," evaluate. Asking God to lead me, I evaluated my thinking in light of God's truth. I realized I believed that I needed to be married to be happy and that God was cruel to withhold marriage from someone who craved companionship and affection as much as I did. I believed that marriage was the only means by which I could get my affection needs met and that my worth would be greater if I were married. I had "bought into" some of the cultural standards prevalent in the conservative evangelical subculture – that marriage was a sign of greater maturity and value. I had also "bought into" what the current Western culture dished out in regard to sex being the primary means by which adults get their affection needs met. In addition, I believed that God was not interested in my emotional well-being, but was cruelly withholding what I wanted most in order to make me into a "better person." I was back to my "God is mean" belief.

In contrast to these erroneous beliefs, God brought to my mind Scripture passages that assured me that he really did care about me and was interested in providing for my needs – even my need for affection. And I remembered that my worth was not dependent upon my marital status but on what Christ did for me on the cross.

Now it was up to me to make a decision, the "D" of "REED." In light of God's assurance that he meets my needs, I started purposely looking for how God was providing me with affection. Suddenly I realized how much affection I was receiving from my friends, co-workers, and fellow church members through their hugs, attentive listening and eye contact, thoughtful cards and notes, and small gestures such as a touch on the arm or a pat on the back. I also decided to agree with God about my worth and started having thoughts such as: *It is perfectly fine to be single – it's people, not God, who might judge me according to whether I'm married or not*, and *I'm special because of how unique it is to be my age and single*.

Soon the need to take a snack to bed went away. I never had to consciously concentrate on not snacking at bedtime. I just noticed one day that I wasn't doing it anymore. From time to time, I still find myself wanting to get a bedtime snack even though I don't feel physically hungry. Having already thoroughly prayed and thought through this behavior in the past makes it much easier to recognize it for what it is now even though the reasons are a little different now that I'm married. (My husband works a night shift.) I continue to invite God to speak to me about what is going on in my thinking and beliefs.

To the degree that we realize that God provides us with a means to respond in a healthy, godly way to our emotions by turning to him – and deepening our intimacy with him – the need to eat when we feel painful emotions will diminish.

Reflection

1. What are some of the emotions you suspect you are trying to avoid when you eat at times when you're not physically hungry?

2. What are some emotional needs you're trying to meet with food because they don't seem to be met in other ways?

3. What would happen if you felt your emotions rather than avoided them?

4. What are some ways God may be meeting your needs that you just didn't previously recognize?

What Others Have Experienced

- What are some emotions you're avoiding through eating? What are some emotional needs you're trying to meet with food?

I've stopped being surprised when women in each new small group come up with different emotions they are stuffing and different emotional needs they're trying to meet through eating. Of course, a common theme is that women are "swallowing" their anger when they binge or constantly snack. Here are some other comments that have been made about how food helps women cope with or avoid their feelings.

- *I'm afraid of being deprived. If it's there, I need to eat it now because it may not be there tomorrow. Too many good things are gone before I get them.*
- *It's my way of procrastinating. I'll get to whatever it is after I eat.*
- *It's like "biting the bullet." I want to be in control and too many things are out of control. I can control the fact that I get to eat the food I want.*
- *It's my way of dealing with my husband's rejection. He doesn't want me, so I turn to food for comfort.*
- *I hate to be told what to do. My husband expects me to be a certain way and do certain things. I guess my eating is my little rebellion.*

For every woman who struggles with overeating, there is an emotional reason to eat.

For every woman who struggles with overeating, there is an emotional reason to eat. But, for every woman, the food is only a very temporary "fix" and usually adds guilt and shame to the emotional mix. And, how do they deal with their guilt and shame about their overeating and overweight? They eat some more!

Most women don't believe there's an alternative to their "emotional eating" that will really work for them. They feel trapped into eating as a coping mechanism. They also are very focused on eating as the horrid outcome of having emotions, so they get more determined to avoid the emotions – and end up eating more! It's a vicious cycle. The solution is to redirect the attention from the emotions and overeating to the underlying thinking and beliefs the emotions are alerting them to. Rather than concentrating on "fixing" the eating or avoiding the feelings, seeing emotions as the "red light on the dashboard" and turning to God for a "tune-up" gives women the freedom to accept their emotions and use them as a catalyst for changing their beliefs and the resulting negative feelings.

However, there is often a great deal of fear that "if I feel my emotions, I'll be a basket case." This leads us to the next question.

- What would happen if you felt your emotions?

We see our emotions as being potentially totally out of control. This is where building trust in God is crucial. If you see God as someone who is not only capable of handling your feelings, but also willing to listen and provide you with the strength and means to move through them, you will venture forth and start expressing how you feel to him. It often feels like going out onto thin ice and taking some baby steps in order to test just how solidly you're being supported. But look who's been out there skating before us! In the Psalms, many of the writers virtually hollered at God in regard to their fears and frustrations. And God helped them through it all. Almost every psalm that starts out with despair or railing against God ends with hope and praise for him.

If you see God as someone who is not only capable of handling your feelings, but also willing to listen and provide you with the strength and means to move through them, you will venture forth and start expressing how you feel to him.

Actually feeling and expressing to God our emotions need not result in meltdown. Even spending a period of time engaged in hysterical crying won't kill you. Women feel that, once they start feeling an emotion – or start crying – they'll never stop. But you do stop. There's always some task that comes up that you have to do. Also, you just get tired of crying or it comes to its natural end, especially if you're letting God in. His desire is to lead you into hope and light (Jeremiah 29:11; Ephesians 5:13-14). If you let yourself feel your emotions and express them fully to God, the worst that will happen is you'll feel bad for a while, but then you'll feel much, much better and the "need" to eat will have been met because that "need" was really a need to avoid or cope with emotions, not to actually eat.

In fact, when we feel our emotions, it's usually very difficult to eat at that moment. Most emotions cause your throat to constrict, making swallowing difficult. I remember the first time I realized this. Shortly after I started recognizing I'd been using food to avoid feeling my emotions and determined to start feeling them, a friend took his life. For several days, I was horribly upset, feeling anger, guilt, and grief very acutely. And I just could not eat. It felt as though if I ate, I'd choke. Prior to this time, I'd always eaten my way through difficult circumstances. This time, I was full of anguish and rage and couldn't eat a bite. Yes, it was a painful experience, but with prayer, time, and the comfort of friends, the emotions grew less intense. If I had "stuffed" them through eating, I'm convinced it would have ultimately taken me much longer to come to terms with what had happened to my friend and to all of us who knew and loved him.

- What are some ways God may be meeting your needs that you just didn't previously recognize?

Many woman are so focused on how they want to get their needs met that they don't recognize the ways that God is providing for them. For me, the need I was constantly complaining to God about was affection. However, when I was willing to see how God was already providing, rather than insisting he provide for me as *I* wanted, it became apparent that God had been overwhelming me with affection for years. I had been "adopted" by several older couples, constantly welcomed to take part in their family gatherings. I had many friends and they showed me affection in a variety of ways – kind notes, listening, gentle and appropriate touches, hugs, interested eye contact. My co-workers regularly

Many woman are so focused on how they want to get their needs met that they don't recognize the ways that God is providing for them.

extended love and kindness toward me. My boss even gave me gifts once in a while for no special occasion, just because he saw an item he thought I'd like. His wife treated me like a daughter, asking questions that "checked up" on me like a mom would do. An older woman I'd met in church had for years been a "mothering mentor." Once I was willing to see it, I stopped feeling that I was deprived when it came to affection.

Most of the women in Weight of Grace groups want their *husbands* to meet certain real and perceived needs. It's understandable that we would have expectations about the role our husbands should play in our lives. Our culture – and the Christian subculture – set us up for *high* hopes in regard to what marriage will do for us. But, husbands are faulty people with their own sets of needs and problems. Ultimately, only God can be the perfect husband (Isaiah 54:5). Often, God uses husbands to meet the needs of wives. But, there are many times when husbands either can't or won't meet our needs.

When women insist that only their husbands meet certain needs, they miss out on enjoying God's provision and the intimacy with him that surpasses what a husband can offer.

When women insist that *only* their husbands meet certain needs, they miss out on enjoying God's provision and the intimacy with him that surpasses what a husband can offer. Yes, husbands can and do disappoint. But, when they do, the opportunity is there to look to God to fulfill where husbands fail. Of course, this can all be seen as very "pie in the sky." "God doesn't cuddle up to me at night." That's true. However, such a statement is evidence of a narrow view concerning how needs are met. If you insist that your needs must be met through an affectionate bedmate, you miss the other ways in which God is meeting the needs you're seeking to meet in this one way. When we ask God to reveal his provisions for us, he does reveal them. We don't need to substitute food for what we're not getting. We need to ask God to show us what we *are* getting – from *him*.

Homework

1. At least once this week, make use of the "REED" concept when you feel negative emotions or find yourself eating when you're not hungry. Use the following page to write what you experience through engaging in this process.

"R E E D" – TAKING YOUR EMOTIONS TO GOD[4]

RECOGNIZE: Acknowledge your emotions; don't suppress them. Ask God to help you identify what emotions you are feeling.

_____

_____

EXPRESS: Write to God how you feel.

_____

_____

_____

_____

EVALUATE: Consider, and ask God to reveal to you, what your emotions say about your thinking on the issue at hand. How do your behavior and feelings reflect what you are thinking and believing? What false beliefs about yourself and God are your emotions indicating? How does what you think and believe compare with God's Word?

_____

_____

_____

_____

_____

DECIDE: Choose to agree with God's truth concerning the issue at hand. Then, choose to act on that truth, knowing that the Holy Spirit will empower you. For example: "Father, I feel anxious about my husband possibly losing his job. It's hard for me to trust you in this area when I think of our family's needs. Thank you for listening and caring about how I feel. I know you promise to meet all our needs (Philippians 4:19), so I am casting all my cares on you (1 Peter 5:7). Therefore, I choose to go about my life, not focusing on the potential problem, but trusting you to work this out for the good and to meet our needs in your way and in your timing."

_____

_____

_____

_____

_____

_____

_____

2. Complete the following Bible study.

EMOTIONAL INTIMACY WITH GOD

Is God emotional? When you think about how emotional God is, what do you usually think?

_____

_____

_____

_____

After you are clear about your thinking regarding how emotional God is, look up each of the following passages and jot notes about what each says concerning God's emotions.

Genesis 6:5-6 _____

Exodus 32:10 _____

Psalm 25:6 _____

Psalm 145:8 _____

Isaiah 62:5 _____

Jeremiah 31:20 _____

Mark 10:21 _____

Luke 13:34 _____

Luke 22:44 _____

John 11:35 _____

2 Corinthians 1:3-4 _____

Hebrews 5:7 _____

How do these passages compare or contrast with your sense of God's emotions?

_____

_____

_____

_____

_____

How does God feel about your emotions? What do you think his opinion is about how you feel?

_____

_____

_____

_____

Once you've thought through how God feels about your emotions, look up the following passages and make notes about how God responded to and/or accepted people's emotions.

1 Samuel 1:12-20 _____

Psalm 51:17 _____

Psalm 55:16-17, 22 _____

Psalm 56:8 _____

Matthew 11:28 _____

Matthew 12:20 _____

John 20:24-28 _____

Hebrews 4:15-16 _____

1 Peter 5:7 _____

How do these passages compare or contrast with how you usually think God feels about your emotions?

_____

_____

_____

_____

_____

_____

_____

_____

_____

_____

_____

BEFORE YOU GO ON TO THE NEXT CHAPTER

Homework Follow-up

1. As a result of doing the "Emotional Intimacy with God" Bible study, in what ways did your beliefs about God's emotions and his attitude toward your emotions change?

2. Through using "REED," what did God reveal to you during this past week about your underlying emotions and beliefs when you wanted to eat at times when you weren't really physically hungry?

Comments on the Homework

- As a result of doing the "Emotional Intimacy with God" Bible study, how did your beliefs change about God's emotions and his attitude toward your emotions?

Most women assume God is rather unemotional and stoic.

The overwhelming majority of women who have answered this question had not previously thought of God as particularly emotional at all. Most women assume God is rather unemotional and stoic. For others, only God's "wrath" came to mind. However, these ideas about God's emotionality came from sources other than Scripture – such as how their parents acted or what they'd heard in a scary sermon. The Bible reveals that God's emotional palette consists of many colors and hues. God is passionate, feeling deeply such emotions as grief, joy, elation, anger, and delight. It is no wonder that we, who are created in his image, also experience a broad array of emotions.

Not only does God feel emotions, but also he accepts that we feel emotions too. When Hannah cried out for a son, God didn't say, "Get over it, woman. Be grateful for what you do have!", although that is what her husband basically said to her! No, God took pity on her and granted her the desire of her heart (1 Samuel 1:15-18). When Thomas doubted and wouldn't believe Jesus had risen from the grave unless he had concrete proof, Jesus didn't rebuke him or turn him away. He took the initiative in allowing Thomas to obtain the tangible proof he wanted (John 20:24-27). We have a Savior who is able to "sympathize with our weaknesses" ! (Hebrews 4:15-16)

Most women in Weight of Grace small groups expect God to feel fed up with their emotions and lack of emotional control. And most of these women have experienced parents, husbands, or other significant people in their lives losing patience with them or being very rejecting of them when they had "emotional displays." It is easy to transfer to God what we have experienced with people, but it is not accurate. God understands why we feel the way we do better than even we can. He accepts how we feel and can handle our expressions of emotion better than anyone else. And he knows that he has the truth that will bring us peace in the midst of even the most intensely troubling feelings.

- What did God reveal to you about your underlying emotions and beliefs when you ate at times when you weren't physically hungry?

Often, emotional eating is never analyzed and certainly never analyzed with the help and guidance of the Holy Spirit. Realizing what we're really feeling and why we want to eat when there's no physical hunger definitely brings us at least half way to no longer using food to avoid or allay emotions. This is the "R," "E," and "E" of "REED." But, the most important part is the "D." Once we start deciding that God is indeed interested in meeting our needs; once we start looking for how he *is* meeting them; once we start communicating with God about our feelings, believing he wants to hear and wants to comfort and change our perspective, the emotional craving for food gradually diminishes. It isn't necessary to directly address the eating because that's not the real problem. What's necessary is to lift the hood and let God play master mechanic – changing our old, worn-out, damaged thinking and beliefs for his freeing truth.

It isn't necessary to directly address the eating because that's not the real problem.

7   SOME SPECIFIC EMOTIONS WE "SWALLOW"

My colossal binges almost always started at Dunkin' Donuts® with a baker's dozen that I carefully chose – fat and greasy pastries that were cream-filled and chocolate covered. The next stop was usually Long John Silver's™ for some fried fish to go, along with a dozen or more hushpuppies. Then I continued up – and then back down – the five-mile stretch of Northwest Expressway where nearly every fast food chain had a franchise. I'd stop and buy cookies, ice cream, shakes, burgers – constantly munching along the way – but making sure to buy enough food so I'd still have plenty left by the time I got home. Having already busted my budget, I then proceeded to bust my gut. But usually the food I'd bought wasn't enough. So, once the good stuff was eaten up, I'd start making "rough cookies," a concoction of whatever was on hand – chopped up corn flakes if there was no flour, pink packets of sweetener if there was no sugar, extra baking soda if I had no eggs. Whipped all together and cooked till golden brown. Then I'd gobble them up without even really tasting them. I ate and ate until I felt physically ill. I ate and ate until I lay on my back on my bed and started crying, crying because I was sooooo ANGRY!

In the last chapter, we looked at emotions in general. In this chapter, I'll concentrate more specifically on the most common emotions with which women cope through eating: anger, frustration, depression, anxiety, loneliness, and boredom. You can probably immediately think of times when you've eaten because you were feeling one or more of these emotions – or because you were trying to avoid feeling one or more of these emotions. Most women take it for granted that they *will* eat if they feel any of these common emotions. Television shows and movies portray women as coping with these feelings by consuming copious quantities of ice cream, mashed potatoes, and/or chocolate. However, most of those sitcom and cinema characters are stick thin, leading me to imagine them throwing up off camera! We have been conditioned to think that we can "medicate" ourselves with food in just about the same way we might take aspirin or Prozac®. We refer to some foods as "comfort foods," or we make comments such as, "I think I'll go take it out on a quart of Häagen Dazs®." But, the positive effects of this "medicine" are minimal and short-lived. And the side effects are worse than what we were "treating," because not only does eating in the face of negative emotions result in guilt, self-condemnation, shame, and self-loathing, but also it doesn't help resolve the underlying issues that brought about the feelings of anger or anxiety or boredom in the first place.

It was always the same on the day after one of my monumental binges. I told myself I'd never do it again and I'd always stick to my diet. I worked out a schedule that included more exercise. I planned low-calorie meals for the next several weeks. But, mostly, I hated myself. And, of course, within a week or so, I binged again. There came a point in my life, however, when I realized that, rather than directly attacking the eating with self-recriminations or attempts to crack down on myself with more discipline, the long-term and truly effective solution is to learn godly ways to think through and pray through difficult emotions. In general, the reminder of "REED" is appropriate for addressing any

In this chapter, I'll concentrate more specifically on the most common emotions with which women cope through eating: anger, frustration, depression, anxiety, loneliness, and boredom.

negative emotion. More specifically, let's look at the emotions that seem to most frequently trigger overeating.

Because of the guilt associated with feeling angry and the beliefs many hold that experiencing anger is sinful, it is an emotion women frequently try to "stuff" by eating.

Anger is probably the most powerful and uncomfortable emotion many women feel. There is an abundance of overt, as well as subtle, messages within our culture, and especially within the evangelical Christian subculture, that condemn women – much more than men – for feeling, let alone displaying, anger. Because of the guilt associated with feeling angry and the beliefs many hold that experiencing anger is sinful, it is an emotion women frequently try to "stuff" by eating. For years, I unconsciously believed anger to be so totally unacceptable that I didn't even feel my anger, but in response to any incident in which someone offended me, I bypassed feeling angry altogether and went straight to "eating the world."

As I started to look into a new way of thinking about my eating, I found in my own life – and with many women I know – that a better understanding of what motivates anger brings about a greater acceptance of the emotion and a decreased desire to suppress it through overeating. The following is a helpful diagram regarding the usual progression involved in feeling and harboring anger, which results in bitterness, which leads to a downward spiral of negative attitudes and emotions.[1]

EXPECTATIONS, ANGER, AND BITTERNESS[2]

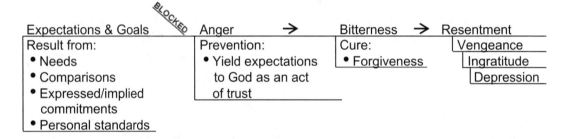

Anger has its roots in the expectations we have, and we form our expectations through various means. Our own sense of need for love, appreciation, worth, affection, comfort, etc., leads to developing expectations about how these needs should be met and by whom. For example, if I feel a need for affirmation, I may have an expectation that my husband should commend me for my accomplishments.

Also, we look around and see how life is for others and, through comparison, formulate expectations. Just about anyone who grew up during the early 1960s and watched television developed certain expectations about parents – that they should in some way resemble Andy Griffith of Mayberry or the Beaver's mother, June. I used to feel terribly disappointed that my father hadn't come up with a nickname for me similar to the ones that Robert Young of "Father Knows Best" used for his daughters, "Kitten" and "Princess."

Another way expectations are developed is in response to the commitments people really do make or make by implication. When a husband vows in a public ceremony to be faithful until "death do us part," the wife's understanding of faithfulness may result in an expectation that he won't look approvingly at other women. When a couple adopts a child, although there are no public vows spoken to the child, the implication is that the couple is making a commitment to faithfully care for him. Family members and the child himself would naturally expect kind and loving treatment to be extended to the adoptee.

As natural as it is for us to have expectations about the people in our lives, it is just as common for us to run into occasions when those expectations are sadly disappointed, when they just are not met. The usual knee-jerk emotional reaction to unmet expectations is anger.

In addition to expectations, another first step toward anger is experiencing blocked goals. Each of us has a set of personal standards, which provide the basis for all our goals, large and small. An example of a goal is the desire to have the house cleaned up before guests arrive. When there is an impediment to reaching that goal, such as two active toddlers dragging all of their toys out of the closet into the living room, a common reaction is anger. What young mother hasn't screamed at her children – or worse – when they've foiled her plans by just being kids?

All our expectations of people and all the goals we have for ourselves set us up for experiencing anger from time to time. Wouldn't it be nice if there were a way to prevent even getting to that point of feeling angry? Well, there is a way to cut off anger at the pass, at least some of the time. The best preventative for anger is to relinquish our expectations and goals to God. Often, as we grow older, we begin to realize that many of our expectations and goals developed in youth were unrealistic and overly idealistic. These are pretty easy to give to God. But just as often, goals and expectations are extremely hard to relinquish. Many times, we don't even realize we have expectations, or the perceived "rightness" of an expectation or goal is taken so for granted that it is not even open to question. Examples of hidden expectations might be believing it's only right that your husband praise you when you dress up for an evening out, feeling your parents should unconditionally accept you, or being sure your children should consistently obey. In order to uncover the goals and expectations we are not even aware we have, we can turn to a wonderful Counselor, calling upon the Holy Spirit to reveal to us the expectations and goals to which we cling and to provide us with the grace to surrender them to God.

When it comes to yielding our goals and expectations to God, it's important to remember that "there is a way that seems right to a man, but in the end it leads to death"! (Proverbs 14:12) Yes, a certain goal may seem very right, but insisting upon its achievement can sometimes be the death of us. Demanding that things go the way we want sets us up for a tremendous amount of anger when they don't. However, when we shift our focus to "all things work together for good" (Romans 8:28, KJV) for God's children, we can more easily relinquish our demand that "it really ought to be this way" and trust that, whatever happens, God will ultimately make it a plus in our lives. In fact, when circumstances don't "go right" for us, this is an excellent opportunity to seek God and put trust in him, to experience a deeper personal intimacy with him. This is in part why an emphasis early on in this book is the need to have an accurate view of our loving heavenly Father. The more

All our expectations of people and all the goals we have for ourselves set us up for experiencing anger from time to time.

you are able to trust God, the less difficult it is to give up on expectations and to be willing to see even the most well intentioned and godly goals sidetracked or delayed.

But, let's face it, we don't always perfectly trust God and we don't always know we have expectations or goals until we've already come face to face with a whopping dose of anger. You just can't anticipate or prayerfully discover ahead of time every single expectation and goal. So, what do you do when preventative measures weren't taken and you find yourself experiencing feelings of anger? Well, there's a cure! It's two-fold: forgiveness and trust. If you're angry at a person, forgiveness is the cure – and true forgiveness involves trust in God. If you're angry over circumstances or unrealized goals, trust in God is the cure.

Let's look at forgiveness first. It is very important to make clear what forgiveness is *not* before most people can find extending forgiveness possible and even natural. Forgiving is *not* the same as condoning. Some women think, *If I forgive him for criticizing me, it's the same thing as saying it's okay that he does it*. But, actually, forgiving implies that the act for which you're extending forgiveness was *wrong*. If the person had done nothing to offend, he or she would need no forgiveness! If you believed what the person did to be right, if you condoned his or her behavior, you would not then need to forgive.

Forgiving is not the same as condoning.

Also, forgiveness does *not* mean you automatically feel good about what has happened. Love does not rejoice over evil (1 Corinthians 13:6). Evil deeds are very sad indeed. We can rejoice in how God makes everything work to the good (Romans 8:28), but we can still know and feel that the offense was a sad, even horrible event. There is a powerful story of a man who forgave the woman who murdered his sister and became friends with her while she was on death row. His forgiveness of the murderess in no way diminished his sense of loss or mourning over his sister's gruesome death. It was sad; it was wrong; it was a terrible loss. He did not have to think, *I'm fine with it now*, in order to forgive the offender.

Forgiveness does not mean you automatically feel good about what has happened.

Forgiveness does *not* mean you must trust the offender. If someone embezzles from your company, you need to forgive him, but you would be an idiot to turn around and entrust him with handling your company's funds again! I forgave my stepfather for molesting me, but should I then have suggested he baby-sit a five-year-old girl? No, forgiveness is not the same as trust. But, forgiveness does leave the door open to trust should the offender repent and show convincing evidence of significant change.

Forgiveness does not mean you must trust the offender.

So, if forgiveness is *not* condoning, changing your feelings, or trusting, what *is* it? I personally find it difficult to define – especially succinctly. I've heard forgiveness described as breaking the chains that bind you to your offender. I like to look at forgiveness as entrusting God with the offender and the offense, believing that God will work out your injury to your ultimate good. Excellent examples of people's ill deeds working toward God's ultimate goals for them and others are found in the life of Joseph (Genesis 37 and 39-50).

Forgiveness is a decision and not an emotion. I remember when I was 25 years old, I chose to forgive my parents and stepparents for the many ways in which I felt they had hurt me during the course of my upbringing. I had to admit that I really didn't *feel* like forgiving them. However, I was the one suffering emotionally – not them – because of my bitterness and resentment and resulting depression. At the time, I told God that, as much as I didn't feel like it, I was choosing to forgive them because I believed he was directing me to do so. As half-hearted as that sounds, the results were amazing. Within a few days of making that decision to forgive, I went from feeling deeply depressed and being almost totally withdrawn to feeling hopeful and eager to be with people.

Forgiveness goes back to one's beliefs about God and his character. To the degree that we trust that God will work all things together for our ultimate good, no matter how horrible the offense, we will find it easier to forgive. And forgiveness does become a little easier with "practice." Seeing what God does with our forgiveness makes us more eager to forgive the next time the occasion presents itself.

Even when you make a choice to forgive and to be a person who is willing to forgive, there are still a few times when it appears forgiveness isn't "working." We sometimes think that, because we've forgiven someone once, we should never feel angry with him or her again. However, it is not possible to anticipate future offenses or their impact ahead of time, even when you've had long experience with forgiving someone. This seems to come up often with women and their mothers. "I forgave her for saying that the last time, so why am I angry that she said it again?" The issue here is that she has indeed offended again. You cannot forgive someone for a future offense, even if it's a familiar one. For each new offense, forgiveness is again necessary. It is sometimes helpful, however, to think through why you take it so hard when there is a repeated offense. It seems that, especially with our mothers and husbands, we have difficulty giving up the "they should be..." *She should be accepting and not criticize me. He should be loving and pay attention when I talk.*

We sometimes think that, because we've forgiven someone once, we should never feel angry with him or her again.

We have little power to make people what we feel they "should be." The "Serenity Prayer" provides a good reminder for us in this regard. We need God to grant us the wisdom to know what is beyond our control and to give us the courage to put our lives, relationships, and circumstances into his hands. So it is with the people who are repeat offenders. We need to acknowledge the expectations we have about such people that are better left with God, and rely on Christ in us (Galatians 2:20) for the grace to repeatedly forgive as each offense occurs.

It is also good to bear in mind that it is possible to forgive someone for an offense and then, later in life, have to forgive again for the same offense when it becomes apparent that it is affecting you in a new way. An example of this would be the teenage incest victim who forgives her father for molesting her, but after getting married, finds she struggles with not enjoying sex because of flashbacks to incestuous events. She may need to forgive her father for this new effect of the offense she'd previously forgiven.

Finally, in regard to forgiveness, the question often arises, "What if I'm angry with someone who really didn't do anything wrong?" Rather than go into detail about what types of offenses may or may not be "wrong," the answer is quite simple. Whether the person truly wronged you or you just perceive the offensive act to be wrong, treat it as though it is a real offense – and forgive. In addition, ask God to reveal to you, not the rightness or wrongness of the offense, but the attitudes of your heart and the offender's heart. Ask God if there is an area in which you are overly sensitive and whether you need to change your beliefs regarding that area. Usually our personal sensitivities are born out of erroneous beliefs about ourselves and God's acceptance of us and power within us.

Whereas anger with people is "cured" through forgiveness, anger over circumstances and blocked goals is addressed through turning to God in trust, trusting that God is taking care of us despite our circumstances and is accepting us despite the fact that we haven't reached our goals. Often, the anger we feel in the face of difficult circumstances is directed toward God. At these times, stepping back and asking God to help us see the "big picture" restores our faith that circumstances don't determine contentment or success – God does. Remember Psalm 73 – that guy was a "brute beast" before God until he allowed God to show him an eternal perspective. When we put our trust in God – that he does indeed care for us no matter how circumstances may look at the moment – we stop railing at our circumstances and start looking for how God is blessing us in the midst of them.

Blocked goals may not only lead to anger with God, but also they can result in anger at one's self. After my monumental binges, there were many times when I realized the only person I was mad at was me – usually for not doing as well in my work or relationships as I thought I should. This type of anger is a result of believing one's worth is tied to achieving a goal. So often, for women, the unrealized goal is long-term weight loss, and the anger at oneself is the result of believing that being "overweight" is wrong or unacceptable. In Chapter 11, we will look at why women feel this way and how that feeling can change.

Understanding what causes anger and how to prevent and cure it is a big step toward eliminating the need to eat in order to suppress it. However, understanding is not enough. Yielding expectations and goals and deciding to forgive must be practiced in the context of relying upon the power of the Holy Spirit. It is ineffectual to turn "dealing with anger" into a mental exercise of checking for expectations and goals and then deciding to forgive. Because God created us to require him as our Counselor, his participation in the process is absolutely necessary. When you start eating when you're not hungry, that is a cue to *turn to God* and ask him for guidance and insight into what is going on "under the hood." If he reveals you're angry, that is another trigger – to turn to him for understanding about your unmet expectations and blocked goals and for the grace to forgive the offender or to put more trust in God. It is only the empowering grace of God that enables us to overcome such a painful and difficult emotion as anger.

Whereas anger is often associated with binge eating (although it is certainly associated with other forms of overeating too), frustration is what many women associate with "grazing" or "nervous nibbling." "When I get frustrated, I eat chocolate." "I get so frustrated I just have to do something, and that something is usually eating." We're so used to frustration in our culture that we see it as a totally separate issue from what it really is – another form of anger. Also, for women especially, it is much more acceptable to admit to feeling frustration than to admit to feeling anger, which is seen as a more serious and negative emotion. However, even though it may not be felt as intensely, frustration is just a mild, or perhaps chronic, form of anger. Frustration almost always has to do with blocked goals, either goals for ourselves or goals we have for others, especially family members.

Whereas anger with people is "cured" through forgiveness, anger over circumstances and blocked goals is addressed through turning to God in trust.

For women especially, it is much more acceptable to admit to feeling frustration than to admit to feeling anger.

Most of the frustration discussed in Weight of Grace groups is with husbands. It is much less threatening to admit to being frustrated with one's husband than to admit to out-and-out anger. It is scary to think of being angry with someone you're supposed to love more than any other person and with whom you plan to live the rest of your life. Also, as I previously mentioned was the case for me, many women feel anger will destroy relationships. We usually don't think of frustration as being quite that "dangerous." However, frustration has just as much potential for hurting relationships as does anger, because it *is* anger and leads to bitterness and resentment if not addressed.

I find it's difficult to convince women that frustration needs to be addressed in just the same way as anger. They tend to feel that frustration is rather trivial and, therefore, can be "brushed off." However, as long as that attitude is taken, the nibbling and grazing continue because eating is often the way women keep their anger at the "only frustrated" level. Once women admit that their frustration is indeed anger and that God-empowered yielding of expectations or goals followed by forgiveness needs to take place, the frustration dissipates and so does the nibbling and grazing.

Frustration needs to be addressed in just the same way as anger.

Now that we've looked at anger and "anger lite," when we turn our attention to depression, the emotion usually associated with eating "comfort foods," you might think this is a totally different emotion from the ones we've discussed so far in this chapter. However, whether it's just "the blues" or debilitating hopelessness, depression is very often an emotional alternative to feeling angry. As with anger, expectations have been disappointed, and as a result, the person feels hopeless about getting what she feels she needs. Food, especially sweets and starches, become the "medication" women take in order to soothe the sadness or to get a little pick-me-up from the increased blood sugar level that results from eating such foods. Also, these comforting foods are seen as what can be relied upon in contrast to circumstances and people. Of course, eating comfort food does not alleviate depression. Not only does the weight gain from eating what the body does not need add to a woman's negative self-esteem and therefore increase her depression, but also there is a sugar low that follows the short-lived high.

Depression is very often an emotional alternative to feeling angry.

With the sense of disapproval women feel regarding their anger, it's no wonder they would instead express their disappointment through sadness and hopelessness rather than through rage. Forms of anger-based depression are expressed in phrases such as "I feel hurt" and "I guess I don't deserve good things to happen to me." When we acknowledge that we feel depressed and turn to God for insight into the root issues, it almost always boils down to unmet expectations and blocked goals. Getting God's perspective on which expectations and goals are unrealistic and how he is meeting our needs his way enables us to turn away from the disappointment we feel and find hope in the reality of how good God is to us. Also, since God is a Comforter and Counselor (John 14:16-17; 2 Corinthians 1:3-4), there is no better one to whom we can turn when we are feeling down. And, when we get more and more into the habit of turning to God with our disappointments and asking him for his perspective, we have less and less of a desire to find comfort, such as it is, in food.

Now we *are* switching gears a little when we consider another common emotion that triggers overeating: anxiety. Anxiety is such an uncomfortable feeling that women turn to food to distract themselves from it. Eating is something to *do* when there is nothing that can be done to address whatever is causing the anxiety. Eating is an attempt to apply a soothing "tranquilizer" to one's jangled nerves and to calm that alarming sense of tension in the throat, chest, and stomach.

Many women try to attack their anxiety with what I call "club verses" (as in "hitting yourself over the head with a club"). They reproach themselves for failing to "be anxious for nothing" (Philippians 4:6, NASB), but this is not helpful, because telling yourself it's a sin to be anxious will not stop you from feeling the anxiety. In fact, it just adds a new anxiety about how much you're sinning! Instead, we need to look more closely at the two most commonly quoted verses about anxiety because they reveal its root issue, which is the degree to which we do not trust in God to take care of us.

We need to look more closely at the two most commonly quoted verses about anxiety because they reveal its root issue, which is the degree to which we do not trust in God to take care of us.

First Peter 5:7 says to "cast all your anxiety upon [God] because he cares for you." The reason we have anxiety, which is really a form of fear, is that we believe something horrible or unbearable is about to happen. What's difficult about anxiety is that it's hard to put your finger on what exactly is causing it. As was emphasized in the last chapter with "REED," it is vital to engage in dialog with God, to seek his input regarding what we're feeling, to ask him for insight and perspective – to cast our anxiety on him. Even if you do not determine the exact cause of your anxiety, you can decide to trust that God will work things out and get you through the uncomfortable sense of panic you're experiencing. You can count on him to do this because *he cares for you* – he cares about you and takes care of you. Even when it does not look as if he is doing so, he is. He sees eternity and we see only this one moment in time, and that not too clearly! He knows what will work out best for us in the long run and is carefully weaving together all the messy looking threads of our lives to form an incredibly beautiful tapestry.

Now, let's go back to the verse many people use as a "club" to try to make themselves stop feeling anxious, Philippians 4:6, but let's add verse 7 also.

> *Do not be anxious about anything, but in everything, by prayer and petition, with thanksgiving, present your requests to God. And the peace of God, which transcends all understanding, will guard your hearts and your minds in Christ Jesus.*

Many women say, "I already know that verse," but what they mean is that they just know it rather than *do* it. As was mentioned in the last chapter, the Psalms give us a model for presenting requests to God in a really honest, heartfelt way. We want to get rid of our anxiety instantly, but instead of pushing the emotion away, we need to see anxiety as an alarm sounding. It is telling us to express our fears to God – to tell him all about it – to be willing to hear from him and to decide to believe him, instead of trusting in our own perceptions and negative projections into the future. When we go ahead and feel the anxiety and talk with God about it, rather than try to avoid it through eating, we actually get through it and over it because God's desire is to become intimately involved in our concerns and to show us his love, which casts out fear (1 John 4:18). In fact, Philippians 4:6-7 should always be read in light of Philippians 4:5b, which tells us, "The Lord is near." He is as available as the air we breathe and is truly interested in hearing all about whatever is causing us anxiety.

The last two emotions we'll address in this chapter are related: loneliness and boredom. Both have to do with wanting circumstances to be different to the point of not appreciating all the good that there is in one's life, and both have to do with a discomfort with one's own thoughts. Loneliness leans a little more toward the former and boredom more to the latter.

I have never met a woman who is truly alone in life. I have met a great many women who so long for a "certain someone" or for their certain someone to act in a particular way that they do not even see all the special people God has placed in their lives for them to love and be loved by. A wonderful message that was directed primarily toward married couples but applies to everyone is "The Principle of Receiving" by Jack Taylor. The title says it all. When we're willing to receive the people God has placed in our lives, we can then see the ways in which God is so wisely meeting our needs through them. When we stop insisting that people be the way we want them to be and when we are willing to appreciate the way that they actually are, we can accept what they are able to give. We not only receive who they are, but also we start receiving from them, receiving their unique ways of loving us.

Food can distract you temporarily from feeling lonely – from the uncomfortable thoughts you have about yourself when your perception is that you are "alone" – but loneliness can be cured permanently when you allow God to show you how much love he has placed in your life through your relationships with him and with the people around you.

Boredom is also about wishing one's circumstances were different. But, instead of wanting people to be more to one's liking, boredom is a result of wanting more interesting activities in which to engage. But that desire for something "better" to do – with the "something better" often ending up being a refrigerator raid – is usually a "red flag" that can alert you to the need to ask God, "What am I trying to avoid thinking about?" When you say you're bored, you may really mean that you're afraid of "down time" when you might start thinking thoughts you'd rather not think about. People who say they can't stand being bored are often people who feel the need to stay distracted.

A college friend of mine used to sit at his kitchen table for about half an hour nearly every morning, doing nothing. When I'd hear him talk about this, it made me horribly uncomfortable. I'd ask him, "Aren't you bored doing that?!" And he'd say, "No, I'm thinking." But many of us are not comfortable with what comes to our minds when we're just thinking. When I was in my teens and twenties and my overeating was at its peak, I was constantly distracting myself from my own thoughts, which were dominated by my nearly unbearable desire to have a boyfriend and also my horrible fear of having one.

It took me years to become truly comfortable with having times – when stopped at red lights or waiting in lines – when thinking is all there is to do. But, I did not have to become totally comfortable with my own thoughts to stop overeating rather than face them. In fact, being honest with God about what I was thinking and being willing to feel the negative

I have met a great many women who so long for a "certain some-one" or for their certain someone to act in a par-ticular way that they do not even see all the special people God has placed in their lives for them to love and be loved by.

emotions that accompanied those thoughts made it almost impossible for me to eat. Emotions "choke you up" and make it hard to swallow. The hardest part of getting comfortable with my own thoughts was just getting started down the path. Once I'd tried feeling the feelings and mentally screaming about them to God, this became easier and more and more my habit rather than turning to food.

Not only was my just-sit-and-think friend comfortable with his own thoughts, he also was comfortable with the idea of not actually *doing* anything for several minutes, even as long as an hour! In our culture – and this seems to be especially true for Christians – there is a prevalent message that one must be *doing* something at all times except when asleep. (However, some groups even think you should be prophetically dreaming then!) When you're supposed to be doing something at all times, but you don't want to do all the things that are there to do, it's boring, and an alternative is to eat. Eating is, after all, *doing* something. Eating can be a way of procrastinating, putting off what you feel you should be doing but don't really want to do.

The answer is *not* to crack down on yourself and get busy doing all those dreaded and boring chores. The answer is, instead, to avoid letting yourself be "pressed into the mold" of this culture (Romans 12:2) that insists on constant activity. "Redeeming the time" (Ephesians 5:16, KJV) may mean taking the time to think – to *do* nothing in terms of outward activity – to "be still and know that" God is God (Psalm 46:10). After all, the most important activity we "do" – prayer – does not appear to accomplish anything at the time we're doing it. Scripture encourages thinking about "things above" (Philippians 4:8; Colossians 3:2). And, certainly, we cannot discuss our concerns with God nor hear from him about them unless we take time to pray and prayerfully think them through. Addressing boredom without using food as a distraction usually means accepting the fact that, even when there is much to be accomplished, it is still important to spend time that has absolutely no structure, if only to give yourself a chance to think, even if those thoughts are not always perfectly pleasant. When God is invited into the thinking, he has the opportunity to help us think through and get past our negative thoughts.

Hopefully, you've seen that the constant theme in lessening your desire to cope with emotions through eating is to increase your willingness to acknowledge your feelings, feel them, and turn to God with them. People who do not eat in the face of emotions are usually people who take feeling a wide range of emotions for granted (unless they're engaging in some other compulsive behaviors, such as drinking or shopping, in order to cope). For those of us who have tried to avoid our emotions by overeating, we need to realize that we can turn to God to help us learn how to feel emotions, as scary as that may seem. And that learning process is also the opportunity for us to learn just how very intimately involved and caring God is.

Addressing boredom without using food as a distraction usually means accepting the fact that, even when there is much to be accomplished, it is still important to spend time that has absolutely no structure.

Reflection

1. What do you think and feel about being angry?

2. How did your parents handle anger – yours and their own?

3. How have you believed you were supposed to address anger and how successful have you been at that?

4. What are you depressed about and what expectations were not met in those situations?

5.   What emotions are you coping with through eating?

6.   What alternative(s) do you see to using food as "medication" for your emotions?

What Others Have Experienced

- What do you think and feel about being angry? How did your parents handle anger – yours and their own? How have you believed you were supposed to address anger?

Of all the emotions women feel, by far the one that stands out most often as the one to be shunned is anger. Whereas it is taken for granted that men and boys get angry – even to the point of fist fights – girls and women are expected to be gentle and "quiet in spirit." Girls are even told that "little girls don't get angry." But, of course, little girls do. For many women who struggle with suppressing anger through eating, their parents forbade displays of anger and never addressed their daughters' reasons for feeling angry or frustrated. If you were angry, you were already wrong, regardless of the precipitating factors.

As an adult observing friends and their children, I have seen parents respond to children's anger in constructive ways that both address inappropriate behavior and the child's reasons for frustration. But many women's parents were not so emotionally mature. Instead, their anger was the basis for punishment, the "silent treatment," threats of abandonment, and worse. When we are reared to believe anger is forbidden, it makes sense that we would find ways to totally avoid feeling it, let alone expressing it. This is where the input of the Holy Spirit is so needed. He is willing and able to point out to us what is really going on inside us when all we want to do is eat and eat. He is also able to comfort our disappointment and frustration once we allow ourselves to start feeling them.

The scariest part is that first time of letting yourself feel really angry. It feels so bad. You think you'll explode and scatter into a thousand pieces or that you'll inappropriately

The scariest part is that first time of letting yourself feel really angry.

express your anger toward a friend or family member. However, is it better to stay locked in a pattern of eating and self-loathing – but avoiding feeling your anger – or to ask God to bring you to emotional healing, able to feel your emotions, to present them to him, and to get his perspective so that you can move on? After all, you are only avoiding *feeling* your anger. You're not avoiding the anger itself. It's still there, but it is under the surface, eating at you – and you are trying to eat it away.

- What are you depressed about and what expectations were not met in those situations?

Women who feel depressed rarely believe their own choices resulted in how bad they feel. They usually point to unhappy circumstances or to people who disappointed them as the causes for their depression. "If I were married, I wouldn't be so depressed all the time." "If my husband appreciated me more…" "If I could move to a warmer climate…" "If I could change jobs…" "If I could find more friends…" These are statements that indicate a focus on what is believed to be "wrong" about one's life and not on what is "right." These are statements that indicate unmet expectations and the need to express those expectations to God, entrust them to him, and ask him how he *is* meeting needs. When I feel depressed, I now see that as a "red light" that alerts me to ask God, "What have I wanted that I didn't get?" And the next question is, "Do I need it and how are you providing for me in ways I haven't perceived?"

Women who feel depressed rarely believe their own choices resulted in how bad they feel.

What about physiological factors that can contribute to depression? Sometimes this is a chicken-or-the-egg issue. Did one's disappointment lead to an imbalance in brain chemistry that resulted in depression or did the imbalance in brain chemistry lead to the depression? My own experience is that there *are* factors that can lead to depression apart from just "wrong beliefs," a failure to forgive, or unmet expectations. As I was growing up, I experienced several traumatic events. At age 25, I exhibited many severe symptoms associated with post traumatic stress disorder. One of those symptoms was depression. Over the course of about five years, I gradually recovered, with all of my symptoms lessening and most of them disappearing totally. Yes, the stresses of my childhood did contribute to my having some physiological deficits and being more susceptible to depression. But, I found the ultimate cure in applying the principles I would apply if the depression had been completely the result of erroneous thinking about God and my circumstances. No matter what the reason for the depression, turning to God and expressing my feelings and thoughts to him, being willing to feel my sadness, and having friends with whom I could discuss my struggles all contributed to overcoming the depression and ultimately the need to "medicate" it with "comfort food."

- What emotions are you coping with through eating? What alternatives do you see to using food as "medication" for your emotions?

Hopefully, you are starting to believe that the most important alternatives to eating are turning to God with, and feeling, your emotions. Sometimes it is just not possible to feel feelings all alone. I, like many women, often need a friend with whom I can air my frustrations and disappointments. Talking with a friend does not automatically mean you're turning to a person rather than to God. You can turn to God and ask him to use your friend to help you hear from him. However, it is not only possible, but also gratifying, to hear directly from God, either through that "still, small voice," through a passage of Scripture, or even through a dream or vision, in regard to what's wrong "under the hood." When it comes to our emotions, there's no better Master Mechanic!

Homework[3]

1. List any incidents in your past that cause you continual hurt. List each person who has contributed to your hurts.

2. Ask God to make you willing to forgive these people – and even yourself – and to trust him to work all things together for the good.

3. By faith, choose to forgive the offenders by an act of your will, apart from what your emotions or reason are telling you. Write out this choice to God. Trust God to change your feelings of anger and hurt in his timing. Read Matthew 6:25-34 and Matthew 18:21-35.

4. Sometime in the next few days, when you experience a negative emotion or when you notice you're eating but are not physically hungry, prayerfully fill out the following "REED" pattern.

Recognize

Express to God

Evaluate

Decide

BEFORE YOU GO ON TO THE NEXT CHAPTER

Homework Follow-up

1. Did God reveal any forgiveness that you needed to extend? What did you do as a result?

2. What did you experience in going through the "REED" exercise? How did your perspective change and how did that affect your emotions and eating?

Comments on the Homework

*   Did God reveal any forgiveness you needed to extend?

Do you trust that God will take care of you even though you've been sinned against?

It is likely you find it difficult to forgive certain people, especially those who are unrepentant or prone to repeat their offenses. But who is this really hurting? Are *they* suffering from your refusal to forgive? Are they changing because you won't forgive? No, but you are – you're growing heavier as you stuff down that anger and bitterness with an éclair or, as I once did, two pounds of carrots so that I could technically stay on my diet. (My skin turned orange for a few hours.) Look to the root issue. Do you trust that God will take care of you even though you've been sinned against? If you don't, tell God why you don't and ask him to help you see your circumstances from his point of view. Even if you're not sure about God providing for you, it is wise to forgive anyway. God has commanded it (Matthew 18:21-22; Ephesians 4:32), not because he makes the rules and demands we obey them, but because he knows how we are made and knows what will work best for us. We were created – especially as new creations in Christ – to forgive. It is part of our very nature, because Jesus is part of our very nature (Galatians 2:20). Going against our nature only throws us out of whack, and one symptom of being out of whack is overeating.

- How did the "REED" exercise change your perspective, emotions, and eating?

There has never yet been a Weight of Grace participant who said her perspective was totally unchanged after praying through an emotional time using "REED" as a guideline. When God is invited into our struggles, he uses that opportunity to reveal his character to us and to redirect our attention from our problems to his goodness and provision. Sometimes, however, our own bitterness and insistence on having our own way are barriers to hearing from God. There have been many times when I so wanted to be involved in a romantic relationship that I just didn't want to see how God was providing for me in other ways. It was going to be what I wanted or nothing. So, you know what that meant: I got nothing – or, worse, a rotten boyfriend. But, God would work on me, usually through wise and caring friends or passages of Scripture that I came across even when I refused to open the Bible. In my case, it was hard to avoid Scripture when I was working at a biblical counseling ministry, but I bet there are all sorts of creative ways in which God gets his Word into your line of vision. As he does with all of us, God wanted me to go to him with my disappointments and to hear from him about how he was providing the best for me, which far surpassed what I was willing to settle for.

God wanted me to go to him with my disappointments and to hear from him about how he was providing the best for me, which far surpassed what I was willing to settle for.

8   RETURNING TO TRUE HUNGER – PART 1

"What do you think is the main issue involved in overeating?" Over the years, many people have asked me this question. The answer isn't a simple one because there is not just *one* main issue.

The reasons why women overeat involve three layers of issues with one bedrock factor underlying them. The diagram below provides a visual for the different layers of issues, represented as water that gets deeper and darker until you hit the earth underneath.

Represented in the diagram as the deepest, often overlooked layer is the need many women feel to stay large or "fat." This is the layer that most women have no idea exists, but women who overeat have deeply held beliefs about themselves and what it means to be "fat" and "thin" that serve as tremendous motivators for their overeating, canceling out even the strongest desire to be "thin."

Next, there is a more obvious layer of issues that contributes to overeating – the "medicating emotions" layer. Here food is used to comfort, distract from, suppress, or calm unpleasant emotions.

The layer that is closest to the surface, that is most obvious, is one's relationship with food and dieting, which is what most women tend to believe is the "real issue" and where they usually concentrate their greatest efforts to "solve the problem" of overeating.

In addition to these three layers of issues, there is an underlying bedrock factor – a woman's relationship with God and her understanding of his character and intimate, loving involvement with her and her struggles, even her struggles with overweight and overeating. Seeing God as a participant in each layer of issues is crucial to experiencing healing and freedom.

LAYERS OF ISSUES

Obvious Layer: Food/Dieting

Deeper, Less Obvious Layer: Eating to Medicate Emotions

Deepest, Often Overlooked Layer: Need to Stay Large/Fat

Bedrock Factor: Relationship with God

Chapter 2 addressed one's perspective about God (the "Bedrock Factor"). This topic was discussed very early on in the book because of its influence on every aspect of one's struggle with food, overeating, and overweight. Chapter 3 explored the underlying beliefs many women have about themselves that motivate them to stay large – or "fat" – and defeated, even though they so intensely desire to be "thin" (the "Need to Stay Large/Fat" layer). Chapters 6 and 7 addressed the use of food in coping with emotions and the alternatives that are found in one's relationship to and communication with God (the "Eating to Medicate Emotions" layer). No matter how much you try to control your food intake or weight, you will not succeed for any length of time until you have prayerfully considered and sought God's input on these deeper issues involved in overeating.

Although the less obvious, "deeper" layers of issues are extremely important to address, in order to experience freedom from overeating, one's relationship to food and dieting (the "Obvious Layer") needs to be overhauled as well. In this chapter and the next, we will look at developing a healthy perspective regarding food and hunger. In Chapter 10, we will explore the issue of dieting and why dieting is especially unsuccessful for Christians.

Most women believe that the answers to over-eating and over-weight are found in controlling their eating (dieting) and not giving in to their hunger.

Most women believe that the answers to overeating and overweight are found in controlling their eating (dieting) and not giving in to their hunger. Women in our diet-crazed culture have been led to believe that, without rigid controls, they will always want to eat more food than what is "good" for them and that submitting to hunger is a guarantee of weight gain. Women often think, *If I were to eat everything I'm hungry for, I'd never stop eating,* or *If I ate every time I was hungry, I'd be a blimp.* Thoughts such as these reveal: 1) ignorance of the natural mechanisms we possess for knowing when to eat and when not to eat, and 2) a confusion between eating for emotional reasons and eating in response to physical hunger.

There are many Scripture passages that clearly show that there is an assumption made in the Bible that people naturally eat when they're hungry and stop eating when they have satisfied that hunger. The hunger mentioned in the following passages is true *physical* hunger, and it is assumed that eating food or wanting to eat food is the natural response to that hunger: Deuteronomy 8:3, Nehemiah 9:15, Job 5:5, Psalm 146:7, Proverbs 25:21, Isaiah 29:8 and 58:7, Matthew 12:1 and 25:35, Mark 11:12-13a, Acts 10:10 (and, no, his hunger isn't what put him in the trance).

A verse that addresses both physical hunger and satiation is Proverbs 27:7:

> *He who is full loathes honey, but to the hungry even what is bitter tastes sweet.*

For years, my single friends and I used the latter half of this verse to joke about why we'd sometimes settle for less than perfectly desirable boyfriends, but this verse actually speaks volumes about a normal, healthy relationship with food. It assumes that, if you've had enough to eat and are no longer physically hungry, even the most luscious dessert loses its appeal. And, if you're overly hungry, you're not all that discriminating about what you choose to eat. Many women say that even though they don't feel physically hungry, they still go ahead and eat certain foods, often explaining, "I just like the taste." Proverbs 27:7 certainly contradicts them. Wanting to continue to eat after hunger is satisfied is not in our design. This means that if a person still wants to eat after physical hunger is satisfied, no matter how tasty the food is, the eating is for emotional reasons having to do with issues in the deeper layers shown in the diagram on page 107.

Look at Ephesians 5:29:

> *After all, no one ever hated his own body, but he feeds and cares for it, just as Christ does the church.*

It is assumed by the writer (Paul, under the inspiration of the Holy Spirit) that everyone loves his or her body and cares for it properly. In Titus 2:11-12, we read that God has given all believers the grace to live "self-controlled, upright and godly lives." This is the *norm*. It is normal and natural to do what is right for yourself physically and to be moderate and godly in your behavior, including your eating. It is not normal to "never stop eating" or to eat until you "become a blimp." Women have been brainwashed by the diet mentality of our culture to believe a lie about themselves – that they do not come by moderation naturally, that it must be imposed on them by a structured diet of "legal" or "fat free" or "healthy" foods in certain restricted quantities. Also, this same pervasive diet mentality convinces women that they must ignore their hunger, that hunger is, in fact, their enemy. But all the Scriptures listed above imply that hunger is, instead, one's friend. It tells you when you really do need to eat. And, when the hungry feelings end, this tells you when it's time to stop eating.

Read Genesis 2:9, 16. God commanded Adam and Eve to eat of the fruit of the garden and he made food tasty. Food is meant for nourishment and for pleasure, when you're hungry, and any other use of food is not what God intended (e.g., to avoid feeling emotions or to keep yourself "fat"). In fact, eating food for reasons other than to satisfy physical hunger is an attempt to meet your needs in your own way and not in God's way. As you'll remember, meeting your needs in your way is a definition of "the flesh," and living in the flesh is a departure from what is normal for a Christian. Living in the Spirit is the norm for "new creations in Christ." The Spirit indwells us and brings forth fruit in our lives. One of the fruit listed in Galatians 5:22-23 is "self-control." Unlike what many women believe, it is *not* natural to be "out of control" regarding food and eating.

Eating food for reasons other than to satisfy physical hunger is an attempt to meet your needs in your own way and not in God's way.

Even if this point hasn't been proven to your satisfaction from Scripture, all you have to do is look at people you know who never have to worry about weight gain. These people have never dieted! Look at small children of normal weight. You know how difficult it is to get a two-year-old to eat when he's not hungry. No way! When I was reconsidering my attitude toward hunger, my roommate served as a model for me of how "normal" people behave toward food. Karen and I were about the same height and age but, unlike me, her weight didn't constantly go up and down significantly. And Karen never dieted. On some days she would eat a ton of food and on some days she ate almost nothing. On some days she ate all sorts of the "healthy" stuff and on some days she ate pretty much all "junk." How did she get away with this? It took me months of stringent dieting to get down to

Karen's weight, and then I had to constantly fight to stay at that weight – and I always eventually lost the battle!

The way Karen "got away with" her eating habits was that she was just doing what came *naturally*. She ate when she was physically hungry. She ate what she really wanted. And she quit eating when she was no longer physically hungry, when she reached that "just full enough but not too full" point.

It is apparent that we have been designed with many physical cues that prompt us to action. Physically healthy people know when they need to go to the bathroom. Although many ignore the physical signals, physically healthy people can tell when they need to sleep and, given the chance, quite naturally wake up when they've had enough sleep. Most people respond promptly to thirst. But when it comes to responding to the physical cues of hunger, many women have "lost touch" with what is natural. Our culture discourages us from "listening to our bodies" to tell us what we need. And as long as we believe our bodies will steer us in the wrong direction, we will fail to take advantage of the God-given mechanisms that enable us to eat moderately.

When it comes to responding to the physical cues of hunger, many women have "lost touch" with what is natural.

Even if you do believe that physical hunger and satiation are the signals for when it is best for you to eat and to stop eating, the trick is learning to read those signals and respond to them. Years of ignoring hunger and eating past "full" have left many women without a clue about when they really are hungry and satisfied, as opposed to just wanting to eat for other reasons. I'll be honest – learning to become responsive to physical hunger takes time and effort. I started experimenting with how my own hunger felt in October 1984. During that process I often overate and often ate when I was only emotionally, not physically, hungry. But I don't think I could have rediscovered my true hunger signals without missing them a few times and realizing what *wasn't* real hunger. By August 1986, I was very consistently differentiating between physical and emotional hunger. By October 1987, making that differentiation was almost always unconscious. I had become the person I was created to be, a person who very naturally eats moderately without having to think about it much, just like my roommate Karen.

Doing some exercises offered in a few of the anti-diet books I read really helped in finding what was and was not a hunger signal *for me*. (Your homework will provide exercises similar to those I did.) In Weight of Grace small groups, different women report having different sensations that alert them to their hunger. And these sensations change with the degree of hunger. I know I'm beginning to get hungry when I start to feel a tiny bit light-headed and there's a bit of pressure in my throat. This is followed by a hollow sensation in my stomach and then that sinking feeling usually associated with low blood sugar. I've learned that responding to the very first sign of hunger results in not being hungry enough to eat a whole meal, so I try to wait a little while and eat just before that shaky, low-blood-sugar feeling hits. I don't have an exact moment of just-so-much hunger every time I eat, but that doesn't really matter because no matter when in the hunger progression I eat, I stop eating when I no longer feel hungry, even if that means eating just a bite or two.

That's the really hard part – the stopping! When I was still dieting and overeating, I used to dread starting to eat. I used to postpone eating each day till I absolutely could not stand it anymore, because I knew that once I started to eat at all, I'd keep eating and eating and eating. Of course, part of the problem was that I'd wait so long to eat that I'd end up horribly hungry. But the other problem was that I didn't pay attention to how it felt to be satisfied and I was eating for reasons other than physical hunger.

Learning that "just full" feeling also takes experimentation. And it takes something else that's foreign to most women – the assurance that you will get to eat what you really do want to eat every time you feel hungry. If you believe that whatever meal or snack you're eating is "illegal" or the last tasty food you'll have for a great while because you really should be dieting, you will eat as much as you can right now, no matter how awful you feel physically as a result. Eat, drink, and be merry, for tomorrow we diet! But if you take all the "legal," "illegal," "fattening," etc., labels off all your food and allow yourself absolutely whatever you want whenever you're physically hungry, there is no need to eat a whole lot right now. It will be there again later when you get hungry again.

This can be very scary. Eat cookies? Eat ice cream? Eat fried chicken? Any time I'm hungry? Hmmm. That just doesn't sound right. Those foods make you fat! That's not healthy! No, it isn't healthy if that's all you ever eat. But, as we'll see in the next chapter, if you're eating in response to true physical hunger, what you'll eventually crave is what is good for you. And my experience over the past 20 years is that no food is fattening – what's fattening is eating when you're not hungry.

Learning when I was satisfied and then not eating another bite took a willingness to spend the time needed to concentrate on how I was feeling physically whenever I ate – but I had to do this for only about 21 months. Once I got used to the "just full" feeling, I didn't need to always consciously think it through. It became more and more natural to just know when I was finished eating. Getting to that point was not just a matter of paying attention to when the hunger was no longer there, I also had to learn to leave food on my plate, which wasn't what I was taught to do when I was a child. I learned to ask for doggy bags almost every time I ate out. I started seeing that the price of a buffet was paying only for the food I actually ate in response to my hunger, not for all the food I could possibly stuff into myself while I was at the restaurant. (I've since decided that eating at buffets isn't my favorite dining experience because I just don't get my money's worth.)

Part of acknowledging when you're hungry and when you've eaten enough is being willing to buck the system. I find that I tend to eat five small meals or snacks a day, not three big meals. This is what feels physically good for me. But, for you, it may be different. I know a naturally slim man who usually eats only one big meal a day. Acknowledging hunger and satiation can mean sitting at the dinner table with your family and taking only a couple of bites because you aren't hungry at that moment. It can mean deciding that not every scrumptious dish at a dinner party or potluck has to be tasted. There will be another party with another spread – and, when you're hungry again, you can eat something just as scrumptious at home. Paying attention to physical hunger and satiation means people may think you're crazy and that you've just given up on ever overcoming your "weight

Learning that "just full" feeling takes experimentation. And it takes something else that's foreign to most women – the assurance that you will get to eat what you really do want to eat every time you feel hungry.

problem," but you'll know that you're really doing the only truly sane and natural thing there is to do when it comes to eating.

Reflection

1. Do you fear feeling hungry? Why? (What do you think would happen if you let yourself get hungry?)

2. What are the benefits of feeling your hunger?

3. How does hunger feel for you? Where in your body do you sense hunger?

4. How does it feel when you have reached the point of satisfying your hunger? How does it feel when you go past that point?

5. What are the obstacles to eating when you're hungry?

What Others Have Experienced

● Do you fear feeling hungry? Why?

Most women who struggle with overeating have never even considered how they feel about experiencing physical hunger. They either try very hard to avoid ever feeling hungry, or they force themselves to ignore hunger when they do feel it. For many women in Weight of Grace small groups, answering this question awakens them to the fears they do have about hunger.

Many women are afraid that, if they go ahead and feel physical hunger, they will be far more tempted to eat what they believe they shouldn't and in nearly limitless quantities. For these women, hunger equals the potential for, at the very least, breaking a diet, and, at worst, going on uncontrollable eating binges. As a result of this fear, they plan each day's allowance of food (based on fat grams, calories, or other measurements, depending on their diet plan) and apportion the food in such a way to never go very long without eating and, thus, avoid ever feeling hungry.

On the other hand, many women have learned various ways to just tune hunger out so that they can stay within the parameters of their "eating plans." Once when a co-worker and I both heard her stomach growl, she dismissively said, "In 18 minutes, the hunger goes away." She then busied herself more intensely with her work. She didn't eat until her predetermined mealtime. She saw herself as an extremely "disciplined" person, congratulating herself on conquering her own bodily urges.

Both of these ways of dealing with hunger are products of the massive brainwashing that has taken place in our culture. Since Satan is the "prince of this world" (John 12:31; 16:11), it is no surprise that he would make use of various programs and publications to try to convince us that our own bodies are the enemy. He doesn't want us to accept that the way God created us naturally results in moderation and an appropriate relationship with food. And, he certainly doesn't want Christians to know that, since the Holy Spirit indwells them, it is part of their very nature to be self-controlled. Once women become open to the possibility that their bodies won't betray them and may even provide them with the guidance for when it is appropriate for *them* to eat (not when some program tells them to

Most women who struggle with overeating have never even considered how they feel about experiencing physical hunger.

eat), it is then possible to start exploring how their hunger feels and what amount of food satisfies it.

Again, think of the people you know whose size seldom varies and who never diet. These people respond naturally to inner physical cues. They don't think about it very much. Women are always telling me how "disciplined" I am when I don't eat even though there's a lot of appealing food in the room. It's not clench-your-teeth-and-resist discipline. I've just returned to the way I was as a small child. I eat when I'm hungry, and there's no food on earth that tempts me to eat when I'm already feeling full!

- What are the benefits of feeling your hunger?

Many of the women in Weight of Grace groups who have begun to eat in response to their hunger say that a big benefit for them is that food tastes much better. In fact, they find that one sign that they're no longer hungry is that food begins to taste flat.

If you start eating when you're not hungry, the "full" signal will never come on because it was already on at the outset.

Another benefit frequently mentioned is that eating when you're hungry makes it easier to determine when you're satisfied. A problem for those of us who have dieted very much is that we usually start eating either when we are not physically hungry (because a diet or our emotions tell us to) or when we are overly hungry and feeling terribly deprived (because a diet told us *not* to eat). If you start eating when you're not hungry, the "full" signal will never come on because it was already on at the outset. Therefore, the only signal to quit eating will be getting horribly uncomfortable, which is way past the point of physical satisfaction. When you're overly hungry to begin with, the tendency is to gulp and wolf and not even taste your food. It is easy to go right past the "I'm satisfied" signal when you eat really quickly just to quench that painful physical need.

When you learn to recognize your unique signs of hunger and eat in response to them, you will be better able to discover your unique signs of being just full enough. As a result, you can truly enjoy eating but still feel physically comfortable and, maybe more importantly, happy with your God-given moderation in regard to food.

- How does hunger feel for you? How does it feel when you have reached the point of satisfying your hunger?

There are a variety of physical cues that tip women off to their hunger. This is certainly what each woman must discover for herself. It will not do to determine how someone else recognizes hunger and then assume those cues will be the same for you. Although there is not a vast variation in how hunger feels from person to person, there are very unique nuances to each person's sense of physical hunger. Just to give you some ideas of what to look for, here are a few descriptions of hunger that Weight of Grace group members have given:

- *I start feeling a little tired and notice it's been a while since I last ate. Then I wait a few minutes and I feel that yearning feeling in my lower chest and stomach. That's when I'm hungry but not too hungry.*
- *If I get a little shaky, I've waited a little too long to eat.*

- *My stomach starts rumbling, but sometimes that's nothing. When it stops rumbling and then I get a feeling in my mouth and throat that feels like food will make it go away, then I know I'm hungry.*
- *I feel an emptiness in my stomach, almost like it's caving in a little.*

These are comments women have made about feeling they've had enough to eat:

- *The emptiness is gone.*
- *The food stops tasting as good as it did at first.*
- *There's a feeling in my throat that another bite will be too much.*
- *There's no more sense of aching or weakness. I feel good, energized.*

Sometimes it's difficult for women to concentrate all the attention on themselves that's required to discover how hunger and satiation feel for them. They consider this too self-centered or selfish. However, it's really a way to eventually no longer have to worry about every bite of food they eat. The investment now is worth it because of the freedom for years to come.

- What are the obstacles to eating when you're hungry?

For married women and for mothers, the obstacles to eating when they're hungry can seem insurmountable. Throughout the entire time that I was learning to listen to my own hunger, I was single and had a lot of flexibility regarding when I could eat. However, most of the women in Weight of Grace groups are married and/or have children. Also, there are many women whose work situations don't allow eating except at set times.

First, let's look at the "I have a husband and children and gotta eat at mealtimes" situation. Women who prepare and serve meals to family members have to be brave and not always eat everything the family eats or every time the family eats, especially when first learning to "get in touch with" their hunger. This may mean sitting with family members while they eat and "playing with" your food. What's important, especially until you are very familiar with your feelings of hunger and satiation, is to eat only when you're hungry and to stop eating as soon as you stop feeling hungry. This means *not* eating just because it's "time to eat" or to be social. With some family members, you can explain what you're trying to do and why. However, it's odd how, many times the family members who don't struggle with overeating or overweight are the very ones who get alarmed when you don't stick to an eating plan of some sort. Just because they don't have to diet doesn't mean they haven't bought into the diet mentality so prevalent in our culture.

Eating only when you're hungry may look very odd at first – to you and to your family members, especially if you've dieted quite a bit. You probably won't eat at the same times every day. You won't have the same amounts of food each time you eat. Sometimes you'll eat quite a bit of food and sometimes you'll eat only a bite or two. When you're letting hunger take its natural course, there is no way to make yourself feel hungry to certain degrees at certain times. Although this process requires effort at first, the result will be that you will later never have to work at it again. When you diet and ignore when you're hungry and what you're hungry for, as nearly all the diet programs out there tell you to do,

Women who prepare and serve meals to family members have to be brave and not always eat everything the family eats or every time the family eats.

you have to work at staying on your diet or maintenance plan for the rest of your life. They may call it a "lifestyle change," but it's really adopting the unnatural activities of imposing mealtimes when your body doesn't want food and depriving yourself of food when you really are hungry.

What if it's just not possible for you to eat whenever you feel hungry? This would be the case for cashiers, factory workers, mothers of toddlers, department store sales people, and anyone whose job doesn't provide many breaks or prohibits food in the workplace. First, whenever you possibly can – on your days off or when the kids are with their grandparents for the day – be sure to work at eating only when you're hungry. But, when you just can't do that, you will need to experiment with anticipating your hunger. First, try eating only when you're hungry and then see just how hungry you get by the time you have a chance to get to some food again. Then try eating a little food before your shift even if you aren't hungry. See if that amount gets you through to your next break and if you were hungry by then. Through trying different amounts of food and different kinds of food, you can find an amount of food to eat before you start working that will result in your feeling just the right amount of hungry at your meal breaks.

What if it's just not possible for you to eat when-ever you feel hungry?

Sound like too much effort? How much effort have you been putting into addressing overeating and overweight through dieting? How much energy goes into guilt over, and obsession with, food? At least the effort to learn to respond to your own body will eventually lead to "doing what comes naturally." What you're currently doing will never be natural.

Homework

1. For the next few days, use the following chart to keep track of every time you eat, even if you eat the tiniest amount of food. Note the time and what you ate and whether you were physically hungry. If you weren't physically hungry, prayerfully discern what triggered the eating. If you were hungry, use a one-to-ten scale to rate just how hungry you were. Don't try to eat only when you're hungry. Just observe how you really do eat and for what reasons.

EATING WHEN YOU'RE HUNGRY

Date/ Time:	What you ate:	Were you hungry? If not, what was going on?	How hungry?

2. After you've kept the "Eating When You're Hungry" chart for a few days, use the following chart to keep track of how it feels when you stop eating. Note the date and time, what you ate, and whether you were physically hungry to begin with before you started eating. When you stop eating, use a one-to-ten scale to assess how full you felt and then make notes about how it felt physically to be that degree of full. Do not try to make yourself do the "right thing." Just observe your own behavior as dispassionately as you can so that you can see how different degrees of fullness feel to you.

HOW IT FEELS WHEN YOU STOP EATING

Date/Time:	What you ate:	Hungry when you started eating?	How full when you stopped eating?	How did you feel physically when you stopped?

BEFORE YOU GO ON TO THE NEXT CHAPTER

Homework Follow-up

1. What insights about what triggers your eating did you gain from keeping the first chart?

2. What did you discover by rating your hunger?

3. What did you discover about satiation from keeping the second chart?

4. How convinced are you that your body knows when to eat and when to stop eating? Why?

Comments on the Homework

- What insights did you gain from keeping the charts? What did you discover by rating your hunger? From rating how full you were and how that felt?

On and off for many years, I kept charts of what I ate in order to keep track of whether I was eating the correct amounts of different food groups as outlined in the diet program I was on. So when a book I was reading about discarding diets suggested that I keep a chart to track when I was eating in response to hunger, it was not my idea of fun. Nevertheless, I kept the chart for a couple of weeks, remembering that I was not judging myself but only observing myself[1]. The charts in your homework are useless if you alter your behavior in order to make the contents of the charts look better. However, if you stay honest with yourself and let yourself observe and record with an uncritical eye, keeping the charts for a while will help you start to distinguish between physical hunger and wanting to eat for emotional reasons, as well as help you discern the hunger and satiation levels that "work" for you.

After keeping track of my eating for a while, I started realizing at what level of hunger my body was most "happy" to eat.

After keeping track of my eating for a while, I started realizing at what level of hunger my body was most "happy" to eat. Later, when I tried rating how I felt after I stopped eating, I found the point at which I was most comfortably satisfied without being overly full. You may want to continue to use the charts for a few weeks. As you continue to rate your hunger and satiation, you will find your own points of *Yes, I'm really hungry and would very much enjoy eating right now,* and *This is just the right amount; if I eat one more bite I'll be uncomfortable.*

- How convinced are you that your body knows when to eat and when to stop eating?

Discovering that your body knows best when to eat requires taking a leap of faith.

For some women this is a hard sell. But, they usually have confused the physical signals of hunger with the desire to eat for other reasons, such as those that were discussed in previous chapters. Discovering that your body knows best when to eat requires taking a leap of faith. I found that it helped a great deal to do two things when I took that leap. I looked to the Holy Spirit to guide me in distinguishing between physical hunger and "emotional hunger," and I told myself I'd try this hunger/satiation thing only until it was apparent I'd gone down a dead-end street. I'm still traveling down that street, and it turns out it was the road to becoming the person God created me to be, someone who quite naturally eats in moderation and, therefore, stays about the same size all the time.

9   RETURNING TO TRUE HUNGER – PART 2

If convincing women that eating only when they're hungry is a hard sell, especially for inveterate dieters, that's nothing compared to convincing them that they can eat *whatever* they're hungry for. Don't we all *know* that certain foods are "fattening"? You just think about them and put on weight, right? And, aren't there a lot of unhealthy foods that, really, no one should eat? What about fried foods? Everyone knows those are bad for you! In fact, isn't it common knowledge that we all need to change our lifestyles so that we cut out sugar, fat, junk food, and processed foods?

When you watch TV or read women's magazines, there appear to be all sorts of "givens" about what foods are good for you, what foods are bad for you, what foods make you gain weight, and what foods help you lose weight. But, are these God-ordained rules about food – or might these rules fall into the category of "the way that *seems* right..."? (Proverbs 14:12, emphasis mine.)

We know that in the Old Testament, there were many detailed dietary laws. However, in Mark 7:19, we read that Jesus declared all foods "clean." Since the advent of Christ, no food is considered by God to be "unclean" or off-limits. Nevertheless we label certain foods "illegal" or "bad" or "cheating" and tell ourselves that if we eat these foods we are bad, cheaters, and gluttons. Why? Because we believe that using these guilt-laden labels will motivate us to "behave" and that if we don't "guilt ourselves" into avoiding certain foods, we will overindulge in them. We believe the threat of guilt serves as a deterrent to overeating.

Since the advent of Christ, no food is considered by God to be "unclean" or off-limits. Nevertheless we label certain foods "illegal" or "bad" or "cheating."

The problem with this line of thinking is that guilt works for only a short time, especially since it is not the way we are designed by God to be motivated. As Christians, God motivates us through the indwelling Holy Spirit and the presence of Christ's love in our hearts. The Holy Spirit directs our thinking and points out to us when we are choosing according to "the flesh." Our true inward desire is to do what is right in God's sight (Ephesians 4:24; Philippians 2:13). Guilt only brings condemnation and causes us to focus on the negatives. The Holy Spirit brings truth to light and empowers us to turn from sin and to live as God desires us to live. In fact, all condemnation was suffered by Christ on the cross over two thousand years ago. For new creations in Christ, trying to drum up guilt and the condemnation that goes with it is far less effective than living in the Spirit.

Not only is categorizing food with guilt-inducing labels not necessary for enforcing healthy eating, the Bible makes clear that we are designed to quite naturally take good care of our own bodies (Proverbs 27:7; Ephesians 5:29). Unlike the messages our culture broadcasts about how our tendency is to always go for the "bad" foods if we don't monitor ourselves really closely, God created us to naturally desire what is healthy and moderate. Sin and the flesh, which were not part of our original makeup, draw us into behaviors that are unhealthy. As a Christian, your true, inner nature has been returned to holiness, indwelt by God's Spirit. You are no longer a "slave to sin" (Romans 6:6) but rather have the option to choose to act in line with your new nature. You have a choice about whether you act out of your own ideas about how to take care of yourself or turn to God's power and direction.

All this theology about our new nature is great, but giving up on choosing foods based on labels such as "illegal" and "bad" seems quite frightening to most women who struggle with overeating. The thinking is, *If I don't follow rules that tell me which foods are bad, how will I ever know what I should and should not eat? Won't I just eat foods that are bad for my health and make me even fatter than I already am?*

The Bible clearly addresses what does and does not enable us to engage in behaviors that are beneficial for us. Paul makes two amazing statements in 1 Corinthians 6:12 where he quotes a common and misused saying of the day and then elaborates upon it.

> *"Everything is permissible for me" but not everything is beneficial.*
> *"Everything is permissible for me" but I will not be mastered by anything.*

As scary as this may sound, I have found from personal experience that the first step to eating what is healthy *for you* is to understand that, in regard to food, *everything* truly is permissible. It is impossible to distinguish for yourself what is or is not beneficial *until you agree that all food is permissible.* It is also impossible for you to experience "not being mastered" by food until you accept that all food is permissible. As long as you adopt rules about what foods are allowed or not allowed, food will continue to be an issue, even an obsession, in your life.

The problem with making rules about food is made clear in Romans 7:7b-8:

> *For I would not have known what coveting really was if the law had not said, "Do not covet." But sin, seizing the opportunity afforded by the commandment, produced in me every kind of covetous desire. For apart from law, sin is dead.*

It's the "do not touch" sign that makes us crazy to touch and see how it feels. It's our "laws" about food that arouse our desire to break these "rules." When do you most crave chocolate or fried chicken? When your diet says you can't have them, of course! When you adopt the culture's pronouncements about certain foods, you set yourself up for obsessions with what has been labeled "wrong," "illegal," or "off-limits."

In order to experience freedom from obsessions with food that result from dieting and culturally-imposed restrictions, it is necessary to take what, for many, is a very big leap of faith – set aside all the negative food labels and decide that *all foods are truly permissible.** Once you are convinced that everything is truly permissible, then you are able to find out which foods are really not beneficial *for you.*

When you are permitted to choose from every food available, you can then make choices based on how your body reacts to different foods.

When you are permitted to choose from every food available, you can then make choices based on how your body reacts to different foods. If you don't let yourself eat fried chicken, you'll never find out that it makes your stomach ache or makes you feel as though you have less energy. Instead, you'll just long for that "forbidden fruit," fried chicken. If, however, you experience a few times for yourself some negative consequences from eating

---

*There are, of course, very necessary dietary restrictions that some people must follow, as in the case of diabetes, hypoglycemia, or food allergies. These are not the same as restrictions imposed by weight-loss diets, which declare "bad" many foods that are not necessarily harmful for most people.

fried chicken, you'll find that you really don't want to eat it very often. Or – and this is just as important a discovery – you could find out that you feel just fine when you eat fried chicken. Then, as a result of knowing you can have it any time you want, you'll eat it only when you're really hungry for it, which won't be all that often because there are a lot of other tasty foods you'll feel hungry for. If you think that fried chicken is a food you should never eat, you'll eat it only when you're "cheating," and the guilt over eating it, as well as the pleasure of indulging in something so "sinful," will distract you from how your body really feels when you eat it.

As long as I told myself chocolate donuts were off-limits, all I thought about was eating chocolate donuts. But, when I said I could have all the chocolate donuts I wanted – as long as I was hungry for them – I got to the point where I wanted to try other foods and, for months at a time, didn't eat any chocolate donuts at all.

The key is not eating what is "right" or "wrong." The key is eating *when you are physically hungry and what you are truly hungry for*. Once we remove the labels, once we remove the guilt, we are free to try different foods and see for ourselves what is "beneficial." Given my tendency toward insomnia, it isn't hard for me to avoid caffeinated drinks and to refrain from eating chocolate after about 2:00 in the afternoon. If I had kept these foods on my "forbidden" list and hadn't tried them and seen for myself their effect on me, I would have forever craved them and felt deprived because I couldn't have them. Now, I know I can eat chocolate and drink colas as much as I want, but having experienced the negative results enough times, I truly don't want those foods very often. This isn't out of guilt or because some study told me these foods are "bad."

The key is eating when you are physically hungry and what you are truly hungry for.

Actually, it boils down to a form of conditioning. When I ate certain foods, I felt physically uncomfortable or suffered in some negative way (e.g., indigestion or insomnia). These uncomfortable experiences made those foods less attractive to me. And there are so many other wonderful foods I can eat without negative consequences that I don't feel deprived by omitting a few that are obviously not beneficial *for me*.

When you eat whatever you really want – at times when you're truly *physically* hungry – it tastes fabulous and it rarely takes a large amount to feel satisfied. When you know you can have that food again just as soon as you're hungry for it, why gorge yourself on it now and make yourself feel sick or uncomfortable? Why not wait and have it again when you'd really enjoy it? When my whole life was spent either on a diet or breaking one, each time I prepared to start on my diet program again after getting "off the wagon," knowing that I wouldn't be allowed to eat certain foods once I started dieting, I ate way more of those foods than I was hungry for. Now that I know I'll never be restricted again, I never want to overstuff myself. It will all be there when I'm hungry for it. Or food that's just as good will be there – various foods do go out of season or spoil or are available only while you're at Grandma's.

When I first started eating what I really wanted to eat whenever I got hungry, for several weeks I always made sure I had a glazed devil's-food donut within reach. After several weeks of a pretty donut-heavy diet, I started craving other foods, such as raisins and cooked carrots and turkey sandwiches. Over the next several months, I moved from one special craving to another. First, I ate one or two of those chocolate donuts nearly every day, then it was a bag of M&M'S® every morning, then Twix® bars, then popcorn, then ice cream, then bagels with butter, then bagels with cream cheese. It seemed I had to make my way through all the foods I'd always believed were absolutely off limits. All the while, I was also eating other foods because I got hungry for them, and many of them were foods I thought I'd never want again because they were what I used to think of as "diet foods."

After about a year and a half of periods of craving certain foods, I reached a point where I no longer had any special cravings. In fact, now I'm hard pressed to say what my favorite foods are. I *can* tell you what I almost never eat, and I avoid most of those foods because I just don't like how I feel after I eat them. They really don't appeal to me anymore, even though they used to be some of my most desired "forbidden" foods. They're no longer forbidden – they are permissible – but they sure aren't beneficial *for me*!

Look at the people you know who stay slim without working at it. How many of them stick to only the "good for you" foods? None that I know of. In the last chapter, I mentioned my roommate Karen as a model for me regarding eating in response to true physical hunger. Observing another friend helped me quite a bit regarding eating the food I really wanted.

Chuck is an attractive man who is my age and whose size never changed throughout the 20-plus years during which we maintained an active friendship. Because our birthdays are two weeks apart, there were many years when we celebrated together with a nice dinner out. We had one of those dinners during the period of time in 1985 when I was first experimenting with eating only when I was hungry and eating only what I was hungry for. We went to one of my favorite restaurants, where every item on the menu is luscious. Before the meal was served, special wait staff came around to each table, serving up as many small, warm, powdered sugar covered apple fritters as you could eat. I had always found these fritters to be irresistible. My usual pattern had been to eat quite a few of the fritters and then eat my entire dinner even though it meant leaving the restaurant feeling overstuffed and uncomfortable. This time, however, I noticed that Chuck didn't eat even a single fritter. I asked him why and he said that even though he liked fritters, he *really* liked what he ordered and didn't want to in any way ruin his enjoyment of it. This prompted me to think about what I enjoyed more, the fritters or my entrée, and I realized I actually did like the fritters more. I decided to eat several fritters and then I sort of pushed the food in my main course around on my plate and asked for a doggie bag. The next day, the leftovers made a great lunch and at neither meal did I feel physically uncomfortable. I felt quite satisfied after both meals. I'd eaten only as much as I was hungry for and exactly what I really wanted at the time.

If you've bought into the diet mentality that is so pervasive in our culture, eating what you really want to eat can seem very, very scary because you associate certain foods with weight gain. But, the issue is not really *what* you eat; it's *how much* and whether you're physically hungry. What is also scary for many women is the idea of not eating a "balanced diet" every day. But I've found I quite naturally eat a balanced diet; it just gets balanced over about a one- to two-week period, rather than balanced every single day. Given a

Look at the people you know who stay slim without working at it. How many of them stick to only the "good for you" foods?

If you've bought into the diet mentality that is so pervasive in our culture, eating what you really want to eat can seem very, very scary because you associate certain foods with weight gain.

chance, your body will not crave only "junk food" all the time. Your body needs various nutrients – but they're not just in all the foods you've been brainwashed into believing they're in. When you give yourself a chance, you'll naturally select what makes your body run best. Think of how many times you've experienced constipation, diarrhea, or missed periods when you've been on some diet. Diets are not the natural way to eat. They don't allow you to respond to *your* body.

In addition to eating the food we really want, there are a couple of other things which pertain to overweight and for which we "hunger" and require that we "listen to our bodies": thirst and exercise.

In our diet-crazed culture, there are a lot of "rules" about drinking fluids, especially related to weight control – how much to drink and what kinds are "good" or "bad." And, it's easy in our busy lives to ignore the often subtle physical cues that indicate that our bodies are asking for water or juice or even a carbonated beverage. Sometimes we can even mistake thirst for hunger. I've found I need to not only check if I'm physically hungry before I eat, but also I need to check if what I'm craving is food or liquids. Also, despite the barrage of television and magazine articles that insist everyone should drink eight glasses of water per day, I've learned through experience to drink water and other beverages in the same way I eat food – based on my physical cravings. When I forced myself to drink 64 ounces of water per day, I experienced some uncomfortable physical side effects. When I drink only what I physically crave, my bowels, blood pressure, and hydration are all healthier.

Sometimes we can mistake thirst for hunger.

When it comes to exercise, there is also an assortment of "guidelines" to which we've all been exposed. But, getting exercise is as individual as our food preferences. When we give ourselves permission to "do what comes naturally," when we ask God to direct us in even our forms of exercise, we will indeed find what is right for us. Unfortunately, the word "exercise" has attached to it many negative connotations, such as "no pain, no gain" and "just do it." Yet there is that need in each of us to move, to be physically active, to make use of the marvelous mechanisms that are our bodies. Our muscles, joints, and tendons all want to do some sort of activity some of the time, and there's a wide variety of activities they can do. Each person can find not only enjoyment and the physical release of tension that comes with movement, but also personal expression through that movement.

There is that need in each of us to move, to be physically active, to make use of the marvelous mechanisms that are our bodies.

Not only do you need to engage in physical activities that are right for *you*, they should be right for you *at this particular time*. As our lives change, our movements change too. Whereas taking walks feels good during the spring, going for a swim may feel better in the summer. Running may have felt great in youth and then be a problem as knees and feet age. Some of us have movement built into our lives – team sports, physical labor in our jobs, mowing the lawn – and for these people it is important to respect the need to rest from movement. However, for all of us who have avoided exercise or forced ourselves to exercise in ways we didn't enjoy, there is a need to prayerfully listen to our bodies' ache to move around and expend energy, and to look for those activities that best fit us.

I remember a time when I was first becoming aware that, even when I no longer forced myself to work out three times per week, I still wanted to engage in some form of regular physical activity. I was spending a week with a friend and her small child. She was eight-and-a-half-months pregnant with twins, so we were mostly house bound. Even though I'd never been much of a dancer, nearly every day I found myself dancing around the living room throughout two of the toddler's favorite TV shows, both of which included a lot of sing-alongs. My body just seemed to say, "Gotta dance!" Since then, as I've prayerfully listened to my body and experimented with different forms of exercise, I've discovered what feels good, both physically and emotionally, to me, and some amount of exercise has quite naturally become a regular part of my lifestyle several days a week year-round.

Reflection

1. What are the foods you consider to be "forbidden" and why do you consider them to be so?

2. How do you determine what is not beneficial for you in non-food areas of your life?

3. What types of physical activity do you most enjoy? What types fit well into your lifestyle? Do you deserve to spend the time that it takes to engage in physical activity?

What Others Have Experienced

- What are the foods you consider to be "forbidden" and why do you consider them to be so?

Women *love* to answer this question. It's like finally talking about a secret love. They get to express their deepest desires, their naughtiest food fantasies. It's proof of the power rules have to make the ordinary seem wildly desirable. Of course, the reasons these foods are forbidden usually have to do with "common wisdom" or diet plans. Also, there are foods about which individual families develop taboos. I remember a number of times when my mother saw me eating peanuts, she said, "You know, that's what farmers feed pigs to fatten them up." Of course, since peanuts were "wrong," when I did eat them, I overate. Now that peanuts are perfectly okay to eat, I rarely want to eat them. They just aren't a favorite, but it has nothing to do with making pigs fat. As a matter of fact, I found out from a pig farmer I know that the only reason pigs would be fed peanuts is if the farmer grew peanuts and it was therefore cheap feed.

With all the studies, news segments, and print and Internet articles circulating about food and health, it's understandable that you would be worried about certain foods clogging your arteries, raising your blood pressure, or leading to colon cancer. We all have to make choices about what studies we believe and how we'll act upon that information. Making food choices for health reasons is not the same as proclaiming certain foods off-limits because they're "fattening." But, when women are totally honest, most of their food no-no's are based solely on a fear of gaining weight.

Making food choices for health reasons is not the same as proclaiming certain foods off-limits because they're "fattening."

When I decided to eschew dieting and try the "eat when you're hungry/eat what you're hungry for" approach, I also decided to, at least for a time, not consider most food-related health studies for a while. If I wanted real butter on a bagel, or real cream cheese, that's what I ate. What was interesting was that my cholesterol stayed well under 200. When I could have foods with fat in them, I no longer gorged myself on them. Within just a year or so, my body's own "intelligence" surfaced, and I started craving foods I always considered to be a total chore to eat: fish (especially tuna), cottage cheese, and lettuce. These were foods my diets usually required and, when I discarded dieting, I swore I'd never even look at them again. Never say never. Once every food became "legal," even these foods were what I occasionally craved. In fact, a lettuce salad (but with regular dressing only – none of that fat-free stuff) is one of my favorite meals.

There was a time when I did decide to eliminate certain foods for health reasons. I was determined to share an apartment with a woman who had three cats; and although I love cats dearly, I am also terribly allergic to them. A friend had overcome some allergies by going on a special diet, so I consulted his nutritionist. For six months, which was the amount of time the nutritionist prescribed, I avoided milk products, sugar, aspartame, whole wheat products, citrus fruits, caffeine, and peanut products. I also took some special mega-vitamins. I found that, given my motivation to overcome the allergy to cats, it was absolutely no problem to go on this particular "diet." I was in no way restricting myself in hopes of weight loss. In fact, throughout the entire time I was on this diet, my size didn't change at all.

At the end of the six months, I was still allergic to cats, but my symptoms were lessened. However, my somewhat milder allergies to dogs and horses were gone. It turned out that another friend, who owned a dog, needed a roommate also, so the anti-allergy diet had not been for naught. I had started this diet three years after I gave up all weight-loss dieting, but when I started it, I still feared I'd binge-eat if I proclaimed certain foods off limits. However, I never binged once. I knew I could have absolutely every food other than the ones the nutritionist said I should omit. I knew that I could quit the diet at any time and eat whatever I wanted. And, I wasn't on the diet to lose weight. All of these factors meant that giving up some foods for a while didn't automatically lead to binge-eating. Food restrictions for valid health reasons (e.g., diabetes, high blood pressure, food allergies) need not have the same negative effect that weight-loss diets do. There is not the same sense of deprivation when you are convinced your health is truly at stake.

- How do you determine what is not beneficial for you in non-food areas of your life?

There are a number of areas in life in which we seem to quite naturally live by "all things are permissible, but not all things are beneficial" (1 Corinthians 6:12).

There are a number of areas in life in which we seem to quite naturally live by "all things are permissible, but not all things are beneficial" (1 Corinthians 6:12). Certainly, there's no law that enforces brushing your teeth. It's perfectly legal to never ever brush your teeth. However, you just have to go a couple of days without doing so and you know why you don't need a law to tell you brushing your teeth really is beneficial! It's the same with bathing and washing your clothes. We learned many disciplines from our parents, and most of us have tried breaking family rules in areas such as tidiness and hygiene only to find we returned to them after learning through experience why they were practiced by our parents in the first place. You don't think of yourself as being highly disciplined because you avoid grabbing casserole dishes out of the oven without a potholder. You probably have had an experience with the pain of a burn that long ago convinced you that, yes, all things are permissible, but not all things are beneficial when it comes to reaching for baking dishes in the oven. By the time we reach adulthood, there are many areas in which we have learned, either "the hard way" or by observing others learning the hard way, that certain behaviors are just not beneficial.

Learning what's beneficial about foods is similar. It's important to learn what foods are beneficial for you through your own experience, not because someone told you a particular food would "make you fat." I'm convinced that no food is "fattening." It's just the quantities of food we eat when we're not hungry for them that cause us to gain weight. When the decision is made that your body can be trusted to crave what it most needs, it's possible to become the person you were created to be, someone who does not need rules and regulations to determine what's "good" or "bad." You can find out for yourself what does and doesn't work best for you.

- What types of physical activity do you most enjoy? What types fit well into your lifestyle? Do you deserve to spend the time that it takes to engage in physical activity?

Many women have been so bombarded with our culture's rules about exercising that they are absolutely repelled by the idea of engaging in any physical activity beyond what's required in their regular day-to-day lives. Even those who would enjoy engaging in some form of exercise feel their lifestyles just won't allow them the time needed. It *is* sometimes difficult to be creative about how and when to get exercise, to fulfill your body's craving for movement. Certainly, the best place to start is with prayer, but you need to be open to what God might reveal. Also, if your concept of God is that he would never permit you to be so selfish as to take time for yourself, you probably won't feel comfortable doing any enjoyable physical, recreational activity. But, you weren't given all those moving parts just so they could atrophy!

It may help to discuss this issue with your family. There may be activities all of you can do together, such as bowling, dance lessons, playing tennis, or joining the YMCA and taking swimming lessons. This could be a way to do activities together instead of you just driving family members to their activities.

If you have an activity in mind that appeals to you, see if God will grant you that desire when you ask him. He can be very creative about providing the time, resources, and opportunities, even when you're not. As was mentioned earlier, you don't have to stick to just one type of activity. Different seasons and different stages in life lend themselves to different forms of exercise. When you decide on activities based on what you really want to do, you'll be much more likely to do *something*. When you set up exercise rules for yourself, it's very likely you'll do little or nothing.

If your concept of God is that he would never permit you to be so selfish as to take time for yourself, you probably won't feel comfortable doing any enjoyable physical, recreational activity.

Homework

1. Read the following article[1] about "intuitive eating" and highlight the parts that stand out to you or with which you identify. Also, make notes, below, about those statements you just can't believe are true and why you don't believe them.

USA TODAY • WEDNESDAY, APRIL 26, 1995 • 5D

By Nanci Hellmich
USA TODAY

HEALTH AND EDUCATION

Intuitive eating satisfies body, mind

You're craving strawberry shortcake. But instead of indulging, you try to fend off the yearning by eating a rice cake with a strawberry on it.

"If you eat a rice cake with a strawberry on it and call it strawberry shortcake, I guarantee you're going to eat the real thing in the near future," says nutritionist Evelyn Tribole, 35.

"We've got to bring the pleasure back to eating. If you've had a pleasurable eating experience, you'll be a satisfied eater. And if you're a satisfied eater, you're less likely to overeat," she says.

Tribole and Elyse Resch, both registered dietitians in Beverly Hills, Calif., don't prescribe specific day-by-day diets for their clients, who include actresses, CEOs of major companies, successful business people and ordinary folks.

Instead, they try to get their clients to stop fretting about food every minute and learn to enjoy it. The two nutrition therapists explain their techniques in a new book, *Intuitive Eating: A Recovery Book for the Chronic Dieter* (St. Martin's Press, $21.95).

The authors point out that diets often fail and dieting can be

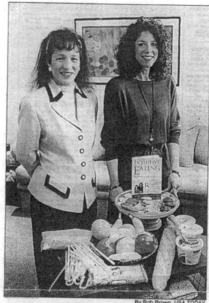

By Rob Brown, USA TODAY
BREAKING OLD EATING HABITS: Dietitians Evelyn Tribole, left, and Elyse Resch advise against specific day-by-day diets.

Different dietary habits, characteristics

Evelyn Tribole and Elyse Resch outline some eating styles in *Intuitive Eating*. Many characteristics of unhealthy styles could get in the way of becoming an intuitive eater.

Careful Eater
 ▶ Trigger: Fitness and health.
 ▶ Characteristic: Appears to be a perfect eater, yet anguishes over each morsel.

Unconscious Eater
 ▶ Trigger: Eating while doing something else.
 ▶ Characteristic: This person is often unaware that she/he is eating, or how much is being eaten. There are many subtypes.

Chaotic Unconscious Eater
 ▶ Trigger: Overscheduled life.
 ▶ Characteristic: This person's eating style is haphazard – gulp 'n go when food is available.

Refuse-Not Unconscious Eater
 ▶ Trigger: Presence of food.
 ▶ Characteristic: This person is especially vulnerable to candy jars or food present at meetings.

Waste-Not Unconscious Eater
 ▶ Trigger: Free food.
 ▶ Characteristic: This person is susceptible to the all-you-can-eat buffets and free food.

Emotional Unconscious Eater
 ▶ Trigger: Uncomfortable emotions.
 ▶ Characteristic: Stress or uncomfortable feelings trigger eating – especially when alone.

Professional Dieter
 ▶ Trigger: Feeling fat.
 ▶ Characteristic: This person is perpetually dieting, often trying the latest commercial diet or diet book.

Intuitive Eater
 ▶ Trigger: Biological hunger.
 ▶ Characteristic: Makes food choices without facing guilt or an ethical dilemma. Honors hunger, respects fullness.

a steppingstone to an eating disorder. Their plan is designed to help people discover the intuitive eater in themselves. Intuitive eaters are people who listen to their bodies to determine if they're hungry, says Tribole. Most toddlers do just that if there is not too much interference from outside forces such as well-meaning parents or a bombardment of TV commercials.

Intuitive eaters ask themselves: "Am I hungry? Am I full? Does it sound good? Is it what I really want? Does it really taste good?"

But many people have become chronic dieters – people who are at war with food and their bodies, the authors say.

Chronic dieters are preoccupied with food. They consider a good day one when they undereat. But that often backfires: They feel deprived psychologically and biologically. They enter the primal hunger state and eventually the undereating triggers overeating – and they'll eat anything in sight, says Tribole. "When you are starving, you are vulnerable. If you're in front of the vending machine, you'll grab the Snickers bar."

Resch agrees. She says for years she prescribed specific diets for her clients. They would lose weight after several months on her plan. But when they came back the next year, they had regained all the weight they lost. "My insides were hurting" from the stress of watching clients regain weight, says Resch.

Now she counsels her clients to listen to their bodies. Eventually, they learn to eat when they're hungry and stop eating when they're full. And they choose healthier foods because "your body feels better when you eat healthy foods."

Resch, 50, says her weight is completely stable after years of struggling with 20 pounds. She

eats French fries and bacon occasionally, but they do not constitute the majority of her diet because "I don't feel good if I eat a lot of greasy food." If you really pay attention to how you feel after you eat these foods, you won't want them as often, she says.

When you know you can eat anything you want and you truly believe that, then you can start looking at the nutrition guidelines and follow the food pyramid, Tribole says.

Resch says as her clients become intuitive eaters, they often achieve a natural healthy weight, but intuitive eating won't help people maintain an abnormally low body weight, which many people want.

You have to accept your body type, Tribole adds. You can't go from size 8 shoe into a size 6, no matter what you do.

With intuitive eating, "you're making peace with food and making peace with your body. Having a healthy relationship with food is just as important as eating healthfully."[1]

Change your attitude toward food and weight

To become an intuitive eater, Evelyn Tribole and Elyse Resch outline these 10 principles in their new book:

▶ **Reject the diet mentality.** Throw out the diet books and magazine articles that offer you the false hope of losing weight quickly, easily, and permanently. If you allow even one small hope to linger that a new and better diet might lurk around the corner, it will prevent you from being free to rediscover intuitive eating.

▶ **Honor your hunger.** Keep your body fed biologically with adequate energy and carbohydrates. Otherwise, you can trigger a primal drive to overeat. Once you reach the moment of excessive hunger, all intentions of moderate, conscious eating are fleeting and irrelevant.

▶ **Make peace with food.** Call a truce; stop the food fight! Give yourself unconditional permission to eat. If you tell yourself that you can't or shouldn't have a particular food, it can lead to intense feelings of deprivation that build into uncontrollable cravings and, often, bingeing. When you finally "give in" to your forbidden foods, eating will be experienced with such intensity, it usually results in Last Supper overeating and overwhelming guilt.

▶ **Challenge the food police.** Scream a loud "No" to thoughts in your head that declare you're "good" for eating under 1,000 calories or "bad" because you ate a piece of chocolate cake.

▶ **Feel your fullness.** Listen for the body signals that say you are no longer hungry. Observe the signs that show you're comfortably full. Pause in the middle of eating and ask yourself how the food tastes and what your current fullness level is.

▶ **Discover the satisfaction factor.** When you eat what you really want, in an environment that is inviting, the pleasure you derive will be a powerful force in helping you feel satisfied and content. By providing this experience for yourself, you will find that it takes much less food to decide you've had enough.

▶ **Cope with your emotions without using food.** Find ways to comfort, nurture, distract and resolve your issues without using food… If anything, eating for emotional hunger will only make you feel worse in the long run. You'll ultimately have to deal with the source of the emotion, as well as the discomfort of overeating.

▶ **Respect your body.** Accept your genetic blueprint. It's hard to reject the diet mentality if you are unrealistic and overly critical of your body shape.

▶ **Exercise.** Forget militant exercise. Just get active and feel the difference. Shift your focus to how it feels to move your body, rather than the calorie-burning effect of exercise.

▶ **Honor your health – gentle nutrition.** Make food choices that honor your health and taste buds while making you feel good. You will not suddenly get a nutrient deficiency or gain weight with one snack, one meal, or one day of eating. It's what you eat consistently over time that matters.

2.   Read the following excerpt from *The Psychologist's Eat-Anything Diet*. Then, over the course of the next few days, use the chart on page 133 to gauge the degree to which the foods you eat "hum" or "beckon." Use a one-to-ten scale to indicate the degree to which each food hummed or beckoned.

Foods that "hum" to you are those that you really crave and love—quite regardless of immediate availability.

Foods that "beckon" to you are those that you had not been craving. It is a food that's available now. "It looks good," "it will taste fine," it starts to appeal to you, to invite you.

When a certain food hums to you, you yearn for it. When a food beckons, it calls out to you. They are two distinct, quite different events.

The image of humming derives from its similarity to a tune that you can't get out of your head. Foods that hum can almost be heard inside your head. It's as if a message is coming up from inner depths, directing you toward a particular food, persisting until you respond.

Beckoning foods aren't on your mind. Quite often, even the idea of eating isn't on your mind—until you look in that bakery window, get a whiff from that candy kitchen, or notice delicious-looking food being served at the next table.[2]

To summarize the differences between humming and beckoning:

Humming Food	*Beckoning Food*
1. You think of the food without seeing it, or before seeing it.	1. This food wasn't on your mind until you saw it.
2. You yearn for the food.	2. The food calls out to you.
3. The food may not even be immediately available.	3. It's immediately available.
4. A food you feel a craving for, right now. Desire for the food comes from inner depths.	4. It looks good. You'd enjoy it, but you don't crave it.
5. It satisfies "hunger."	5 It tastes good but doesn't satisfy. Or you have to overeat to get the satisfaction of fullness.[3]

GAUGING HUMMING AND BECKONING

Food Item and Circumstance	Hummer or Beckoner?	To What Degree?

BEFORE YOU GO ON TO THE NEXT CHAPTER

Homework Follow-up

1. What in the article "Intuitive eating satisfies body, mind" did you find hard to "buy"? What did you like in the article?

2. What did you learn from the "humming" and "beckoning" exercise?

3. What do you long for, what do you crave, that is not food and for which you're using eating as a substitute?

4. What are some of the non-food ways you can "feed" yourself and add satisfaction to your life?

Comments on the Homework

- What in the article did you find hard to "buy"? What did you like in the article?

Most of the women who have attended Weight of Grace small groups find the "intuitive eating" article pretty palatable. By the time they read it, they are starting to have a little bit of hope that their bodies could actually inform them about when to eat, what to eat, and when to stop eating. The biggest obstacle to really believing this is captured well in the article: "If you allow even one small hope to linger that a new and better diet might lurk around the corner, it will prevent you from being free to rediscover intuitive eating."[4] There are many women who just will not give up on dieting altogether. The women who have experienced little freedom from overeating after attending Weight of Grace groups have been those who decided they'd diet down to an "ideal weight" and *then* start eating in response to physical hunger. The problem however is that, once they get to that goal weight (and very few do), they feel so deprived by the dieting that they start overeating. Or, they're terrified of regaining weight so they remain on their diet to some degree just in case eating in response to physical hunger doesn't really work. Dieting is a trap and will be addressed fully in the next chapter. It's a shame, but most women who struggle with overeating and "fat" have to learn the really hard way, through many weight losses followed by re-gaining the pounds, that diets are part of the problem and *not* the solution, and some women never come to see this.

- What did you learn from the "humming" and "beckoning" exercise?

Most women heartily agree with author Geneen Roth's statement, "Most of us eat beckoning foods most of the time."[5] Most of us 1) don't take the time to think through whether we're really hungry and what we really want to eat, and 2) rush around quite a bit and, therefore, hurriedly eat whatever is available and easy to eat quickly. "Whatever is available" food is almost always a "beckoner." It's the bag of chips that's already open, the Pop-Tart® that you don't even bother to toast, a can of cola and a candy bar from the vending machine. It seems that everything else is much more pressing than your need to stop and really think through what you're hungry for. And, yet, most naturally slim people actually do take the time to carefully decide what it is they really want to eat. Many of the naturally slim people I know are also people who do not feel compelled to constantly be on the go.

Most naturally slim people actually do take the time to carefully decide what it is they really want to eat.

For many women, there's an underlying belief that says, *I don't deserve to spend time on myself,* or *It's selfish/not Christian to spend time thinking about what I want to eat and taking the time to obtain and/or prepare it.* How much more "Christian" is it to eat in an unhealthy way? Isn't it pretty selfish to be constantly obsessed with food and dieting, even if you are getting a lot done for other people? Consider how learning to eat in the manner that you were created to eat might be okay with God. If it takes a little time and a little "selfishness" now, it pays off later with how very little you have to think about it once you're back in the groove of naturally responding to your hunger and personal food preferences.

- What do you long for, what do you crave, that is not food and for which you're using eating as a substitute?

Most women who try to assuage their cravings in life with food are longing for change in their relationships, especially in terms of affection, acceptance, and unconditional love. I get a tense uncomfortable feeling when I think back to how deeply and for how many years I longed for a genuinely affectionate relationship with a man. And for years, eating sweets and starches was my substitute for that affection. Even now, because my husband and I work opposite shifts, I sometimes long for affection in the evenings when I'm home alone and he's at work, and my emotional habit is to think of cookies, chocolate cream pies, and ice cream. But those foods distract me only briefly from the longing. They don't satisfy it at all.

Women in Weight of Grace groups have mentioned longing for respect from their children, wanting to receive affection from their husbands that doesn't always have to lead to sex, desiring to have a nicer home in which to live or new furniture or chic clothes, wishing for a life that has fewer demands or for a different job or for the financial ability to stay home instead of working outside the home. One woman longed for the baby she aborted and kept trying to fill the void with more and more food.

The answer is not in getting all that we crave, but in letting God show us what we already have.

Of course, the food never gets you what you long for, but we tend not to think this through. We just eat and distract ourselves from our desires or give ourselves a little consolation through a "treat" since we can't have what we really want. The consolation bites us back though when we end up hating ourselves for overeating and being "fat" – and we still don't have what we long for. The answer is not in getting all that we crave, but in letting God show us what we already have. Our concentration on our desires blinds us to the ways God has already provided. When we turn to him and ask him to show us how he is meeting our needs and even our desires *in his way*, we find the fulfillment that we can never provide for ourselves through food or even through getting what we want.

- What are some of the non-food ways you can "feed" yourself and add satisfaction to your life?

So, if eating isn't going to get it for us, what are some of the ways to find emotional and sensual satisfaction without turning to food? As was mentioned above, turning to God with our longings is the very first step. Then, being open to see how he is providing for us in ways we may not expect is the next step.

If you long for respect from your children or parents, look for how God is providing you with respect from your Christian family. Or, perhaps, God is helping you learn that respect is not a prerequisite to happiness. Ask him why you feel such a strong need for respect. See if there is a deeply held belief that is not valid in light of Scripture, such as *I must have respect in order to feel worthy.* As mentioned in a previous chapter, my cravings for affection were greatly relieved when I was willing to see how God was providing me with affection through my friends and co-workers rather than through a boyfriend. The affection I craved was in a different package than I thought I needed, but when I saw all the forms of affection that were actually there, the one that wasn't there didn't matter as much. This is not to say I never again longed for an affectionate relationship with a man. But, when the longing became painful again, I was better equipped to get past the pain because of the practice of prayerfully thinking through the provisions God had already made for me.

Not only do we need to be open to the creative ways God is providing for us, we also need to become aware of the myriad ways he brings joy and satisfaction to our lives and how these "feed" us. For people who diet and/or overeat, there is a tendency to try to get most of one's pleasure in life from food, thus missing out on the pleasures present in a variety of experiences. It's easy to get into ruts or to stay in a familiar box of routine activities and not notice all that's wonderful and fulfilling in one's life. We can ignore the numerous ways emotional and sensual satisfaction is available. Do you ever go to art galleries – or auto races? There are certain pieces of art that literally give me goose bumps when I stop to take them in. And the thrill of fast cars and someone crossing a finish line can provide a rush that might even compete with chocolate!

I love those old Doris Day/Rock Hudson movies, and there's a scene in one that reminds me of how we can overlook the everyday pleasures that are around us. Rock Hudson's character erroneously believed his death from some rare disease was imminent, and he confided this to his friend, played by Tony Randall. While pondering the brevity of life, Tony realized he had taken a lot for granted and started running his hand over a coffee table, caressing the wood and commenting on how cool and smooth it felt and how he had failed to appreciate such experiences enough.

As silly as it sounds to get a charge out of a table, it's true that smooth wood does feel good. There are all sorts of sensual pleasures we don't appreciate or allow to "fill" us. Daffodils come in many beautiful shapes and colors and smell fabulous. Birds and squirrels in the front yard are fun to watch. Sheets feel and smell wonderful when you first take them out of the dryer. A band playing a John Phillip Sousa march can make your heart swell, and a good R&B singer can take your emotions all over the map. Colors, textures, fragrances, melodies are all experienced through our senses. Remember the John Denver song, "You Fill up My Senses"? God has provided us with a world full of legitimate sensual delights.

I have found that my appreciation of the sights, sounds, smells, and textures in my life reduces my desire to try to get most of my pleasure from eating. Also, fully savoring the taste of the food I eat means finding satisfaction with smaller amounts of food. Our physical hunger is not the only hunger we have, but it can, unfortunately, often be the only hunger we feed.

Our physical hunger is not the only hunger we have, but it can, unfortunately, often be the only hunger we feed.

10 WHY DIETS DON'T WORK, ESPECIALLY FOR CHRISTIANS

Each January the diet ads are everywhere – TV, magazines, radio – because the companies that offer diet programs are hoping to cash in on women's New Year's resolutions to really try this year to lose that weight and keep it off this time. When I see these ads, I feel very sad and also very angry. Starting at age 12, dieting became for me a source of great pain, shame, and hopelessness. Yes, I've often succeeded at dieting. But for every success, there was the corresponding failure – usually regaining all the weight I'd lost and often gaining even more. Every time I hear a friend or co-worker talk about the latest diet she's on, I cringe. I feel sure, especially if the dieter is a Christian who truly seeks God's will, that the new diet may "work" for a while, but there's heartache ahead. Why am I so sure? Not just because of my own experience and that of hundreds of other women who have gained back as much weight or more than they lost from dieting, but also because of what the Bible says about legalism and its affect on all people – and especially on Christians.

To start to see why diets are especially unsuccessful for Christians, let's look at a passage from Colossians. See if parts of it sound really familiar to you.

> *Since you died with Christ to the basic principles of this world, why, as though you still belonged to it, do you submit to its rules: "Do not handle! Do not taste! Do not touch!"? These are all destined to perish with use, because they are based on human commands and teachings. Such regulations indeed have an appearance of wisdom, with their self-imposed worship, their false humility and their harsh treatment of the body, but they lack any value in restraining sensual indulgence.* Colossians 2:20-23

Remind you of anything? How well I remember the lecturer at a diet program class I attended telling us to avoid having certain foods in our homes, to avoid even touching or seeing these foods. Rules, rules, rules. Diets, even those that are called "lifestyle changes" rather than "diets," consist of varying amounts of rules by which the dieter is to regulate herself. But look at how that passage in Colossians ends. "Such regulations...*lack any value in restraining sensual indulgence*" (v. 23, emphasis mine). The rules don't work! But why? In this chapter, we are going to explore why diets do not work, especially for Christians. In order to understand why this is, we will look at an overview of the concept of legalism, an often subtle and insidious opponent to our walk with God and to living in dependence upon him.[1]

We are going to look at three main concepts involved in legalism: "the Law," "religious legalism," and "standards." First, when referring to "the Law," this means all the rules and regulations that are spelled out in the Old Testament. In Romans 7:12, the apostle Paul tells us that the laws of the Old Testament are "holy, righteous, and good." Paul also says of the Law that its purpose was to point us to Christ: "So the law was put in charge to lead us to Christ..." (Galatians 3:24a). How did the Law lead us to Christ? By proving to us that we

"Such regulations ...lack any value in restraining sensual indulgence."

were incapable of keeping it and thus incapable of living up to God's holy standards. Therefore, the Law brought us to the realization that we were in desperate need of a Savior. No one (but Jesus) has ever been able to totally fulfill all the requirements God laid out for a holy life. Therefore, no one has ever been able, through keeping the Law, to achieve the righteousness that would allow him or her to live in union with a holy God. Without special intervention on God's part – without the sacrificial death and miraculous resurrection of Christ – we cannot achieve holiness and righteousness. We could not do this on our own, no matter how hard we tried to follow all the rules. The rules were right, but we went wrong. The rules actually pointed out to us how far afield we were from holiness. And that is good, because it creates in us an awareness of our need for Jesus.

With the advent of Jesus Christ – in light of his atoning death that, through faith, enables us to enjoy his righteousness and an eternal union with God – how are we then to view the Law, the Old Testament rules and regulations? First, we can see that the Law is an outline of how life was intended to be lived. The Law provides us with wisdom and understanding about the parameters of life as God created it. (See Deuteronomy 4:5-8.) We realize that God never intended for us to worship anyone or anything other than him. We understand that God made us in such a way that it is healthy for us to engage in sex only within the confines of marriage, that lying to one another and stealing from one another is harmful to all involved, that getting rest on a regular basis and stopping to worship God is absolutely necessary to our well-being, along with many other guidelines for living. As Bill Gillham says, the Bible is the "manufacturer's handbook" for how people were designed to run smoothly.[2]

In looking at the Old Testament dietary laws from a New Testament perspective, we see that Jesus himself rescinded them. See Mark 7:18-19 and Acts 11:7-9. And, all of the sacrificial laws are completely fulfilled by the "once and for all" sacrifice of Jesus Christ on the cross. See Colossians 2:13-14 and Hebrews 10:1-12. All of the moral and ethical laws are totally fulfilled by Christ living in us and having written his laws on our hearts by means of the Holy Spirit. See Galatians 2:20 as well as Hebrews 8:10 and 10:14-16.

For the believer, the Law gives us understanding about life and is fulfilled, summed up, and lived out by and through Jesus Christ.

So, to summarize this first concept regarding legalism, "the Law": For the believer, the Law gives us understanding about life and is fulfilled, summed up, and lived out by and through Jesus Christ.

In turning to the second concept, "religious legalism," we see in 1 Timothy 1:8 that the Law can be used improperly. The improper use of law is religious legalism. Religious legalism occurs when a person believes that acceptance by God is available only through keeping the Law. This makes performance the basis of obtaining God's acceptance rather than the finished work of Jesus Christ on the cross. Religious legalism puts the emphasis on self-effort and promotes the belief that man actually can fulfill God's righteous standards. The Pharisees of Jesus' day engaged in religious legalism. They even added their own laws to the Law of God in order to make sure they would stay well within the parameters of the Law. As Jesus pointed out, though, they failed to actually keep the Law because their hearts were not right. They appeared compliant on the outside, but they were still corrupt on the inside. Not only that, but also they had so much faith in their adherence to the Law that many of them totally missed the fact that they needed a Savior – even though he was standing right in front of them!

What happens with religious legalism and those who practice it is, because no one can possibly live up to God's Law, they have to contort the laws to fit what they *can* fulfill. Religious legalists emphasize the rules they are able to keep and turn a blind eye to others that they fail to keep. Look at the Sermon on the Mount in Matthew 5. When Jesus said, "You have heard that it was said..., but I tell you...," he was telling the religious legalists that they were keeping only part of the Law and not all of it. Haven't you known someone who, for religious reasons, refused to go to movies but thought nothing of watching television or renting DVD's? This is an example of how religious legalism engenders inconsistent behavior and hypocrisy.

When you read the Bible as a set of "oughts" and "shoulds," you get caught up in trying harder and harder to do all those "oughts" and "shoulds." Eventually, you either fail and give up completely by leaving what you perceive to be "the faith" or you have emotional problems from the stress of trying to live the Christian life in your own strength. This is exactly what happened to me when I was in my early twenties. I tried desperately to adhere to all the "laws" I felt I had to keep in order to be a "good Christian." I couldn't do it. I collapsed. But, before I came to the end of myself, I experienced all of the typical symptoms of legalism: panic attacks, bitterness, workaholism, depression, resentment, and being hyper-critical.

I tried desperately to adhere to all the "laws" I felt I had to keep in order to be a "good Christian." I couldn't do it.

Finally, to understand legalism, it is important to examine a third concept, "standards." Standards are the rules people have for themselves that may or may not be based on Scripture. These rules are what people feel they *must* do in order to gain acceptance from others, God, or just from themselves. Standards are usually "caught" from our families, the culture, peers, authority figures, the media, and religious training. We are often told, either directly or tacitly, that when we do "thus and so," we will be thought of as a "good" person. The basic belief is: *I must be accepted and approved of by others in order to feel good about myself; therefore, I must do "this."* A prime example of standards is how women believe they must be reed thin in order to be acceptable to themselves and others. Many women even feel this is one of God's standards.

Symptoms of legalism – either the religious kind or the kind that's based on keeping one's own standards – include smugness (*I keep my standards but others don't.*); high expectations of others (*If I have to, so why don't they have to keep this standard too?*); being critical of others (*They really don't have very high standards, do they?*); a low tolerance of people making mistakes (*He should have been able to keep that standard!*); fear of failure (*I'll hate myself if I fail at keeping this standard.*); and self-punishing behaviors (*I didn't keep that standard, so I deserve to eat a ton and make myself fat.*). These symptoms are very often evident in women who are on diets.

Even for those who become convinced that legalism is negative and not productive (even counterproductive), it is difficult for them to let go of their standards because they believe their legalism is what's keeping them in line, keeping them from going off the deep end and getting totally out of control. But just the opposite is true. Not only do laws and

It is difficult for them to let go of their standards because they believe their legalism is what's keeping them in line.

rules "lack any value in restraining sensual indulgence," as Colossians 2:23b says, but also they actually lead us to sin more, not less. As we saw in the last chapter, according to Romans 7:8-9, there's nothing like a "Do Not Walk on the Grass" sign to arouse a strong desire in us to tromp on that grass! As Paul said, "when the commandment came, sin sprang to life..." (Romans 7:9), and "the power of sin is the law" (1 Corinthians 15:56b). Think about how totally luscious everyday foods such as butter and mayonnaise seem when you're on a diet that forbids or limits those foods.

So, if rules, laws, and standards don't enable us to live a godly, moderate life, what does? Read Galatians 3:3, 5, 10-14 and 5:16-25. The alternative to legalism is living life "in the Spirit," living in constant and total dependence upon the indwelling Christ, humbly asking him to guide us and being confident that he will and does. The emphasis at the beginning of this book on understanding one's new identity in Christ as a "new creation" was to serve as the underpinning for grasping why we can trust that the Holy Spirit is at work in us to guide us into right behavior. We do not need to constantly crack the whip and toe the line in order to make sure we live as we "ought." Instead, we need to humbly rely upon God and his work within our lives. We can accept that he has given us a new heart, that we are motivated from within to be holy and moderate. We can follow the promptings of the Spirit, who directs us, for example, to pause and ask God for help in figuring out why we want to eat even when we're not physically hungry. As Galatians 5:16 (AMP) tells us, "...walk and live habitually in the (Holy) Spirit – responsive to and controlled and guided by the Spirit; then you will certainly not gratify the cravings and desires of the flesh – of human nature without God." "Where the Spirit of the Lord is, *there* is freedom" (2 Corinthians 3:17b, emphasis mine).

So, why don't diets work, *especially for Christians*? Because diets are a form of legalism, and legalism is the polar opposite of how we, as new creations in Christ, are designed to live our lives. When we try to follow a set of rules and regulations, we cut out the Holy Spirit and we engage in legalistic self-effort. Women who struggle with overeating and overweight have prayed and prayed that God would enable them to stick to their diets. But God doesn't answer their prayers as they'd like because he wants us to *fail* at *self*-effort. He wants us to realize that the only way to live life as he designed it is to live in constant communication with and dependence upon *him*. He didn't design you to control your eating through rules. He created you to respond to inner urgings – not only physical, but also spiritual – which perfectly and individually direct you far better than any one-size-fits-all diet program possibly can.

The alternative to legalism is living life "in the Spirit," living in constant and total dependence upon the indwelling Christ.

Reflection

1. In what areas of your life do you currently have discipline and why do you think you have it in those areas?

2. What are some of the reasons you are motivated to "do right" (avoid sin, do loving acts, pursue a relationship with God, treat others with kindness, etc.)?

3. What would happen if you never, ever dieted again? What would happen if you continued to diet?

What Others Have Experienced

*   In what areas of your life do you currently have discipline and why do you think you have it in those areas?

Many of the women in Weight of Grace small groups give a knee-jerk answer to this questions, saying, "I don't have any discipline," which indicates that they are focusing almost totally on their eating and dieting and that they are failing to see the bigger picture of their life as a whole. Among those same women, none fails to brush her teeth regularly, bathe regularly, do laundry as it is needed, pick the kids up after school and other events, get the shopping done so that there's enough food in the house, and comb or brush her hair nearly every day. Most women take these activities for granted and don't realize they are part of the discipline in their lives.

Now, are people disciplined in the areas of their hygiene and taking care of the needs of their families because there is a set of rules that says they must do so? Usually not. Usually,

They are focusing almost totally on their eating and dieting and failing to see the bigger picture of their life as a whole.

people are motivated to brush their teeth and groom their hair regularly because they enjoy how it feels when they do and they dread the consequences of not doing so. They like feeling clean and don't like feeling grungy. And most people are motivated to engage in activities that meet the needs of family members because of their love and loyalty, wanting to do what's best for people who count on them for nurture and care.

The truth of the matter is that if rules were in place regarding the routine "disciplines" of our lives, we would probably resent them. As long as my husband doesn't tell me he expects me to pack his lunch each day, it's a joy and a gift to get to do so. I can well imagine that I'd frequently find excuses to avoid making his lunch if I knew he believed it to be my "duty." If there were monitors who checked our teeth every day for cleanliness, don't you know we'd find ways to cheat and bluff?! It's the same with trying to motivate ourselves to "eat right." As long as the rules say we ought to, who wants to? And this doesn't even take into account that our motivations for wanting to lose weight are based on less than godly principles and, therefore, create inner conflict over whether we really "ought" to be "thin."

As long as the rules say we ought to, who wants to?

Now that I no longer try to use rules and regulations to keep my eating in line, I'm as motivated to avoid feeling overly full as I'm motivated to keep my teeth clean. I don't like the way it feels when I'm overstuffed. I like how I feel when I've eaten just the right amount of food to satisfy my hunger. I feel energized and content when I've eaten to that "just right" point. I feel sluggish and bloated when I overeat. Since I know I can eat whatever I want the next time I get hungry, why overeat now? There's no diet around the corner that motivates me to "eat now for tomorrow we diet." There are so many activities other than eating that I want to do. When the rules said I couldn't eat, that was all I wanted to do. Now that there are no rules and I can eat whenever I want and whatever I want, I have the freedom to assess what I really do *want* to do, and I don't want to overeat. It just doesn't feel good. And that's evidence of my return to the "real me," the new creation in Christ who allows the Holy Spirit to direct her.

- What are some of the reasons you are motivated to "do right"?

There are times we are faced with rudeness and we choose not to react in kind. There are times when we are very tired and we choose to help a friend with her garage sale anyway. There are times when we really want to spend time praying or reading the Scripture and don't even think of turning on the TV. What gives us that "umph" to do what is right, especially when doing right is to some degree difficult or inconvenient?

There are two basic categories of motivators for all the "good" that we as Christians do. One motivator is self-centered, doing what is right because it will somehow get us what we want. Many of our "good deeds" are done for very selfish reasons. (In fact, given the fallen condition of our souls without Christ, all good deeds done by those who do not believe in Christ are done, ultimately, for selfish reasons.) This is where doing good because the "rules" say you should can come in. There is a personal satisfaction we can enjoy when we "do as we ought" or follow a rule. Of course, there can also be other rewards of various types and sizes for "doing good": the appreciation of a recipient, the smugness of knowing we're better than others, the recognition of those who notice our not-so-random acts of kindness. Christians are not exempt from this form of motivation. When we as Christians act out of the flesh, even when we do "good," the motivation is always selfish.

On the other hand, for new creations in Christ, the greatest motivators in the universe are within us, the Holy Spirit and the love Christ puts in our hearts (John 14:16; 2 Corinthians 5:14). Because God indwells us and has changed our hearts, it is indeed our nature to act in godly ways. When we turn to God for his power to motivate our behaviors, we act in ways that are Christ-like. Why should our eating be any different than other areas of our lives? The Holy Spirit is at work in us to make us more and more like Christ in *every* area of our lives.

For new creations in Christ, the greatest motivators in the universe are within us, the Holy Spirit and the love Christ puts in our hearts.

- What would happen if you never, ever dieted again? What would happen if you continued to diet?

There are usually two distinct camps when it comes to how Weight of Grace small group participants answer this question: those who are terrified and those who are tired. The terrified ones are those who say they will experience extremely negative consequences if they give up dieting. They expect to become "blimps," to start eating and never, ever stop. They feel they are facing the death of a dream, of a goal for which they have striven for years. One woman answered, "I'll never weigh what I want to weigh." When I asked her if in all the 20 years she'd been dieting she had ever weighed what she wanted to weigh, she said she had once, but that lasted only a few months and was one of the most stressful times of her life. Almost all that women feel they'd be giving up by not dieting they never achieve by dieting anyway – and certainly for no significant period of time. At some point, such dreams and goals need to be recognized for what they are, fantasies.

Another answer that came from the "terrified" camp was so very telling: "I'd have to accept myself whether other people do or not." Yes, as long as you're dieting, you can tell yourself you're going to get "better," and you can accept yourself later. And you can believe that others will accept you later too, so it doesn't matter that they don't accept you now. Not dieting does mean going ahead and accepting how you look right now, and others who have minds polluted by this world may not accept you at this point. Not dieting also means putting faith in God and in *his* assessment of you, which is not dependent on your size. It means you get to exercise faith that God will enable you to be your best self, your true self, regardless of whether that person looks the way the culture considers ideal.

Not dieting means putting faith in God and in his assessment of you, which is not dependent on your size.

The small group participants who are in the "tired" camp are the ones who see the end to dieting as the beginning of freedom and rest. They answer this question with comments such as, "I'll have more peace of mind," or "I won't think about food so much and I'll have less guilt." They've dieted a long time with not much to show for it but self-condemnation and two or three wardrobes to match their constantly changing size. Many times, those in the "tired" camp are women who have had some experience with the grace of God and release from legalism in other areas of their lives. They just haven't before seen grace applied to eating and weight. So, it starts clicking with them. One of the best ways to prime yourself for accepting that dieting doesn't work is to expose yourself to God's grace. Prayerfully read the book of Galatians and ask God to show you how this applies to you in areas where you're still trying to "live up to" standards and rules. There are numerous books available that have "grace" in the title or with grace as the theme. A few of my favorites are *Grace Walk* by Steve McVey, *Grace Works* by Dudley Hall, and *Tired of Trying to Measure Up* by Jeff Van Vonderen. There are also many books that address how to live in the power of the Spirit, rather than by keeping rules. I especially like *Lifetime Guarantee* by Bill Gillham and the *Be Transformed* workbook by Scope Ministries International.

This question of what would happen if you never dieted again is often the "make it or break it" question for members of Weight of Grace small groups. If they really can't accept the diets-don't-work thinking, then this material is just not helpful to them. My prayer is always that women will catch the vision of how God desires to work in their lives to allow them to be themselves, their true selves, which means quite naturally eating in moderation after a transition time of a few months to a couple of years of learning what that feels like for them.

Homework

1. Read the transcript of Malcolm Smith's message, "Self-Disciplined Religion," provided with permission in Addendum Two, starting on page 255. The title is a little misleading – that's what Mr. Smith is preaching *against*. Highlight those parts of the transcript with which you particularly identify.

2. Complete the following study.

LEGALISM AND DIETING

1. Look up the following verses and, in your own words, write what each of the verses says about what motivates Christians to act in a godly manner.

   a) Romans 2:4 _____

   _____

   b) 1 Corinthians 6:12 _____

   _____

   c) 2 Corinthians 5:14 (see the NASB or Amplified translations) _____

   _____

   d) Galatians 5:16 _____

   _____

   (continued)

---

2. Read the following summary of what was said in other Weight of Grace small group discussions about what motivates women to be self-controlled.

   a) It was noticed that we all have discipline in several areas, such as work, brushing our teeth regularly, following traffic laws, doing laundry, pursuing college degrees and continuing education, etc. The reasons for having this discipline varied. The following are some reasons given by group members:

      • Recognizing what the consequences will be if we don't follow through.
      • Having a desire to "work as unto the Lord."
      • Wanting to achieve our goals (in education, career, salary, etc.).
      • Having a love for others and wanting to be conscientious for their sakes.
      • The Holy Spirit motivating us to "die to self."

   These are all valid reasons for doing "what is right" and can apply to why we would do what is right for ourselves in terms of our eating for the right reasons.

   b) In discussing what would keep us from being totally out of control if we gave up dieting forever, these were mentioned as factors that engender self-control:

      • The Holy Spirit empowers us.
      • Our new nature in Christ includes a desire to be moderate and to be conformed to Christ's image.
      • When we don't have a bunch of rules, then we don't have to keep fighting the urge to break them all the time.
      • Knowing we can have whatever we want whenever we want it means we don't have to have it all now.
      • We don't really want to feel so uncomfortable after eating.
      • We can allow ourselves to feel our emotions and communicate with God about them so that eating is not the way we deal with them.

3. Look over the list in #2a of five reasons we have discipline. For each reason listed, give an example from your own life when you have had discipline for that reason.

   _____

   _____

   _____

   _____

4. Look over the list in #2b of six factors that facilitate self-control. For each one, give an example of a situation in your own life where that reason could apply or has applied.

   _____

   _____

   _____

   _____

BEFORE YOU GO ON TO THE NEXT CHAPTER

Homework Follow-up

1. What stood out to you in the transcript of Malcolm Smith's message? With what did you identify and how did you see it relate to dieting and overeating?

2. Is there already evidence of self-control in your life? Does this give you hope regarding your eating?

Comments on the Homework

- With what did you identify in the transcript and how does it relate to dieting/overeating?

When we try to control our lives through our own efforts – through the flesh, no matter how "godly" our actions may appear – we ultimately fail.

I especially like the opening of Malcolm Smith's message because Titus 2:11-12 is the passage I use in Weight of Grace Ministries literature to summarize my understanding of God's solution to overeating. It is the grace of God – the unmerited gift of salvation and our ongoing transformation into the likeness of Christ through the power of the indwelling Holy Spirit – that teaches us, instructs us, to live sensibly! When we look to the Holy Spirit to guide us, he really does do that. When we try to control our lives through our own efforts – through the flesh, no matter how "godly" our actions may appear – we ultimately fail. And we miss the true joy and victory of what it means to be a new creation in Christ and to have an intimate, dependent relationship with God.

Many of the women who have read the transcript of Malcolm Smith's message immediately pick up on his reference to dieting and how it arouses in us the desire to break the diet, as well as fails to provide a workable way to live apart from the diet. But many are also struck by Mr. Smith's attacks on the "religious." We are so often taught that being "spiritual" actually consists of gritting our teeth and following the rules of whatever sect or denomination we're a member. Or we are told that our gratitude to Christ for our salvation should be an adequate motivator to engage in right behavior. Personal willpower and even overwhelming gratitude are not sufficient to enable us to live godly lives. It takes God to be godly. Apart from reliance upon the Holy Spirit, try as we might, we cannot live Christ-like lives.

Many women have tremendous difficulty with a conflict they feel over the religious "oughts" and "shoulds" they have been taught, sometimes since early childhood, and the challenge to take the perspective that these very rules may be the enemy that's defeating their Christian walk. My approach in addressing this is to suggest that women give this concept of "walking in the Spirit" a three- or four-month trial. As a result, women discover that they live up to many of their long-held standards because they are just like the hippies-getting-hair-cuts example in Mr. Smith's message. God has no objection to certain standards. It's what's going on in the heart that matters. If our motivation is to maintain rules out of our own efforts to prove to ourselves or to God that we're "good enough," this will not be permitted to succeed. It's contrary to God's design for Christians. If, however, we ask God to direct our steps and empower our behavior, we may end up looking as though we're being very disciplined and obeying rules when we're actually "walking in the Spirit."

An example of religious rules that can be passed off as "godly" is found in how some church groups dictate, blatantly or tacitly, how women should dress. One church I visited occasionally over the course of several years had an unwritten, but very well-understood rule that all the women wear the very modest, loose-fitting, floral print "Laura Ashley"-type jumpers and dresses. The generally accepted understanding was that any article of clothing that clung in any way to one's figure was just forcing the men in the church to lust and, therefore, to sin. One of the women I knew in this church got fed up with the pressure to conform to the church's "dress code" and started dressing in ways that would assure disapproval from fellow church members. In fact, she seemed to be working very hard at looking downright sex-pot-ish. It was no surprise that in short order she felt criticized and unwanted at this church. She left that congregation about the same time that she started taking classes elsewhere on new identity in Christ and the Spirit-filled life. A few months later, this same woman was wearing all her loose-fitting clothes again, saying that she just didn't feel comfortable in that "tight-fitting stuff" anymore. The rule about clothing had been lifted. The freedom had been granted. And she went back to what was comfortable, as well as less provocative, but not because the rules told her to do so.

Getting out from under the rules is only a part of the solution to legalism and dieting, but it is not at all enough. The more important part of the solution is relying upon the Holy Spirit and believing in who you are at the core of your being as a new creation in Christ. It is necessary to go ahead and step out in faith, and then you will see that God provides you with the *grace* to live sensibly and righteously.

If our motivation is to maintain rules out of our own efforts to prove to ourselves or to God that we're "good enough," this will not be permitted to succeed. It's contrary to God's design for Christians.

- Is there already evidence of self-control in your life? Does this give you hope regarding your eating?

By the time women get this far in their Weight of Grace small group experience, many of them are already experimenting with letting go of diets and looking to those inward physical signals and promptings of the Spirit that enable them to eat in accordance with physical hunger instead of in response to their emotions and/or need to be "fat." However, others are still struggling with whether the spiritual fruit of self-control will manifest itself regarding their eating. For these women, I suggest that they make an assessment of their overall Christian experience and recognize that God is already at work in many aspects of their lives, with dieting and eating constituting only a fraction of the areas in which God is transforming them into the image of his Son. Upon reflection, many women realize that they have had victories already thanks to the work of the Holy Spirit within them. They tell of how they sought God's help in controlling their tongues, especially with children or husbands, and saw dramatic success and change. Or they realize that God had enabled them to manage their money and/or time better as they've matured in their relationship with him.

A friend who doesn't have a struggle with food or weight gain spent years trying to set up rules and self-punishments so that she would arrive at work and appointments on time. It was when she finally gave up on her own will power and threw herself on the mercy of God that she started arriving on time at work and appointments more and more often. It is several years later now, and she'd never think of being late for work. She's practically forgotten what a struggle that once was. Another friend could never seem to keep her apartment clean or in any way orderly. This created a problem when she wanted to have people over for a visit. She could invite only those friends she knew would overlook the mess and pick their way through the clutter in order to sit down or walk across a room. She looked to God to change this habit and gradually became more and more tidy until she found she was actually uncomfortable when her apartment reached a certain level of disarray.

You don't need a diet to keep yourself in line. In fact, that diet is sabotaging not only your ability to eat moderately, but also your relationship with God.

Look at some of the areas of life that the Bible says are most important – demonstrating love through action, forgiveness, returning good for evil, praying, giving, seeking opportunities to get to know God better, sharing the Gospel with unbelievers. It is very likely that you have gradually made progress is several of these areas. This is because the Holy Spirit indwells you and you have the new heart of a new creation in Christ. If God is at work in you to change you in these areas, why wouldn't he also work in the area of eating? You don't need a diet to keep yourself in line. In fact, that diet is sabotaging not only your ability to eat moderately, but also your relationship with God. This is why God doesn't let Christians succeed at dieting. Succeeding at diets is failing at trusting in him.

11 SQUEEZING INTO THE MOLD

I can remember that, at age 12, I loathed myself because I wasn't thin. And I kept on loathing myself for being "fat" until I was 31, when I started reading some books and articles about how women are objectified in our culture and base their value upon their appearance. A passage of Scripture that I had previously memorized suddenly came to life for me regarding my own self-image. In Romans 12:2, there is an interesting word that seems to apply only too well to what our culture does to women.

> *Do not* **be conformed** *to this world—this age, fashioned after and adapted to its external, superficial customs.* (AMP, emphasis mine)

As was mentioned briefly in Chapters 4 and 7, the word translated here as "be conformed" communicates the idea of being pressed or squeezed into a mold.[1] My own paraphrase of the beginning of Romans 12:2 is: "Do not let yourself get squeezed into the shape this world wants you to be in." What our culture is trying to do to women is to *squeeze* them into an unrealistic, uniform ideal of thinness. I call this the "thinness gospel." This gospel proclaims that if you're thin, you're happy, men want you, you'll marry a handsome man, you can wear any clothes you want and look good in them, you're universally admired, people will look up to you, and on and on and on. This message is so prevalent in our culture that most women don't even question it. The need to be thin, the virtue of being thin, is a given. It is carried right over into the Christian subculture as if it were God's idea to begin with.

What our culture is trying to do to women is to squeeze them into an unrealistic, uniform ideal of thinness.

But, who is it that runs this "world" that is putting the squeeze on women? John 12:31 tells us that Satan is the "prince of this world," and we know that his desire is to "steal and kill and destroy" (John 10:10). Of course, Satan wants to find ways of making us hate ourselves, and he wants to provide ways to distract us from the important concerns of life by getting us to focus on the superficial. If he can set a standard and get all of us to believe that standard is right and good and achievable, knowing full well it's outside the reach of 99 percent of us, wouldn't that fit in well with his destructive plans? And all the better if he can convince Christians his standard is actually godly!

What is very interesting to note is that the standard that reigns today has not always been *the* standard and, in fact, is not a universally held standard throughout the world even now. One of my favorite novels is *Jane Eyre*. In it there is a passage in which Jane, a very slim and small woman, bemoans the fact that she is not "plump" like the beautiful Blanche, a rival for the affection of the man Jane loves. Of course, today, the tables would be completely turned and Blanche would be envying Jane. Look at art books that show nudes painted by Rubens or Renoir. For these artists of another era, the ideal woman was round, curvy, and what our Western culture would now call "fat." As recently as the 1940s and 1950s, Americans idolized women like Marilyn Monroe, Maureen O'Hara, Jane Mansfield, and Jane Russell, all of whom would have to lose weight to be considered sex symbols today.

Not only have standards for beauty changed with time, but also the standard of "thin equals beautiful" is not universally held in our day either. Today in many Third World and developing countries, the larger the woman, the more beautiful she is considered to be. For those who have little, having some fat on one's body is associated with wealth and affluence. A Weight of Grace small group participant, who is of Anglo-Saxon descent, said her Hispanic husband was in absolute dread of her losing weight. He was reared in Central America and highly valued his wife's full, round figure.

Values regarding body size and appearance are culturally determined, not set by God.

Values regarding body size and appearance are culturally determined, not set by God. What we regard as beauty changes constantly. The one constant is that, in any given culture, what is valued is usually what most of the people cannot achieve. This is evidence of how the standards of "the world" are manipulated by Satan. In contrast, God's value system is not based on surface appearance. According to passages such as 1 Samuel 16:7 and 1 Peter 3:3-4, God values a person's inner motivations, his or her heart.

First, Satan tries to get Christians to believe in the thinness gospel that lures us into accepting a one-size-fits-all standard instead of reveling in the infinite variety of God's creations. Then, Satan manages to throw us into greater turmoil by creating conflicting messages about thinness and food within the Christian subculture. On the one hand, we believe that being/staying thin is a sign of godliness. But, on the other hand, we as "good Christian women" are not supposed to be overly tempting to men, right? It's hard to be thin in a culture that calls thin sexy and, at the same time, also remain less than alluring. And isn't food a way of expressing love and a focal point for many of our Christian gatherings and "fellowship"? So we are constantly around it, preparing it, giving it to others to show we care for them. It's hard to be the only one who doesn't get to have any of all that "love" we're dishing out. The conflicting messages are not only within the Christian subculture. Just look at the cover of most women's magazines. On the same glossy page is a woman who lost has over 100 pounds on a diet right next to a headline about a new recipe for red velvet cake.

It's difficult to sort it all out. One way to cope is to just bail out and be "fat." Then you don't have to deal with the potential of being a temptress or of being proud about how you look. Yes, some may think you're a "glutton," but isn't that better than being a "Jezebel"? Being fat keeps you out of trouble. In fact, being fat is actually more godly than being thin, right?

Neither being fat nor being thin is, in and of itself, godly.

Wrong. Neither being fat nor being thin is, in and of itself, godly. Being the person you were created to be, a new creation in Christ, motivated by the Holy Spirit, in constant communication with God about every aspect of your life, staying open to his guidance and promptings – that's godly. Being that person may result in having looks that get praise in our culture – or in having looks that would only get praise in another culture or in another time. Have you adopted the standards of this world? Have you done so without really even analyzing where you got your ideas about what's beautiful and what's not? Who and/or what has defined beauty for you and how do you determine if someone is truly beautiful?

If you find you have adopted the "pattern of this world," if you're brainwashed, so to speak, how can you change the way you perceive and feel about what is attractive or not? Isn't it automatic to feel repulsed by "fat" and attracted to "thin"? Let's look at Romans 12:2 again, the entire verse this time:

*Do not conform any longer to the pattern of this world, but **be
transformed by the renewing of your mind**. Then you will be able to test
and approve what God's will is—his good, pleasing and perfect will.*
(emphasis mine)

The way we change – the way we are transformed out of the mold and into God's
viewpoint – is through the renewing of the mind. The fact that we are new creations in
Christ means that we have the potential to experience the "mind of Christ" (1 Corinthians
2:16). The indwelling Holy Spirit is working from within to make us more and more like
Jesus (Romans 8:29). As we prayerfully think through what we believe and ask God to
show us his perspective, he does so through his Word, through that inner "still, small
voice," and through his Body, the church. (But it's important to realize that many within the
church have totally accepted the worldly view of thinness. Nevertheless, God leads us to
those within his Body who will join us in resisting the unbiblical messages of this world.)

I remember well the first time I decided to accept the fact that, no matter what size I
was, I was beautiful and that the cultural standards did not define my beauty, God did. I
was much larger at that time than I had previously believed to be acceptable, and I was
pretty sure I was going to get larger because I had just given up all dieting. Then, shortly
after making this decision, I started "keeping company" with a man who made it clear to
me that I was larger than any women he'd ever been interested in before. (This man didn't
ever call our relationship "dating," but we spent quite a bit of time together.) He was fairly
slim at the time, having just lost weight through dieting, and he was very conscious of the
fact that I wasn't dieting and, in his mind, badly needed to. On one occasion when this man
made a comment that seemed to say, "You're the largest woman I've ever hung out with," I
believe it was God who put it in my mind that I was also the most beautiful, intelligent, and
interesting woman he'd ever hung out with! Making the decision to allow God to give us
his mindset opens the door to totally changing how we view ourselves and our culture's
standards.

But it isn't a one-time decision. That's why I said I remember the *first* time I made the
decision. With a culture that screams at you that you need to be thin, thin, thin, it's
sometimes necessary to decide daily – or several times each day – to resist the world's lies.
There are many days when, at some point during the day, I think to myself, *You really are
getting fat*, or *You sure could stand to lose about five pounds*. When I hear myself think these
thoughts, I also start to think, *Who says you're getting fat?!* and *Who are you going to lose that
five pounds for?!* Then I realize I'm being lured into "the mold" and fight back with, *I'm a
sexy, curvy girl who is an absolute piece of art!*

I get very hot under the collar over the bombardment of messages that are constantly
thrown at women saying that they just don't measure up. Oh, and all of those commercials
that come out and tell you if you'd just go on this or that diet, you could finally achieve real
happiness. Yuck! What bunk! What you'll achieve is a ton of frustration when you lose
weight for a while and then gain it all back and then some. What you'll achieve is a
temporary, self-centered lifestyle that's not only impractical, but also contrary to God's

*With a culture
that screams at
you that you need
to be thin, thin,
thin, it's some-
times necessary
to decide daily –
or several times
each day – to
resist the world's
lies.*

design. I believe the anger I feel when I encounter these cultural messages is, at least in part, the righteous wrath God feels toward the lies Satan tells women.

Yes, many of the people around us are, and may remain, strongly influenced by the "thinness gospel" that bombards them daily. Husbands, boyfriends, parents, and peers may not join you in your new perspective, but my experience is that, with time and by just living the truth, many around me – and many around other women who have rejected the thinness gospel – have gradually changed their minds.

Let me challenge you to ask God to open your eyes to the lies that have been told to you by our culture, which is fixated on thinness, and to the *real* beauty that you are in Christ.

Reflection

1. Where did you get the idea that being "thin" meant being beautiful and being "fat" meant being ugly?

2. What are the characteristics you value most about the people you love?

3. What do the people who love you value most about you?

What Others Have Experienced

- Where did you get the idea that being "thin" meant being beautiful and being "fat" meant being ugly?

I often ask women, "Who told you that you are fat?" Sometimes there are specific people who have told them they're fat, usually parents, husbands, or peers. Then I ask, "Who told *them* that you're fat?" The answer is usually, "Everyone knows that I'm fat!" Sometimes when I ask, "Who told you that you are fat?" the answer is, "I just know that I am." These answers reveal the unquestioning acceptance of a cultural standard. A similar question is, "Why do you think you need to lose weight?" For the person who has started to catch on to the idea of culturally-tied beliefs about "fat" and "thin," the answer can't be as simple as, "So I can look better." That would be too superficial. So, I often hear, "I just feel better about myself when I'm thinner." Of course, this begs the question, "Why?" Where do women get the idea that being thinner equals being better?

It is obvious that this message comes from many different aspects of our culture – television, movies, magazines, and one of the hardest ones with which to argue, the medical community. It's easy to say that the glitzy and godless "beautiful people" might not be appropriate models for us to emulate, but it's hard to argue with statistics about mortality and heart disease. Nevertheless, even the standards of the medical community are in constant flux. Some studies say being slightly under weight (according to whatever the charts call the ideal weight that year) prolongs life, and other studies show that women with a little extra fat are the ones who live the longest.

No matter what the medical community says about the value of weight loss, the fact remains that the usual way prescribed to go about that weight loss is dieting. And dieting is 1) not effective for bringing about long-term weight loss, and 2) a legalistic work of "the flesh." Is it healthy to have your weight constantly fluctuate while you lose for a while on a diet and then gain it all back (and more) when you get off of the diet? It seems reasonable that staying alert to the physical signals of hunger and finding ways of addressing emotions through prayer, rather than through eating, would result in a weight that's healthy for each individual. God created a "fearfully and wonderfully made" machine when he created the human body (Psalm 139:14). Even though we know the body will eventually run down and die, it is still able, for nearly all people, to signal its needs for food, fluid, sleep, and exercise. (There are physical disorders which can interfere with the body's natural signaling ability, but they are rare.)

Going back to the perception women have that they're "ugly," it is very difficult to convince women that the way they look would at some time or in some culture be considered absolutely fabulous and desirable. Satan's brainwashing via our culture is that effective. The truth is that the culture is fickle and that what's "in" today or "in" here is "out" somewhere else and will be "out" tomorrow.

- What do you value most about the people you love and what do they value most about you?

I've never *loved* anyone for his or her looks. I've been *attracted to* people based on their looks, but that is never what makes me love or value them as friends. In fact, I've found that

It seems reasonable that staying alert to the physical signals of hunger and finding ways of addressing emotions through prayer, rather than through eating, would result in a weight that's healthy for each individual.

the physical features my loved ones have that are departures from the cultural ideal are often very endearing. I love the wrinkles on my husband's nose. I think the bald spot on one friend's head is cute. I find the roundness of some of my girlfriends beautiful and feminine. I have a full behind that my husband loves to pat and grab. My former roommate and I both like each other's looks better when we aren't wearing makeup.

When we love people, it's usually based upon their character. The world tells us to love someone because he or she is beautiful on the outside, but the Spirit convinces us to love because of the love he puts in our hearts. If someone is so shallow as to disqualify you on the basis of your weight, that person is to be pitied. When you list the characteristics you love about individual people, you know that how they look is very low in priority, if it's even a factor. Look at how little children love. Do they love their mothers only if they look a certain way? We were created knowing in our hearts the way to love – unconditionally. It is this world that sucks us into its mold and convinces us that love and acceptance can be obtained only if we look as the world prescribes. That may be true for the world. The world and the worldly may think those who don't fit their mold don't deserve love. But those with the love of Jesus within their hearts know better.

The world tells us to love someone because he or she is beautiful on the outside, but the Spirit convinces us to love because of the love he puts in our hearts.

Homework

Read the following excerpts from Susie Orbach's book, reprinted here by permission. Highlight the sections that stand out to you or to which you especially relate.

EXCERPTS FROM *FAT IS A FEMINIST ISSUE*
By Susie Orbach
New York: Berkley Books, 1978
Used by Permission

The current aesthetic of thinness forces cruel pressures on the individual women. Few women are naturally thin, or indeed naturally any size. We are a variety of sizes. But the thin aesthetic which has dominated the last twenty years has put women in the impossible position of feeling that they must curb their appetites and their food intake. They must do this at the same time that they feed others and express their caring and concern for them through the food they prepare and serve. In other words, women absorb a powerfully contradictory message vis a vis food and eating. It is good for others, but bad for the woman herself; full of love and nurturance for others, full of self-indulgence to herself.[2]

Much of [a woman's] experience and identity depends on how she and others see her. As John Berger says in *Ways of Seeing:*

Men act and women *appear.* Men look at women. Women watch themselves being looked at. This determines not only most relations between men and women, but also the relation of women to themselves.[3]

This emphasis on presentation as the central aspect of a woman's existence makes her extremely self-conscious. It demands that she occupy herself with a self-image that others will find pleasing and attractive – an image that will immediately convey what kind of woman she is. She must observe and evaluate herself, scrutinizing every detail of herself as though she were an outside judge. She attempts to make herself in the image of womanhood presented by billboards, newspapers, magazines and television. The media present women either in a sexual context or within the family, reflecting a woman's two prescribed roles, first as a sex object and then as a mother. She is brought up to marry by "catching" a man with her good looks and pleasing manner. To do this she must look appealing, earthy, sensual, sexual, virginal, innocent, reliable, daring, mysterious, coquettish and thin. In other words, she offers her self-image on the marriage marketplace. As a married woman, her sexuality will be sanctioned and her economic needs will be looked after. She will have achieved the first step of womanhood.

Since women are taught to see themselves from the outside as candidates for men, they become prey to the huge fashion and diet industries that first set up the ideal images and then exhort women to meet them. The message is loud and clear – the woman's body is not her own. The woman's body is not satisfactory as it is. It must be thin, free of "unwanted hair," deodorized, perfumed and clothed. It must conform to an ideal physical type. Family and school socialization teaches girls to groom themselves properly. Furthermore, the job is never-ending, for the image changes from year to year. In the early 1960s, the only way to feel acceptable was to be skinny and flat chested with long straight hair. The first of these was achieved by near starvation, the second, by binding one's breasts with an ace bandage and the third, by ironing one's hair. Then in the early 1970s, the look was curly hair and full breasts. Just as styles in clothes change seasonally, so women's bodies are expected to change to fit these fashions. Long and skinny one year, petite and demure the next, women are continually manipulated by images of proper womanhood, which are extremely powerful because they are presented as the only reality. To ignore them means to risk being an outcast. Women are urged to conform, to help out the economy by continuous consumption of goods and clothing that are quickly made unwearable by the next season's fashion styles in clothes and body shapes. In the background, a ten billion dollar industry waits to remold bodies to the latest fashion. In this way, women are caught in an attempt to conform to a standard that is extremely defined and constantly changing. But these models of femininity are experienced by women as unreal, frightening and unattainable. They produce a picture that is far removed from the reality of women's day-to-day lives.

The one constant in these images is that a woman must be thin. For many women, compulsive eating and being fat have become one way to avoid being marketed or seen as the ideal woman: "My fat says 'screw you' to all who want me to be the perfect mom, sweetheart, maid and whore. Take me for who I am, not for who I'm supposed to be. If you are really interested in me, you can wade through the layers and find out who I am." In this way, fat expresses a rebellion against the powerlessness of the woman, against the pressure to look and act in a certain way and against being evaluated on her ability to create an image of herself.[4]

BEFORE YOU GO ON TO THE NEXT CHAPTER

Homework Follow-up

1. How do you feel about the way our culture tries to get you to meet its standard of thinness? How well have you kept up with the culture's demands?

2.   Have you used your "fat" to rebel against the cultural ideal and its pressures? How?

3.   If you did not view yourself through the cultural grid, how would you evaluate yourself?

Comments on the Homework

- How do you feel about the standard of thinness, and how well have you kept up with the culture's demands? Have you used your "fat" to rebel against the culture's standards?

Many women feel objectified and even used as ornaments or status symbols.

It is often at this point in the Weight of Grace small group experience that many women start realizing just how angry they are with the expectations that have been placed upon them to conform to unachievable standards. Often there are others around them – usually parents or their husbands – who have added to the cultural pressure to be thinner. Many women feel objectified and even used as ornaments or status symbols and find that it makes sense that they've used being "fat" as a way to resist the control of others.

It is good to become aware of the anger. It is good to express it to God and to talk it over with a trusted friend who understands about "world system" lies. You cannot get over it until you realize it's there. Many women stuff this anger. Not only do they get "fat" to resist the pressures to be thin, but also they eat to suppress the anger they feel about those pressures and the anger they feel toward the people who are exerting the pressure. I've known several women who were for years closely monitored by a mother or a husband, and if their weight wasn't maintained at a certain level, punishments of various sorts were meted out. Affection and approval were withheld; even allowances and needed clothing were denied them.

For most of us, though, the pressure is far more subtle. There are the disapproving looks from others and the constant bombardment of images set up before us that lead us to compare and fall short. Sometimes it's just easier to accept that you're a failure than to constantly yearn for what you seem to never achieve. Why keep hoping? Why keep trying when you just don't ever get there? For many women, the feeling they have most often about cultural standards is hopelessness. And rightfully so. That's the point. Satan wants you to feel hopeless and defeated.

But God is the God of hope. And our hope can't be invested in ungodly ends. Our hope is that, when we seek God's will and live in God's way, we will find there the joy and fulfillment that the praise of this world could never provide.

- If you did not view yourself through the cultural grid, how would you evaluate yourself?

For many women, the "correct" answer to this question seems totally theoretical, unreal. Believing that God says you're beautiful because your heart is set on him and his will doesn't seem as though it will stand up well when you go to the next singles party and see all the men flock to the thin women. The critical mother and controlling husband won't buy that! This is indeed a rubber-meets-the-road issue, and it comes down to what's only practical. Have you ever reached the ideal and stayed there? Do you enjoy life when you're dieting and obsessing about every bite you eat? Has accepting the cultural standard helped you meet it? And is it right to adopt it? Is it God's will for you to be "thin" by hook or by crook? What are the important issues of life to him? Might seeking to be transformed by his Spirit be not only the right thing to do, but also result in your being the person he desires you to be, the best person you can be, who may or may not fit in with the culture's idea of what's good, right, or beautiful, but who will at last have peace?

Believing that God says you're beautiful because your heart is set on him and his will doesn't seem as though it will stand up well when you go to the next singles party and see all the men flock to the thin women.

This seems to be an appropriate point at which to mention one of the ways women tend to keep track of whether they are "succeeding" or "failing" at meeting cultural standards regarding size: weighing themselves. This can be an extremely difficult habit to break. And it is an emotional habit. There is a feeling of control women get from knowing that number, and many believe that if they don't know their weight, their weight will go totally out of control. However, this is not really logical. Measuring is not the same as controlling. That's like trying to control the temperature with a thermometer. In fact, what usually happens is that, as a result of weighing themselves, women actually eat more than if they weren't weighing themselves. If the scale shows that you've "passed" by losing some weight, the tendency is to let up a little on your diet, which usually leads to letting up a whole lot! If the scale shows you that you've "failed" by gaining or staying the same, the tendency is to console yourself with food or to go ahead and blow it big time since you've already failed for that day.

Weighing yourself is a trap. It is evidence that you are still entrenched in having to measure yourself against cultural standards. It is another form of legalism, another way you're trying (in your flesh) to motivate yourself to lose weight. And it doesn't work. What

Weighing yourself is a trap.

works is giving God the chance to show you that the true you, the new creation in Christ who has a spirit of self-control, does not go hog wild if you don't measure yourself every day or every week.

If you're going to give up the fleshly legalism of dieting, that means giving up the yardstick by which dieting is measured, weighing yourself.

Since 1984, the only times I have been weighed have been when I've gone to the doctor's office. Even then, for the first five or six years after I decided to stop weighing myself, when the nurse had me step on a scale, I got on the scale backwards so I couldn't see my weight. The habit to judge myself as a failure or success based on that number was so ingrained that it took years to reach the point where knowing that number didn't throw me emotionally. If you're going to give up the fleshly legalism of dieting, that means giving up the yardstick by which dieting is measured, weighing yourself.

Remember the man I was seeing who thought I was too "fat" for him? When we were seeing each other, he was fairly slim as a result of recent dieting. It was at about the time that we stopped seeing each other (because he developed an interest in someone else) that my weight dropped down to the weight where I've pretty much remained ever since – and his weight started going back up. In fact, he gained more weight than he ever had before. His dieting backfired. He had criticized me for not dieting – and then, after he rejected me, he marveled at how not dieting was what actually "worked" for me. Ha ha!

12   WHAT'S SEX GOT TO DO WITH IT?

Since 1986, when I first spoke publicly about my experiences as an incest survivor, I have discussed with scores of women the topics of sex, sexuality, and/or how they feel about being female. All of these women – in fact, almost all the women I know – have at some time had disturbingly negative thoughts and emotions about these topics. It's probably safe to say that it's impossible to live one's life very far into adulthood without having had some exposure to negative or inappropriate sexual situations. And often this exposure is well before adulthood! In Weight of Grace small groups, for nearly every participant, attitudes and beliefs about sex play some role in the mix of issues that motivate their overeating and overweight.

As was mentioned earlier in this book, as a result of having been sexually molested by my stepfather, I formed beliefs about myself which contributed to my "need" to be "fat." Later, experiences I had while dating only reinforced my erroneous belief that I had to stay "fat" in order to keep from behaving in an immoral manner. *My* fear was that I'd "go for it," but there are many women who instead feel revulsion toward sex. This is an understandable reaction to having been coerced into sex or may be the result of feeling guilty for engaging in premarital or extramarital sex.

For many women, the subject of sex is so sensitive that there has been no way for them to address their emotions, experiences, and struggles in that area except through ignoring or suppressing them. This is very often the one topic women feel they just cannot discuss with God. It may not be a totally conscious belief, but many women have the sense that God is just too pure to think about sex, especially forms of sex that in any way deviate from conventional intercourse within the context of marriage.

When a matter that strikes at the very core of who you are cannot be discussed with anyone, not even with God, and is painful, shameful, and in many other ways emotionally laden, it makes sense you'd want to suppress your thoughts and feelings about it – and one way do that is through overeating. This is one of the two ways women deal with sex through food. This goes back to the "medicating emotions" layer of issues illustrated on page 107. Overeating is used as a way to suppress or distract oneself from the painful emotions associated with negative experiences and beliefs about sex and/or sexuality. A woman may have negative feelings about sex as a result of being coerced into sexual involvement through incest, rape, or molestation, or as a result of engaging in inappropriate or immoral sex of her own volition. She may even have had negative experiences within marriage if there was abuse or insensitivity on the part of her husband. Because of past negative sexual experiences, the very thought of sex, and the thoughts she has about herself, seem unbearable because of the emotions that are aroused, such as shame, self-loathing. and revulsion. Therefore, an escape, a way to sedate the emotions, can be found through eating. Or, overeating unhealthy foods to the point of nausea can be a way of punishing herself for being a "bad person."

The second way women cope with sex through overeating has to do with the "need to stay fat" layer of issues. (See the diagram on page 107.) Because sex and sexiness are so

When a matter that strikes at the very core of who you are cannot be discussed with anyone, not even with God, and is painful, shameful, and in many other ways emotionally laden, it makes sense you'd want to suppress your thoughts and feelings about it – and one way do that is through overeating.

closely associated with thinness, a way to avoid the whole arena of sex and sexuality is to just be "fat" and thus turn oneself into a form of eunuch. Without even knowing why she feels an intense urge to eat when not hungry, a woman overeats in order to be "fat" because she believes being "fat" means she's undesirable and, therefore, sexually safe. For example, you may recall "Lois" from Chapter 4. She did not struggle with her weight until she became promiscuous in her late teens. About a year after she became sexually active, she started to gain weight. Right before she married she lost weight (by dieting) but then became larger than ever shortly after the "I do's." Years later, when she attended a Weight of Grace small group, she realized she had perceived being "fat" as the only way to make sure she wouldn't "sleep around" and this continued even after she married. She believed that her "fat" was making her so unattractive that she would not be faced with the temptation to cheat on her husband.

In addressing the eating-in-order-to-suppress way of coping with negative feelings about sex, the basic principles that were discussed in Chapters 4 and 6 apply (i.e., renewing the mind and "REED"). However, when it comes to sex, it's much harder for most women to express their emotions to God (the first "E" in "REED") than it is when they feel angry or jealous or depressed. Usually their shame stands in the way, and shame about sex is very, very powerful.

For years, I lived with tremendous, withering shame regarding having been what I considered "sexually involved" with my stepfather (although I later realized it was not at all involvement in the adult sense but, rather, molestation that I did not initiate). A turning point for me was when both a female and a male counselor demonstrated their comfort with discussing in relative detail aspects of the molestation I'd experienced. They carefully but openly discussed how I felt about myself as a result of my experiences – that I considered myself to be a "slut and whore" who was very easily lured into "nasty" acts. They used terms such as "vagina" and "penis" and avoided vulgar euphemisms. They managed to discuss sex without being crude or embarrassed and yet were not overly clinical either. Their approach made me realize that if these Christian counselors understood, it was possible that God also understood my sexual experiences and feelings about those experiences.

God has no reason to be embarrassed by sex and is fully aware of every aspect of sex and sexuality, from the wholesome to the grossly perverse.

God has no reason to be embarrassed by sex and is fully aware of every aspect of sex and sexuality, from the wholesome to the grossly perverse. His holiness does not restrict him from looking upon and considering the sexual acts of people, whether or not the acts are sinful. There is a great deal of licit and illicit sex in the Bible. God is aware of it all and concerns himself with it enough to include it in his Word. In fact, it was for every single type of sin that Jesus died. Our sexual sins are as wiped clean by the blood of Christ as are our sins of lying or gossiping.

For me, it took gradual steps of faith in being more open with God about the feelings of self-loathing and shame that I associated with sex. I communicated to him about my feelings through prayer and journaling. In Hebrews 4:16, we are encouraged to *boldly* approach God to receive grace. We can trust God with our most shame-filled feelings and "hang ups." He will listen and help. He is not disgusted with *you*. He is, of course, saddened by all sin. If you sinned in some sexual activity, you are forgiven because of Christ's shed blood on the cross. If you were not the one who sinned, but the one sinned against (such as with incest or rape), God does not see you as "soiled" or "ruined." He knows that the sin reflects only upon the perpetrator and in no way upon you or who you are. He also knows that he is redeeming all of your most horrendous scars and turning them into part of what makes you uniquely beautiful and able to love as he loves.

Many women make the mistake of thinking that all their negative feelings about sex need to be resolved or brought to the surface before they will stop overeating in order to suppress their feelings. This is not true at all. When we start believing that, no matter what we are feeling, even if we don't know why we're feeling it, we can turn to God for his understanding, comfort, and input, the need to eat in the face of negative emotions will continually diminish. It's not that all our hang-ups must be known or addressed. What matters is that we turn to God with any emotions and struggles we may have.

In looking at the second way women cope with sex through overeating, here are some examples of the kind of thinking that may underlie the felt need to be "fat" in order to avoid sex:

If I am fat...
- *I won't have to deal with flirting.*
- *I won't be faced with the temptation to get sexually involved when I shouldn't.*
- *I won't have to worry about how to respond when I'm "hit on."*
- *I won't have to have sex with my husband (because he won't want to).*
- *I won't have to discuss sex with my husband (because he won't want to).*
- *I won't have to think about what I want or don't want when my husband and I have sex (because we won't even be having any sex).*
- *I don't have to worry about having a child right now (because we know it's not healthy for me to do so at this weight).*
- *I don't have to worry about whether I'll make a bad choice about whom I'll marry (because no one will ever want to marry me).*
- *I won't have to say no to someone asking me out (because no one will ask me out).*
- *I won't have to set the sexual boundaries when I'm dating (because no one will date me or because no date will want to have sex with me).*
- *it's less likely someone will try to rape me.*

There are many very compelling reasons that have to do with sex or being female that lead women to feel more comfortable when they're "fat."

So, if you relate to some of these reasons for staying "fat," what should you do to change? Perhaps nothing. There is no edict from God that says you must be thin. There's nothing wrong with being larger than the cultural ideal. The issue isn't that you should stop using your "fat" to cope with your hang-ups so that you can then lose weight; the issue is that you, as a new creation in Christ, *need* to rely on God, not on your own devices, in order to be who he created you to be. Part of our sanctification process is learning to walk in the Spirit instead of in "the flesh." And using your fat to cope with your problems

Many women make the mistake of thinking that all their negative feelings about sex need to be resolved or brought to the surface before they will stop overeating in order to suppress their feelings.

is not addressing your problems God's way. It's *you* dealing with your problems *your* way rather than depending upon the Spirit.

I asked God to direct my thinking so he would expose my underlying motives for staying "fat."

When I wanted to find out how I was going about trying to solve my problems in my own strength through my "fat," I asked God to show me, and he did. One of the ways he did so was through my doing the exercise Geneen Roth provides in her book, *Breaking Free from Compulsive Eating*, and which I assigned you to do as homework in Chapter 4. As I did the exercise, I asked God to direct my thinking so he would expose my underlying motives for staying "fat." The following is the dialog I had with myself when I did that exercise. ("F" stands for my "fat self" and "P" stands for my "real self.")

P: Why are you there?

F: I am protecting you. I am keeping you safe from involvement in areas where you would be very afraid to become involved.

P: But you're making me miserable too. You make me hate to buy clothes and look in the mirror.

F: You were just as frightened of the mirror when you were thin. Maybe more so. You think you *are* me and that *you* are the foreigner.

P: I don't know who I am. I think I am very evil and you keep me in check.

F: In some ways I make it easier for you to keep your desires in check, or at least you seem to think I do. You seem to feel you can just write off men as long as I exist. You're sure they have all written me off. Perhaps they're not just writing me off. Perhaps they're writing you off because you're frightened and angry and these feelings manifest themselves in ways that put men off. If I were gone, you'd have to find out if men have been writing off you or me.

P: I just don't feel I can face that. I'm afraid I'd be out there, raw and vulnerable, and I'd know what a truly unappealing, up-tight, frightened person I am. I feel I have to believe that I am basically loveable, even by fellow humans, but that men can't get involved with me because they don't look beyond the surface.

F: I think you know that's not true. I think you know that your appearance isn't as intimidating to men as your fear of involvement, your lack of trust, and your anger at them and at how society views womanhood, especially for a Christian. You don't want to get angry with someone you care about. You don't want someone to whom you're attracted to find that you are disgusting because of your attitudes.

P: Why isn't there a man who believes women are as valuable as men? Why did God have Scriptures that so strongly imply man's supremacy over women?

F: I don't have the answers, but certainly *I* am not the answer to this problem. I don't think you should use me to shield others from knowing you believe these things. If you really don't want to risk anyone knowing, you do not have to get involved, even if I'm gone.

P: I'm pretty sure I couldn't resist the opportunity, on the slim chance some man might accept me, beliefs and all. I would want the "eggs" [my code word for affection and attention] for however brief a time they were available to me before the "boom" fell. I feel you keep me from the temptation. I don't have to decide whether or not to get involved (and most probably "go for it" and get hurt). The decision is made for me. You stop them coming before there's even a chance of a relationship.

F: I am far from sure that I am the main reason men don't become interested in you. I'll bet you would and could maintain the same defenses that are keeping them away as you do now. I wasn't there when you broke up with Joe. I wasn't there when you didn't get involved with David or John. You don't just jump at every chance you get. If you don't want to get involved and yet you do in some ways too, don't blame me. Don't use me. Don't hide behind me.

P: If I really don't need you in order to stay uninvolved, why have you been there for all those years?

F: Because you've always believed that I keep you from becoming sexually involved.

P: Don't you?

F: Ask Dotty. [Dotty was a very sexually active, 5'4", 260-pound, atheist friend, who seemed to have more than her share of lovers.]

P: So, you're saying *I* keep myself out of sexual involvement.

F: Yes, you have a very solid moral code and are not so needy that you'd go outside that code to try to meet those needs.

P: I have in the past.

F: You have not betrayed the Scripture; and even if you did, we all do err and that's what Christ died for. Basically, I'm asking you to try to live without me and see if you can trust yourself, the person you are in Christ, and the Holy Spirit within you.

God wants to reveal what's motivating you to stay "fat." However, there are times when you're ready for such information and times when you're not. God knows best when the time is right. Whether or not you understand what underlies your need to stay large, turning to God to help you with your fears, desires, shame, and confusion about sex and sexuality is a big step toward undoing the need to eat in order to avoid issues related to sex.

Whether or not you understand what underlies your need to stay large, turning to God to help you with your fears, desires, shame, and confusion about sex and sexuality is a big step toward undoing the need to eat in order to avoid issues related to sex.

Reflection

1. What about being "thin" has to do with sex? What do you want sexually out of being "thin" and what do you fear sexually about being "thin"?

2. What is staying "fat" doing for you in the area of sex and sexuality?

3. Is sex okay? How does God feel about sex?

4. Have you had negative sexual experiences? Do you see a connection between those experiences and your eating and/or need to stay "fat"?

What Others Have Experienced

- What about being "thin" has to do with sex? What do you want sexually out of being "thin" and what do you fear sexually about being "thin"?

For most women, there is a simple equation: Thin = Sexy. And, for many women, there is a second equation: Sexy = Sinful, Shameful, Bad, Wrong, Sluttish, etc., etc. The combination of these two equations does not, however, totally negate another equation that's very deeply ingrained: Thin = What You *Should* Be (for any number of reasons). The conflict between these beliefs about being thin is behind a great deal of yo-yo dieting. For many years in my teens and twenties, dieting was fairly easy. I'd religiously stick with whatever "plan" I happened to be on for long periods of time, and I'd often have dramatic weight-loss results. Then, I'd gain it all back, and sometimes more. I was just not comfortable being what others considered laudably thin. I loved the attention, but I also felt constantly anxious when I was thin. And I didn't know why – until I realized I could ask God about it. When I did ask, it became clear that my desire to be thin was in juxtaposition to my desire to avoid sex and sexual temptation. If you think you'll be sexy when you're thin and if sex is emotionally dangerous to you, then it makes sense that being thin is also emotionally dangerous to you.

On the other hand, if you think you have to be thin to be sexy, you're not looking around at the real world. No matter what the media may try to promote, there are women who are larger than the cultural ideal who are dating, marrying, flirting, and being awfully sexy. When I was at my very largest, the husband of a friend backed me into a corner, got right up against me, and whispered to me about how sexy I looked in the shirt I was wearing. And, believe me, I wasn't trying to look sexy. Don't kid yourself. You can't shield yourself totally from sex by being "fat." And, as a Christian, your refuge and protection is not in your own devices (i.e., staying "fat"), but in the Lord, his love and protection, and in the self-controlled person he has made you to be in the power of his Spirit.

- What is staying "fat" doing for you in the area of sex and sexuality?

Not only do many women feel their "fat" is protecting them from unwanted sexual advances or engaging in inappropriate sex, staying large can also address issues they have with being female. If you're like me, there have been numerous times when both men and women have in some way or other discounted you on the basis of your being female as opposed to male. In high school, I was a straight "A" student in college prep courses, and yet my father felt it absolutely necessary for me to learn secretarial skills and did not want me to attend college. He didn't feel it at all necessary for my stepbrother to learn secretarial skills. He also frequently listened intently to what my stepbrother had to say, even though much of it seemed like nonsense to me. But, Dad wouldn't listen to more than a sentence or two from me without blurting out, "That's a bunch of bull," or a similar comment.

These incidents, whether accurately or inaccurately perceived and interpreted, resulted in my believing that, because I am female, I have less credibility with others than males do. Although I didn't think it through at the time, I later realized that being large gave me a

For most women, there is a simple equation: Thin = Sexy. And, for many women, there is a second equation: Sexy = Sinful, Shameful, Bad, Wrong, Sluttish, etc., etc.

If you're like me, there have been numerous times when both men and women have in some way or other discounted you on the basis of your being female as opposed to male.

sense of gravity, of presence. When it came to "throwing one's weight around," I had some heft. I felt I would be taken more seriously than some "cute little thing." Ironically, being large resulted in my having large breasts, which, with some men, lowered my credibility all the more! I will admit that, to this day, I gravitate toward higher heels, higher hair, very erect posture, and consciously deepening my voice. Not all the "tapes" are erased yet. Intellectually, I know my reputation is in God's hands, that he provides credibility when it's needed. But my "flesh" still sometimes goes into automatic pilot when it comes to wanting people, especially men, to take me seriously.

Many women use their "fat" to provide a sense of physical protection.

Many women use their "fat" to provide a sense of physical protection. My mother once told me she feels safer crossing the street when she's large. I'm not sure if she meant drivers would be more likely to see her and avoid hitting her or, if a car were to hit her, she'd be well-padded and less seriously injured. I don't think she knew why she felt that way either. In talking with women in small groups, I haven't run across a whole lot of them who are afraid of traffic, but I certainly have met quite a few who fear rape. As I've mentioned before, I used to think to myself, *When a would-be rapist sees me, he'll think twice about messing with this "big momma."* The fear of rape, for me, was a hard one, especially because I know of Christian women with enormous faith in God who have been raped. At a point, it came down to whether I should trust myself and my fat to protect me or trust God to never allow anything into my life that he didn't also give me the grace to accept and find victory in. I don't *feel* 100 percent confident in God when it comes to this issue, but I believe the only right choice is to put 100 percent of my confidence in God anyway. This is a continual choice. Having the fears totally resolved isn't the key. Knowing where to take the fears is.

- Is sex okay? How does God feel about sex?

It's understandable that well-meaning Christian parents and leaders have attempted to portray sex as "wrong" or negative in order to dissuade believers from engaging in it inappropriately. However, sex is not bad or wrong in and of itself.

There are very few people who are not conflicted to some degree about sex. Oh, the opposing messages we've all received! And so many of the confusing messages have been part and parcel of our religious training. It's understandable that well-meaning Christian parents and leaders have attempted to portray sex as "wrong" or negative in order to dissuade believers from engaging in it inappropriately. However, sex is not bad or wrong in and of itself. It's just that God created us in such a way that sex is terribly harmful to us and our partner(s) when we engage in it outside of a committed, covenant, monogamous, heterosexual marriage. As speaker and author Bill Gillham says, the Bible is "the manufacturer's handbook."[1] If the manufacturer says to use unleaded gas in your car, you'd better not use diesel. God clearly says in Scripture to totally avoid all sex that is outside of marriage. Just because he says that, it doesn't mean sex is wrong or bad. In fact, God also clearly says to participate in sex if you are married (1 Corinthians 7:3-6). Look at the Song of Songs. There we see passionate, sexual feeling, all there in the Bible, not as a no-no, but as an honest expression of romantic and sexual love. In Genesis 1:26-31 and 2:24, it is evident that the creation of the sexes and sexual activity is part of what God declared "very good."

Beliefs about sex, just as beliefs about every other aspect of life, can be transformed by the renewing of the mind. Since God created sex and sees it all anyway, start talking with him about it. Doing so is exercising faith in his love and character. Ask him to show you his perspective on sex and the role he wants sex to play in your life. Also, ask him how to view the special aspects of being female. You reflect his image in ways that are often different than how a man reflects God's image. How does God uniquely express himself through you being female? He will show you why being who and what you are is perfectly wonderful.

For single women (or for married women whose husbands are sexually dysfunctional), responding to sexual desire apart from food can seem impossible. Because I was single when I changed my mind and behavior regarding food, I know this struggle. Some may disagree with me, but I was totally honest with God and myself about how much I wanted to engage in sex and how often I thought about it. As I mentioned before, I found that appreciating the affection that was already present in my life from friends and co-workers greatly diminished my yearnings for sexual involvement. In addition, I decided not to run away from my sexual desires or even my sexual thoughts. I learned to appreciate the fact that I am a warm and sexual person. When desires and thoughts about sex came to mind, I would think through what it was I wanted and also prayerfully think through how, as an unmarried person, intercourse and other sexual behaviors were harmful. I would often plead with God for a mate, plead with God for the end to my desire for a mate – and then there would be something else to do in life that got my mind off sex. As a result of being honest about my sexual desires, eating to escape my thoughts and feelings about sex became less and less necessary. The less I ran from my feelings and thoughts and the more I prayerfully thought through what I really wanted and believed, the less I ate in order to cope with the whole arena of sex.

As a result of being honest about my sexual desires, eating to escape my thoughts and feelings about sex became less and less necessary.

In the next chapter, we will explore various factors within marriage that can contribute to overeating and being overweight. This will include a discussion of sex – how we avoid it, how we try to get too many needs met through our husbands, and how, when those needs aren't met, we turn to food.

- Have you had negative sexual experiences? What connection do you see between those experiences and your eating and/or need to stay "fat"?

There are those of us who know very well we've had negative sexual experiences. There are also those who have totally repressed their memories of negative experiences and don't even recall that they happened. There are also those who have discounted experiences as "not all that bad" or even "just normal kid stuff." For those who clearly remember inappropriate, immoral, or traumatic sexual experiences, the challenge is to go to God with them and gain his perspective regarding the incidents and how no incident in the past can reflect on your value as a new creation in Christ now. For those who suspect they have repressed memories about traumatic events, my advice would be to *not force anything*. No one knows you as well as God does and no one, not even you, knows when it's best for memories to surface. Ask God to reveal to you what you need to know now and to give you the grace to live in the Spirit, rather than in the flesh, no matter what may or may not have happened in your life.

For those who have in some way "blown off" negative experiences, this is a form of emotional self-protection and totally understandable. However, it doesn't ultimately help you. If you struggle with overeating, don't brush off what you deem to be a mildly inappropriate sexual experience just because it's not as horrendous as the experiences of others. I know a woman whose father gave her compliments regarding her breasts. She felt a great deal of shame and embarrassment and ate to punish herself because she felt she'd somehow brought on this attention. Having played sexual games with my stepsiblings fed into my beliefs that I was a "whore" just as much as my stepfather's inference that I'd "asked for" his molestation. What some psychologists pooh-pooh as "normal childhood play" may not seem normal to you and may be a source of tremendous self-condemnation that needs "punishment" through staying "fat" or overeating. Ask God how that experience of inappropriate touching, for example, has an effect on your thinking and beliefs, if at all. Be willing to accept that it may play a role in your overeating and/or being "fat." Don't decide this for yourself, but seeks God's counsel.

Homework

1. Spend at least one hour of uninterrupted time – just you and God – during which you prayerfully go over the four reflection questions in this chapter again. Then write some decisions God has led you to make about yourself and sex/sexuality.

2. Read the following excerpt from *Breaking Free from Compulsive Eating* titled "Making Friends with Your Body," that is reprinted, with permission. Complete the suggested exercises.

"MAKING FRIENDS WITH OUR BODIES"
AN EXCERPT FROM *BREAKING FREE FROM COMPULSIVE EATING*
By Geneen Roth

We begin with our hips, our breasts, our thighs, our buttocks. And we begin now. There is no reason to wait. It doesn't get easier. If you are looking with critical eyes, you will find flaws in anything: Fat thighs won't be thin; thin thighs will have cellulite. If you are looking with critical eyes, there is no such thing as an acceptable body. Stop waiting for permission to like yourself. No one can give it to you.

• Pick an area of your body that you dislike. Put your hands on it, rub it, massage it, be tender with it. So far, you haven't gotten rid of it by wishing or hating it away. Try talking to it. Try asking it what it needs from you. Touch it as you would a bird's breast. Quietly, carefully, softly.

• Go through your closet and get rid of the clothes that you don't like or that don't fit you. Especially the tight ones, the ones you have to pour yourself into, the ones that dig into your waist and your thighs and the ones that stand when you sit. *Get rid of them.* Give them away or pack them in a suitcase where you don't have to look at them every day and wonder when you'll be thin enough to wear them again. Plan a "clothes" day with your friends: ask everyone to bring clothes they no longer wear, and when they arrive with their bundles, put them in piles on the floor. Look through the piles, let everyone try clothes on. You can all go home with something new to wear.

• Buy yourself some new clothes, silky clothes, pretty clothes, clothes that feel good and look good NOW. I realize that you want to wait until you lose weight to buy clothes that you like. Why, you ask, should you spend money on clothes for a body size that you want to change?

Because your ideal body is in the future. And this body, the one you've got right now, is the one you have to walk around with every day. Every time you dress it in clothes that aren't pleasing to you, in fabrics and styles and textures that you don't like, you are punishing yourself.

Squeezing yourself into clothes that are too tight will not help you lose weight. The discomfort will not motivate you; it will not force you into getting thinner. It will, however, cut off your circulation, make it hard to breathe, make it hard to concentrate. It will also give you cause to feel as if you are spilling out of your clothes. Wearing clothes that are too tight makes you feel like a restricted, breathless slob. And wearing clothes that you don't like, in colors or textures that don't please you, is another way of telling yourself that you've been bad and so you have to pay the consequences.

Think of your clothes as costumes. Use them as antidotes to your moods: When you're lethargic, wear something bright and bold. When you're happy, wear something outrageous. Use clothes to counter your feelings; explore the possibilities in muted colors, subtle patterns, soft fabrics, nubby textures.

• If you can afford it, arrange for a weekly massage with a professional masseuse. If not, trade weekly massages with a friend. Allow your body – all of it – to be touched by someone who does not have a vested interest in your weight. We often don't claim our bodies; we cut ourselves off at the neck, identifying with our thoughts, our feelings, our faces, while our arms and legs remain strangers. Massage helps us reunite us with our bodies; it provides us with physical pleasure that is not sexual. During a massage no one wants anything from you but your enjoyment at being touched.

Having a massage also helps you realize that your body is finite. If a masseuse works on your feet, then your legs, she has to finish with your legs before she works on your torso. That means your legs do not go on forever. (Did you hear that? Your legs do not go on forever.) They have a beginning and an end. Massage gives you a sense of body boundary, and for people who have distorted and hopelessly large body images, this is extremely helpful.

• Gather pictures of yourself from your childhood through the present. Look at your body. Has your image of your body consistently been bigger than your body actually was? Or did well-meaning parents, aunts, teachers tell you were fat? Were you?

• From magazines, cut pictures of bodies that reflect your ideal size. Look at those bodies. Are they truly pleasing? Are they anything at all like your body? Could you ever, in a million years, look like that? When will you stop trying?

• Spend five minutes every day looking at your body in a full-length mirror. Notice where the curves are, notice the recesses, notice the lines of your arms, the shape of your hands. Notice, observe, but *do not judge*. Every time a judgment arises, replace it with an observation – that is, go from "My arms are flabby" to "my arms follow a line beginning at my shoulders; they extend on either side of my torso, etc. ..."

After you do this for a week, begin making a conscious effort at complimenting yourself. "My skin is creamy." "My hair falls in soft curls around my face." "My legs are strong and firm." Each time you look in the mirror, notice *three* qualities that are lovely about your body. At the beginning you may have to stand there for a long time. But it will get easier. And easier. Look at yourself as if you liked yourself.

Liking yourself will follow.[2]

BEFORE YOU GO ON TO THE NEXT CHAPTER

Homework Follow-up

1. If you're going through this book in the context of a small group, discuss with your fellow small group members the decision(s) you made as a result of prayerfully answering the reflection questions in this chapter. Usually, discussing them with others results in finding out that you are not alone in your experiences and thoughts about sex and sexuality.

2. Why don't you want to be "friends" with certain parts of your body? If you were to make friends with these parts, what would that mean?

Comments on the Homework

- What decision(s) did you make as a result of prayerfully answering the reflection questions in this chapter?

I am continually amazed at how personally God speaks to individual women. Here are a few (paraphrased) comments women have made after prayerfully considering the reflection questions in this chapter:

- *I realized I needed to forgive my father for molesting me. I also realized this was his problem and not mine.*
- *I decided that I really don't want to lead men on. I haven't wanted to do that in a long time, but I was still thinking I would if I got thin.*
- *Definitely, I see that my fat is my protection. A guy has to really get to know me and not just my looks. I'm not sure I trust that God will protect me from getting involved with a man who loves me only for surface reasons. I still need to decide to take that step of faith.*
- *I have hated being a woman [because my father used me for sex] and I thought being fat would erase anything feminine about me, but God is showing me how special and beautiful I am to him, without it being a sick thing.*
- *I realized that men notice me even when I'm fat. My method of dealing with male attention isn't working. I'm asking God to show me his way of responding to the attention I get.*

No matter what revelations you had while praying through the reflection questions, my hope is that you made some decisions about trusting God in those areas. Letting God into the parts of one's life that have to do with sex and sexual identity is a big step and takes faith. As one who has walked into this arena before you, I would encourage you to even tiptoe in if you must by opening up a conversation with God in which you admit your embarrassment and shame. I've found that if you can discuss sex with God, it seems there is little else you can't then more easily discuss with him.

- Why don't you want to be "friends" with certain parts of your body? If you were to make friends with these parts, what would that mean?

So often, the very paths we think should lead to the results we want are in reality the means to greater failure! We think that if we hate our "fat thighs," we'll hate them enough to "do something about it." Wrong. What happens with women over and over again is that, when they hate themselves, they either punish or console themselves with *more food*. We buy clothes that are a little too tight so we'll be motivated to finally lose that weight! Wrong. We hate how we look and feel in those clothes and we punish or console ourselves with *more food*. Hate is just not a good motivator. But love is!

Satan and the world system want you to see yourself as ugly and a failure. Where do those critical thoughts come from? From the accuser (Revelation 12:10) and from measuring oneself against the perverted standards of our culture. At the very top of each of my thighs there is a fatty bulge that sticks out, making my thighs wider across than my hips. I used to loathe this about my figure. I often made the comment that I needed a machete to just whack those saddlebags off. And, even now, I sometimes look into the mirror and shake my head in disgust. But, then I think, *Who told you those are ugly?* Those parts of my body are soft and pleasantly grab-able. They provide a nice expanse of creamy skin. They're round and I even like it that they're not perfectly smooth. There's some interest there. I'm not a teenage girl; I'm a *woman*! Okay, no one's going to hire me for a bathing suit layout, but that's their problem. They're just too rigidly caught up in the mindset of this world and don't even know there's a universe of variety that could be richly appreciated.

Satan and the world system want you to see yourself as ugly and a failure.

I like the way Geneen Roth ends the "Making Friends with Your Body" passage: "Look at yourself as if you liked yourself. Liking yourself will follow."[3] This is taking a step of faith. Since God loves you, loving yourself is right, and you need to take steps to go in that direction, despite your feelings. Actually, your feelings about yourself are the result of an emotional habit that needs to be broken. Your true inner self, the new creation in Christ, agrees with God that you are likeable. The best way to break a habit is to do something else instead. Each time you hate yourself or some aspect of yourself, counter that by telling yourself why you should like yourself or that part of you. Ask God to give you his perspective. (I realize I'm repeating myself when I make that statement, but the only way to step into truth and reality is to see life as God does. This cannot be emphasized enough.) Has hating yourself, your looks, and your body worked for you? If it has, you wouldn't be reading this book. Try learning to like yourself and accept yourself on the basis of who God made you to be rather than on the basis of cultural standards – and see if that "works." "Taste and see that the Lord is good" (Psalm 34:8a).

If you choose to become friends with your body, whether or not the areas you have loathed for so long become smaller or less "fat," you will still become more beautiful.

Of course, what we fear will happen if we "make friends" with the "fat" parts of our bodies is that those parts will never go away – or worse, that they will get even "fatter." Wrong again. Hating those areas results in hating yourself and then in more overeating. And insisting that those areas *must* go away shows how brainwashed you've been by the world system and its arbitrary and impossible standards. If you choose to become friends with your body, whether or not the areas you have loathed for so long become smaller or less "fat," you will still become more beautiful. So much of beauty has to do with one's attitude, which is borne out in the way you carry yourself and how you dress yourself. You're not going to act beautiful if you hate yourself, and so you won't be beautiful – to yourself or others. Why wait till you're "thin" to be beautiful? You're already beautiful now if you'll just let God give you the eyes to see that.

13 "FAT" AND MARRIAGE

If you're single, read this chapter anyway! You have probably been married – or will be married – or will be in dating relationships – or even in friendships – that will be the basis for you relating to much of what is covered in this chapter.

So, what if you've made the decision that conforming to the cultural standards of attractiveness and thinness is not only not working for you, but also is contrary to living life as a new creation in Christ, motivated by the Holy Spirit, *BUT* you are married to a man who has never even considered his own internalized values when it comes to female beauty and sexiness? And, actually, why would he question his beliefs? He, like everyone else in our culture, is inundated with images of the so-called "beautiful people" in photos (*Sports Illustrated* swimsuit issue!), movies, and on TV. The women who are lauded as gorgeous and sexy are thin, thin, thin. He doesn't think through how, about 50 years ago, these same women would have been considered *too* thin to be sexy and how, in different parts of the world and in different times, *they* would have been deemed the ugly ones.

Of course, you can't approach every husband, boyfriend, or male friend in the same way on this topic, but let's look at a couple of real-life scenarios for addressing the "world system" beliefs held by the men in our lives. This first example is one of my favorite Weight of Grace success stories regarding a husband coming around to a more godly perspective about his wife's weight. A woman who had been faithfully attending small group weekly sessions was quite struck by the information presented on how very fickle cultural standards of beauty and size can be. So, she went home from the session in which being "squeezed into the mold" was discussed and asked her husband, "Do you think I'd be more sexy if I lost weight?" The next week, she returned to the small group with the report that he answered that, quite honestly, he did indeed feel she would be more appealing to him if she lost weight. How, she wondered, could she cope with this?

I have had similar experiences with boyfriends and male friends. Even if it isn't always directed at me, most of the men I know make comments that indicate that they find "thin" women more attractive. Some even register total disgust toward women who are even marginally what our culture might deem "overweight." Certainly it's easy to understand how they came to this mindset. After all, this is what I thought for many years too. Nevertheless, the "enlightened me" can get pretty indignant when men, especially Christian men, so thoughtlessly adopt the shallow standards of "the world" in regard to what constitutes female beauty. My knee-jerk reaction to the report from this group participant that her husband had so flatly said he'd be more attracted to her if she lost weight was to sharply retort, "He doesn't even know what sexy is! Is there any other woman in the world who knows as much about him as you do and still loves him as unconditionally as you do? Now *that's* sexy!" As I calmed down, I wrote out for her the following series of questions and comments to discuss with her husband in regard to what is truly attractive and sexy:

Is there any other woman in the world who knows as much about him as you do and still loves him as unconditionally as you do? Now that's sexy!"

- *Do you think that any of the women you consider to be very beautiful and desirable would find you to be handsome and desirable if they knew you as well as I do?*

- *Have you ever considered that the very fact that I am different from everyone else out there makes me interesting and special, especially to you since I'm yours?*

- *You could look at various parts of my body as being much more interesting than the bodies of those women who are more like teenage boys than like real women. For instance, grab onto this fold of my stomach and feel how soft and hold-able it is. Try tucking your hand in here and feel how warm I am. (You can just let your imagination run with where "here" was.)*

- *Is there anyone else on this planet who loves you as well as I do and knows you as well as I do and wants to have sex with you? How would it feel to have sex with someone you don't know well and, worse yet, who doesn't even know or appreciate you?*

- *I'm finding out that I'm really beautiful just the way I am, especially because my heart is right with God and I desire to do God's will. God views me as beautiful because God looks at my heart. When you think about how I take care of you and our children, how I tenderly look after your needs and theirs, does that make me any sexier to you? Any more beautiful?*

This particular small group session took place on a Thursday. On the following Monday morning, I got a phone call from the husband. He said he wasn't sure what all was said at our last small group meeting, but he wanted to thank me for his "new wife." Later the participant reported that after she and her husband went over the list of questions I'd provided, they'd had one of their sexiest weekends ever.

But not every man is so easily persuaded. A woman I know is married to a man who for many years was a pretty hard-core believer in "thin = sexy," with no exceptions. His insistence that she maintain a certain weight was a big contributor to her never being able to maintain that weight and, eventually, totally giving up and getting far larger than she probably would have been had he not hounded her. After realizing God was not requiring her to "squeeze into the mold," she changed the way in which she approached her husband's attitude. She decided to agree with God and believe in her own beauty despite her husband's constant disapproval. *And she prayed.*

During the time I've known this couple, I've seen the husband gradually come to accept the value and beauty of his wife and very slowly give up on his idea of what she has to look like in order for him to pronounce her attractive or sexy. She stopped arguing with him. She didn't try to prove her point. She just lived what she believed to be the truth and, in response to his complaints, made statements such as, "I understand that you're unhappy about my looks, but I believe I'm fine the way I am. I've tried for years to be the way you want me to be and have never been able to get there." She has even sympathized with him in his disappointment and expressed how she understands because she's been disappointed in herself for years also. Her disarming honesty, along with the work of the Holy Spirit, is what eventually changed her husband's viewpoint.

No matter what our husbands believe, we still must decide for ourselves what is really true and agree with God about that truth. If your husband wants you to be someone that you are not, ask God for insight into how to hold onto the fact that you have God's approval even while facing disapproval from someone who is so significant in your life.

She decided to agree with God and believe in her own beauty despite her husband's constant disapproval.

No matter what our husbands believe, we still must decide for ourselves what is really true and agree with God about that truth.

And also ask God if you are using your "fat" to make a statement about how you reject your husband's conditional acceptance. This is one of the many ways in which women use their "fat" and overeating as tools to accomplish certain goals within their marriages.

For many years, I've listened to women in Weight of Grace groups discuss their marriages, and I've plainly heard, although often between the lines, how the dynamics of their relationships with their husbands are intermingled with the dynamics of their overeating and staying large. The ways in which women's overeating relates to their marriages appears to fall into three categories: 1) using overeating and "fat" as a form of non-verbal communication, 2) eating in order to cope with disappointments in marriage, and 3) substituting eating for affection and/or sex.

There are many reasons why open communication can be more difficult in marriage than in other relationships. There is more at stake. You don't want to live with someone, day in and day out, who is angry with you or thinks you are a fool because of something you've said. You don't want to risk rocking the boat and maybe causing it to capsize altogether. When there are children, the stakes are even higher. So, what do women do when they have something to say to their husbands but don't feel they can say it? Often, they communicate it anyway, just not through words. For many women that communication can be through their eating or through being "fat."

The most blatant example that comes to my mind is actually that of a man who used to come for counseling at Scope Ministries International and chatted with me frequently because my desk was outside his counselor's office. This man was what doctors call "morbidly obese." He appeared to be about 6'2" and to weigh over 400 pounds. A comment he made to me one day was, "My eating is the one thing *she* can't control," referring to his wife, of course. His wife's attempts to control him were frustrating and extremely irritating to him, and he, in turn, was rebelling against her control by getting very, very "fat" and by eating foods he knew she thought he oughtn't. Often, our non-verbal ways of communicating through eating and being large are not as obvious as this man's, and we usually are not as aware of them as he was.

A friend recently mentioned to me that, although she had freedom from overeating for quite a while after being exposed to principles about legalism and her new identity in Christ, she had again started gaining weight. She said she felt sure it was because she was trying to make herself less desirable to her husband since every time they have sex, he insists that it be "hot sex," that she moan and scream and get terribly excited. She just doesn't want to have to get *that* excited *every* time. She doesn't feel it will do any good to talk with him about it. So she is communicating through her "fat" her desire to avoid having sex with him. Ironically, when I asked her several weeks later if the tactic was working, she told me it wasn't. Despite her increased size, her husband still wanted to have sex just as much as ever. "Fat" often fails to communicate what we hope it will.

Many women enter marriage with a great deal of insecurity. For some women, being "fat" can be a way of "testing" the relationship, of trying to make sure their husbands really do love them "for better or for worse." Or, a woman might so expect to be rejected that she wants to get "fat" to hasten her husband's disgust so that he will more quickly reject her

For some women, being "fat" can be a way of "testing" the relationship, of trying to make sure their husbands really do love them "for better or for worse."

and she can "get it over with now" rather than winding up even more devastated by his abandonment or a divorce after several years of marriage.

"Fat" can also be a way of communicating to a husband that a woman feels she is being taken for granted. A husband may not acknowledge the efforts of his wife in maintaining the household and caring for the children, but he might notice she's gaining weight. When he comments on it, this gives her the opportunity to explain how her very busy life (that he doesn't even notice) makes her vulnerable to snacking, eating on the run, and not getting exercise.

Messages women frequently try to communicate to husbands through overeating and overweight is "I'm angry with you," and/or "I resent you." Since women tend to see their attractiveness as an asset to their husbands, making sure one's husband has an unattractive wife is a way to punish him for his "sins." "Why should I look good for you? You did/didn't/don't _____." Fill in the blank with anything from "...pay any attention to me" to "...cheated on me." That ugly ol' fat is an attempt to make a big statement, one that the woman either doesn't feel she can say aloud or has already said aloud too often to have any effect anymore.

What is more important to address than your communication skills is your willingness to allow God to help you identify if or how you are communicating through overeating and "fat."

There are many excellent books and seminars about communication in general and about communication within marriage specifically, and, certainly, learning how to better communicate is a part of the "cure" for the problem of using your eating and weight to get messages across to your husband.[1] But learning to communicate doesn't happen overnight and, even if *you* become an expert communicator, it still takes "two to tango." What is more important to address than your communication skills is your willingness to allow God to help you identify if or how you are communicating through overeating and "fat." Once you acknowledge what you are doing, then you can ask God how he would have you respond to your circumstances in ways other than overeating and overweight. Very often God does lead women to verbalize to their husbands their concerns, doubts, and feelings. However, sometimes God wants women to just tell *him* and let him change their hearts, their husbands' hearts, or both. Many times, God's answer is inclusive of both honest verbal communication and trusting him to provide in unexpected ways, such as my praying friend whom I mentioned earlier in this chapter.

Overeating is not only used as a means of nonverbally communicating with husbands, but also it can be a way women console themselves when their husbands disappoint them. There are a lot of disappointments in marriage. That's a given because there are a lot of very high expectations in marriage. Since childhood, we have been forming ideas about marriage and what it would do for us. Our culture puts a great deal of emphasis on how much emotional satisfaction, security, and pleasure we are supposed to derive from "falling in love," marrying, and living "happily ever after." As we anticipate marriage, we think, *Finally, I'll get all the fulfillment, affirmation, and affection I ever dreamt of!* We don't usually think, *Finally, I'll live up close and personal with another faulty human being who is focusing on what I can do for him just as much as I'm focusing on what he will do for me.* When, in marriage or in any relationship, we look to another to meet our needs, there will inevitably be disappointment, especially for Christians, because God does not want us to get our needs met through others, but through him.

This is not to say that God doesn't use others in meeting our needs. Problems arise, however, when we expect others to meet our needs in certain ways rather than allowing God to meet our needs, sometimes through others, but in a variety of ways, some of which may not be what we expect. Women are often very focused on exactly how they think their husbands should behave and do not question where they came up with the list of rules they want their husbands to abide by. Many times women express their disappointment with husbands in the same breath as explaining why they overeat:

- *I probably wouldn't snack at night if my husband showed me more affection.*
- *He never approves of me anyway, so why should I even try to lose weight?*
- *While he watches his sports on TV, I'm in the kitchen eating.*
- *He never helps me with anything in the kitchen, and I just eat the whole time I'm in there.*
- *I get so frustrated with how he never helps with the kids that I turn to food to keep from yelling at him.*

The underlying belief behind each of these statements is: *If my husband were meeting my needs better, I would not need to overeat.* As discussed in Chapter 4, many of our beliefs are inaccurate. This is one of those inaccurate beliefs. The truth is that no one *needs* to overeat. That sense of "need" is really a signal that we are trying to work out our problems in our way; that's "the flesh." It's the best way we've come up with to cope. And we often don't consider that there may be an alternative. The alternative is to turn to God with our disappointments and frustrations and ask him to show us how he is meeting our needs even when our husbands are not.

Since Mike and I are relative newlyweds, I'm still in quite the romantic haze when it comes to my husband. Even so, I've experienced some disappointments at times during the course of our marriage. In fact, right after we returned from our honeymoon, I noticed I was often eating a lot of chocolate and sweets and that some of my clothes were getting a little tight. *Wow, I thought, is it true that women just automatically gain weight once they marry?* But then I prayerfully thought through my circumstances. Why did I want to eat sweets constantly? Through bringing thoughts to my mind, God revealed to me that I was coping with a post-honeymoon let-down and trying to recreate the euphoria of our honeymoon by filling with sweets the lonely times of being separated from Mike because of our opposite work shifts. I wanted to continue to feel "spoiled" and "pampered" in the way I had when I was constantly with him. My first thought about a possible solution to this was that I would ask Mike to change from his night shift to working during daytime hours as I do. That would fix things! But then I realized that was *my* solution and, perhaps, not God's. When I asked God for *his* perspective, I suddenly saw all the constructive ways in which I could use the extra time I had that many married women don't have – and I began writing this book! The desire for sweets dropped off. Also, I started to appreciate how our pretty much weekends-only marriage was very much extending that "we're still honeymooners" feeling.

Problems arise when we expect others to meet our needs in certain ways rather than allowing God to meet our needs, sometimes through others, but in a variety of ways.

God wants to reveal to us how extremely creative he can be in meeting our needs in very personal ways. Do you want your husband to help you around the house more? Maybe you're requiring your home be far more perfect than need be. Maybe your husband has a lower energy level than you have, especially if he has a lot of stress at work. There are all sorts of possibilities, and God wants to reveal to you the ways in which *he* (God) is not disappointing you. Then you won't need to expect so much from that faulty person (just like you) to whom you're married.²

Another marriage-related reason women overeat is to try to substitute food for affection or sexual satisfaction. If you've watched movies or television, if you've read novels (especially romance novels, even Christian ones), you very likely think that marriage (or, perhaps, dating) is the ultimate source of affection and acceptance. In fact, you may even believe (perhaps without realizing it) that marriage and romance are the ultimate sources of fulfillment in life. Many women (and men, for that matter) believe they cannot be complete as people unless they are married. And many more believe that completeness comes only when one finds the "perfect mate." This has been the justification for a number of divorces among several acquaintances. "I just married the wrong person." "I didn't discern God's will when I married Joe." However, the beliefs that there is just one Mr. or Ms. Right and that marriage is utopia are not borne out in Scripture. In fact, there is extremely little in Scripture that narrows down the choices regarding whom you should marry. The apparent restrictions are that a Christian should marry a fellow believer and marry someone of the opposite sex. And when it comes to marital love being the be-all-and-end-all in life, even David said there is a love that's greater than that of the love between a man and a woman (2 Samuel 1:26).

Scripture has quite a bit to say about *God* being the perfect "mate" (Isaiah 54:5; Jeremiah 3:14) and our completeness being found in our union with Christ (Ephesians 4:13; Colossians 1:28 and 2:10; Hebrews 11:40). In fact, we as the church constitute the "bride of Christ" (Revelation 19, 21, 22). When we try to find our wholeness through marriage and when we try to get a majority of our needs met through a relationship with a husband, frustration and disappointment are sure to follow – because marriage and husbands were neither designed to make us whole nor to meet most of our needs.

There is no love from a person that can surpass the unconditional love of God, *agape*. This is the kind of love that is described in the familiar "love passage" of 1 Corinthians 13. A husband can sometimes be one of the means by which God expresses that love to you, but the source of such love is always God himself. When we realize that God is the source of the best kind of love, this can free us to welcome whatever love people, including husbands, are able to give us instead of *needing* them to love us in the ways we feel they "should." Having expectations about how our needs for love will be met limits our perception of how those needs are indeed being met, not only through a husband's own unique way of expressing affection, but also through the many other people in our lives.³ Because of the constant focus in our culture on romantic love, we tend to totally miss all the affection that is coming our way through other family members, friends, and co-workers. Also, because so much emphasis is placed on sex and other "touch" forms of affection (kissing, hugging, fondling), we fail to receive and enjoy the affection that's communicated through kindnesses, favors, notes, eye contact, and people giving of their time and attention. When the myriad ways God expresses his love to you through his Word, Spirit, and the people around you are counted, this greatly reduces the need to fill in with food any sense of an "affection gap" you feel your husband leaves in your life.

Many have said that marriage is the crucible in which people's true character is tested. Living daily in intimacy with and dependence upon another person and knowing it's "for the long haul" can quickly force to the surface many issues in our lives that could otherwise remain dormant. And overeating can be a way to cope with those issues. Fortunately, we can choose to see our overeating and "fat" as signals that point out our need to turn to God in order to ascertain how to do more than merely cope. He leads us into the means to come to honesty and true healing that not only solve the overeating problem, but also address the more important issues that lie beneath the overeating.

Reflection

1. What do you perceive to be your husband's attitude about your size and weight? What are your initial thoughts about ways you can best respond to how he thinks and feels about you?

2. How would your husband feel if you lost weight? And how would you feel about that?

3. Are there any messages you are trying to communicate to your husband through your overeating and/or "fat"?

4. Are you in any way trying to discourage your husband's sexual attention through your size/"fat"?

5. Do you feel you are getting all the affection and attention you really need/want from your husband? What are some sources of affection you tend to feel don't really count?

What Others Have Experienced

- What do you perceive to be your husband's attitude about your size and weight? What are your initial thoughts about ways you can best respond to how he thinks and feels about you?

For every woman in Weight of Grace small groups whose husband expects her to be "thin," there have been one or two whose husbands found their wives perfectly lovely and desirable just the way they are, regardless of their weight. I thought it was great when the husband of a friend told her he didn't really like the way she was so rigidly dieting because she'd fallen way below her "f*#!-ing weight." (Yes, he said the "f" word.) In other words, there was a point at which she lost enough weight that she became far less comfortable to have sex with and less desirable to cuddle and fondle. Many women even complain that their husbands aren't "supportive" of their weight loss efforts because their husbands accept them just as they are. Of course, the truth is that acceptance, rather than judgment, is the greater motivator for allowing yourself to be who God made you to be.

Also, there are those husbands who have unhealthy reasons for wanting their wives to stay "fat." Do you remember the song with the lyrics, "If you want to be happy for the rest of your life, never make a pretty woman your wife"?[4] There are men whose insecurities lead them to feel more emotionally comfortable when "the little woman" isn't so little anymore. What if someone better than he is came along and wanted her? There are many articles written about how men want to display a beautiful wife as if she were a trophy, but many women report how threatened their husbands become when they lose weight and start looking more like the cultural ideal. This can be a difficult circumstance. However, a husband's insecurities need not trap you into staying "fat." So often, the husband is really reacting to the changed attitude a woman may have when she feels she's more attractive. It's all tied into the false values of the culture. While you're still larger than the cultural standard, start believing you're attractive and acting as though you're attractive – because you *are*, no matter what the sin-sick culture says. If you do become smaller as a result of no longer eating for emotional reasons, you will not have such a huge, jarring change in attitude. Wear nice clothes *now*. Wear bright colors *now*. Don't wait till you're "thin" to decide you're a "babe." And don't "flaunt it" only if you're "thin." That's buying into the lie that only thin equals attractive.

There are those husbands who have unhealthy reasons for wanting their wives to stay "fat."

You may not be able to quell all of your husband's fears, but you can direct your beauty and sexiness toward *him* without making a public display of it. And, no matter what his hang-ups, living the truth is the only option in line with your new identity in Christ. Staying "fat" for someone else's sake is not being who God made you to be.

- How would your husband feel if you lost weight? And how would you feel about that?

The hard part about your husband loving it if you lost weight is that this means he's not loving it that you are as you are now. This hurts. But he's been brainwashed, so try not to take it so personally. Yes, we think that our husbands should love us unconditionally, but what human being is really equipped to do that? You cannot be "thin" or "fat" to please another person. The only one whom you need ultimately to please is God, and he wants you to be yourself, the true you, the person he created you to be, walking in the Spirit, eating when you're hungry and not for emotional or psychological reasons. If you feel angry that your husband wants you to be a certain way, express that hurt and anger to God and ask him for his perspective. God can and will help you to accept your husband even in the midst of his not fully accepting you. Many times I have seen this very acceptance, offered by wives, used by God to turn the hearts of husbands.

You cannot be "thin" or "fat" to please another person. The only one whom you need ultimately to please is God.

- Are there any messages you are trying to communicate to your husband through your overeating and/or "fat"?

Every married woman who struggles with overeating is not necessarily nonverbally communicating through her eating and "fat." However, when a woman in a Weight of Grace group says, "I can't think of any way I could be sending messages to my husband through my eating," I usually respond with, "Do you ever feel hurt by your husband?" Angry women are often in touch with how they want to punish, control, or communicate with their husbands through their "fat," but women who suppress anger or are fairly reserved tend to internalize that anger as "hurt." They don't feel they can say to their husbands, "You've hurt me," or "I'm mad at you," so they shove their feelings down and, often, use eating to help them do so. Even if they don't intend it, their "fat" screams out their silent wounded-ness. Many of these women claim they feel no emotions at all regarding their husbands. This is a clue also. They emotionally withdraw from their husbands because of the hurt they feel and the fear of being hurt again or more deeply.

In the extreme, these "hurt" wives enjoy playing the martyr. That role becomes part of their identities and they wear their pain like a mantle. Their "fat" is a testimony to how wronged they've been. However, these are the exceptions. I've found that most women who are eating to suppress their hurt don't even realize they feel hurt. They very quickly internalized their pain and then it surfaces through overeating.

If you're angry, let it out with God and don't hold back. Give God a chance to comfort you and to give you the grace to forgive.

If the question, "Do you ever feel hurt by your husband?" brings a lump to your throat or tears to your eyes, this is your cue to turn to God for illumination about what it is you've been suppressing through food. If you're angry, let it out with God and don't hold back. Give God a chance to comfort you and to give you the grace to forgive. Let God show you how he feels about you even if your husband seems not to appreciate or cherish you. It's likely you'll find that, when you face what you've avoided feeling, food will be the last thing you'll want. Experiencing emotions of nearly every sort – truly feeling them fully – is absorbing enough to make food an intrusion and irrelevant.

- Are you in any way trying to discourage your husband's sexual attention through your size/"fat"?

As was mentioned in the last chapter, there are numerous reasons why women feel uncomfortable with sex and want to avoid it. Staying "fat" can be one way of attempting to do that. Unfortunately, being large doesn't really take you out of the running, so looking to God to address your "issues" his way is far more effective than overeating. Coming to grips with this fact is a huge step toward freedom from the felt need to stay "fat."

When women are coping with their own attitudes toward sex, it seems easier to address their issues than when the struggle is with a husband whose attitude about sex is unhealthy, especially when he is insensitive and/or unwilling to discuss the topic. A friend once asked her husband, "Don't you even care that I never have an orgasm?" His answer was, "No." My thought was, *What do you do in a situation like that?!* And the truth is that I don't know what one does other than pray for grace. I do know, however, that eating won't fix the problem and won't ultimately soothe the pain.

Most of the women who say they're eating to have a treat in the face of a deprivation in some other area of life are actually just trying to distract themselves from their anger and disappointment.

If what you want is a satisfying sex life and/or a loving romance with your husband, no amount of food will provide those. You might be thinking, *But at least I can have something enjoyable.* Yes, food can be enjoyable, but there are also many other things in life that are enjoyable and available to each of us. Eating when you're not physically hungry is just not all *that* enjoyable, especially when you compare it to eating when you are truly hungry. And most of the women who say they're eating to have a treat in the face of a deprivation in some other area of life are actually just trying to distract themselves from their anger and disappointment – and perhaps even trying to punish themselves for their anger by making themselves "fat." Because our bodies have such very distinct and perceptible signals alerting us to true hunger, it's hard to believe that food was designed to be used for recreation at times when we're not hungry. The bloated, uncomfortable feeling we get after we eat when we're not hungry is proof of this. That feeling is really not a "treat"!

Yes, we are influenced by our sex-obsessed culture to deeply long for sexual satisfaction within marriage, and we are created to experience sexual satisfaction in the context of marriage. However, sex is by far not the only source of satisfaction in a marital relationship, and marriage is not the only relationship in which emotional satisfaction is available. Our openness to God providing for us in a variety of ways takes the pressure off of us (and our husbands) to get a lot of "needs" met through sex – and it also takes the emphasis off looking for satisfaction through food.

This is in no way a suggestion that you find romantic or sexual satisfaction from anyone other than your husband! Rather, there is a great deal of perfectly godly emotional satisfaction in relationships, such as those with friends, children, siblings, co-workers, and people for whom you are providing discipleship in Christ. When you focus on and cultivate such relationships, rather than focusing on what you don't have, not only do you have less emotional need to overeat, but also you have a lot more joy in life.

Some husbands are not just insensitive; they're abusive. If that is the case for you, you will have to work it out with God and, perhaps, with godly counsel whether it is appropriate for you to engage in the kinds of sex your husband is requesting or demanding. There may be hard choices to make about what you have to honestly say to your husband and what boundaries you must draw with him.

Sometimes what needs confrontation is not out-and-out abuse, but being objectified or used. A woman in a Weight of Grace group told how she came to the point of saying to her husband, "If all you want is a quickie [every time], then just go into the bathroom and take care of yourself." She used humor and a little shock value to make a point that he fully understood and even respected. She had been trying to use her "fat" to say "no" to those quickies. He just didn't "hear" her "fat" telling him "no." She had to say it with her words. You may be afraid that your words won't "work." If that is so, you are still better off to attempt the communication because you will have turned to something other than trying to subtly get the message across through your "fat," which didn't work either.

- Do you feel you are getting all the affection and attention from your husband that you really need/want? What are some sources of affection you tend to feel don't really count?

It seems that the women who feel the greatest need for affection and attention are also the ones who try to get nearly all of that affection and attention from their husbands. That's a lot to put on one individual. Many of us are "set up" for feeling a never-ending need for what we didn't get from our fathers (or even from our mothers). It's like being a bottomless pit. No matter how much affection you get, you still want more. In fact, when you get a little, it makes you want a lot all that much more. There have been many times when I wished a man had totally ignored me rather than offer sporadic tidbits of attention. I wanted *everything* he had! If I'd never seen the carrot dangling, I'd have never started the emotional chase. My husband is a very affectionate man, but I believe, had I married him

You may be afraid that your words won't "work." If that is so, you are still better off to attempt the communication because you will have turned to something other than trying to subtly get the message across through your "fat," which didn't work either.

about 15 years ago, I would have worn him out in the first year. No amount of attention and affection would have totally satisfied, because I would have seen him as the sole source. As I've mentioned before, I was totally discounting the many, many sources of attention and affection that were already freely flowing my way.

Do you *receive* the love of your children, the affection of your friends when they think to give you a call, the attention of your parents even if they're not your favorite people? Do you accept the ribbing you get at the office as people expressing a "safe" form of affection? Are there people who say "hi" and smile when they see you? And are you *giving* affection? This can be just as satisfying as receiving it. Are you taking a moment to write a note of congratulations to a fellow church member who has mentioned a "praise report"? Do you give reassuring, sympathetic pats to your family members when they tell you about their daily trials or victories?

Evaluate whether you're being picky about how your husband displays affection.

Evaluate whether you're being picky about *how* your husband displays affection. A co-worker recently told me that her husband just doesn't think of giving her flowers, but he really enjoys "wining and dining" her on special occasions. She decided to appreciate what he does do – and many other husbands don't – rather than focus on the flowers she has never received. It used to bother me that my boss for 16 years at Scope Ministries International rarely asked me how I was doing or about any aspect of my life. But, what he often did was leave a gift on my desk. He didn't feel comfortable asking personal questions, but he did care a lot about me, so he displayed his affection through the occasional electric frying pan or knick-knack. I have a friend whose husband is not much of a hugger or kisser. This irked her for a long time until she started realizing that he was making all the meals and doing the grocery shopping because he wanted to do it *for her*. He even fussed over the sandwiches he made, never just slapping them together. His meal preparation was one of the ways he showed affection and paid her special attention.

Oh, those movies full of lingering kisses, sweet whispers, and bouquets! They leave out what many men in the real world are doing to display affection. Ever get swept off your feet when your husband swept the kitchen floor? I have. Mike's usual household duties are the vacuuming and dusting, but a couple of weekends ago, while I was shopping, he went ahead and did my chores too! Now that's affection.

Count 'em up. It is likely that God has provided you with a surplus of what a former boyfriend used to call the "three As," attention, affection, and acceptance. When you start realizing you're getting them – from your husband and also from a lot of other people in your life – food isn't as "needed" as a substitute.

Homework

1. If you feel it would be received, go over with your husband the questions and comments listed on page 176.

2. Prayerfully think through the reflection questions in this chapter. Ask God to reveal to you underlying beliefs that you may not have been willing to face before. Ask him for perspective regarding your relationship with your husband, regarding what you're trying to communicate to your husband through your size and eating, and regarding what you're trying to get from food that you wish you could get from your husband. Make notes about what God reveals to you.

BEFORE YOU GO ON TO THE NEXT CHAPTER

Homework Follow-up

1. How did your husband respond to the questions and comments on page 176? What are your feelings and thoughts about his responses?

2. What was the most surprising insight God revealed to you about your overeating/size pertaining to your relationship with your husband (or boyfriend or male friends)?

Comments on the Homework

- How did your husband respond to the questions and comments on page 176? What are your feelings and thoughts about his responses?

Looking at underlying beliefs and motives can be unsettling. It does seem it would be much easier if getting a grip on eating and weight was just a matter of will power and discipline.

Of course, husbands don't always respond as we expect. Many husbands feel quite caught off guard by the entire approach taken in Weight of Grace small groups. They're very used to their wives fretting over their weight and going on and off diet after diet. Looking at underlying beliefs and motives can be unsettling. It does seem it would be much easier if getting a grip on eating and weight was just a matter of will power and discipline. Many of the husbands of Weight of Grace group participants react negatively to all this underlying beliefs/motivations "junk" and think their wives should just stick to a diet and stop making excuses. They especially don't want to have to get touchy-feely and analytical too. Some people – and I've found this more with men than women – just do not relate to the idea of being driven by unacknowledged beliefs. Ironically, these are the very people who often do what they *feel* is right without even questioning their feelings or motives.

If your husband is uncomfortable with analyzing your relationship or helping you explore some of the reasons you overeat, there is no point in pressing the issue. You are responsible only for *your* integrity before God. And you don't want to force issues that your husband may not be emotionally equipped to handle. That's the Holy Spirit's business. Part of the reason why it's helpful for women to pursue freedom from overeating in the context of a small group is that it allows them to realize there are people with whom they *can* discuss struggles and revelations about inaccurate beliefs and thinking. If your husband wants to join you in your journey toward experiencing the freedom you already have, great. If he's uncomfortable, that's great too because God hears you and does care about what is going on inside your head and heart – and there are others who can relate. Appreciate where your husband is in life and what he has to offer, and appreciate the many other resources God has given you.

- What was the most surprising insight God revealed to you about your overeating/size pertaining to your relationship with your husband (or boyfriend or male friends)?

So often we don't believe that God will or actually can speak to us at all, let alone about such a tremendously subjective matter as our own hidden agendas. However, there have been many times when I've asked God to make clear to me what was going on behind my behaviors, and then later I've been reading along in Scripture or writing my thoughts and ideas in a journal and *knew* God was clearly giving me insight. Also, there are a number of Bible studies available that ask provocative questions which facilitate hearing from God about whether what you believe lines up with Scripture.[5] God also communicates through his Body, the church. When we stay in active fellowship with Christians who care about growing in faith, God uses interaction with fellow believers to reveal to us where we're off base in our thinking. The Holy Spirit is more interested in revealing to us the truth about ourselves than we are in hearing it. When we are willing to hear from God, he speaks in a variety of ways to the issues of most concern to him and to us.

If you believe God has not been revealing to you the beliefs and thoughts that are motivating your overeating, start to very regularly read the Bible while asking God to show you personal application. The Bible says of itself that it is "living and active" and "judges the thoughts and attitudes of the heart" (Hebrews 4:12). Also, God has declared that his Word will always have an effect on those who are exposed to it (Isaiah 55:11; John 17:17). Through exposure to Scripture, even if you do not "hear" God speaking specifically to you about the beliefs that motivate your overeating, your beliefs *will* be changed.

The Holy Spirit is more interested in revealing to us the truth about ourselves than we are in hearing it.

14   WHERE DO YOU GO FROM HERE?

Before we look at some possibilities for how you might proceed after completing this book, let's review two key Scripture passages, the internalization of which is pivotal to experiencing freedom from overeating.

> *But I say, walk by the Spirit, and you will not carry out the desire of the flesh.* Galatians 5:16, NASB*

The emphasis of this book has been to point you to how you can "walk by the Spirit" and, as a result, gradually move away from carrying out the desire to go about coping with personal problems and circumstances through eating when not hungry and by staying larger than is natural for you. "The flesh" in Galatians 5:16 is not "lust" for food or, as some want to call it, "gluttony." Rather, "the flesh" is that habit within us to address problems and difficult emotions in our own way. Without thinking about it, we learned to cope with our emotions and difficult circumstances by turning to food. Without thinking about it, we learned to avoid our mixed feelings about the pressures to be "thin" and the real and perceived problems that arise as a result of being "thin" – by staying "fat."

Working out the stresses and pressures of life for ourselves by overeating and staying "fat" is similar to how some people face the fear of loss of self-esteem by lying about their accomplishments. Rather than realizing that God works through us no matter what other people may think about us – rather than walking by the Spirit – the person protects him- or herself by lying. Lying is easier to identify as being "of the flesh" because most of us think of lying as being a pretty bad sin. Overeating, on the other hand, tends to be thrown into the category of "lack of discipline" and perceived as a lesser sin. It is rarely seen for what it usually is: a device of our "flesh," a means we have developed for coping with our lives. What many people do not realize is that the solution is not "cracking down" on oneself by trying to impose more and more discipline through dieting. The permanent solution is, instead, to "walk by the Spirit" – to turn to God for his ways of seeing and his power in addressing the emotions and circumstances we experience.

We are better able to understand how we can "walk by the Spirit" when we realize we are "new creations in Christ," possessing a renewed spirit indwelt by the Holy Spirit. As new creations, we are "alive to God," able to know God's will more and more as our minds are renewed by the Spirit and the Word. (See Romans 6:11, 13 and 12:1-2.) The way to live out being a new creation is to constantly turn to God in prayer – or what I have called "prayerful pondering" or "prayerfully thinking through" – and to expose oneself to God's Word, Christian fellowship, and literature and teachings that acknowledge the new nature

The emphasis of this book has been to point you to how you can "walk by the Spirit" and, as a result, gradually move away from carrying out the desire to go about coping with personal problems and circumstances through eating when not hungry and by staying larger than is natural for you.

---

*I prefer the rendering in the *New American Standard Bible* and other Bible translations that use "the flesh" rather than "the sinful nature" (as in the New International Version) because "the sinful nature" implies we have two natures within us simultaneously. Rather, our nature has been changed to that of a new nature in Christ, but we still war against the flesh, the remnants of our separation from God and the "conditioning" of Satan and the world system to live life our way rather than God's way.

of the Christian, the work of the Spirit, and the renewing of the mind process (often called "sanctification").

Another key Scripture passage that pertains to experiencing freedom from overeating is Titus 2:11-12:

> *For the grace of God that brings salvation has appeared to all men. It teaches us to say "No" to ungodliness and worldly passions, and to live self-controlled, upright and godly lives in this present age...*

It is the grace of God that teaches us how to say "No" to our own "passions." In the case of overeating and "fat," those "passions" are the strong desire to eat when not hungry and the often bewildering "need" to be "fat." If grace teaches us, how do we go about learning the lesson? We learn from grace by acknowledging what has "appeared to all men." ("Men" here includes all people, men and women.). It is most certainly the grace that brings salvation, but it apparently does more than just secure our place in heaven. The grace that teaches us to say "No" is the grace that God extended in changing our inner selves and taking up residence in our very hearts. Some have defined grace as "unmerited favor," which it is, but many also refer to grace as *the power to live the Christian life.*

It is *by God's grace* we can face temptation and flee from it (1 Corinthians 10:13). God has freely equipped us to not only face, but also overcome, the world's attempts to squeeze us into its mold. When we realize who we are in Christ (Galatians 2:20) and how God does indeed lead us through his Spirit (John 16:13), we learn the lesson of grace that enables us to say "No" to overeating, dieting, and making ourselves "fat." God gives us the grace, the power, to reject worldly thinking and behavior and to accept and live out his plan for our lives.

When we realize who we are in Christ (Galatians 2:20) and how God does indeed lead us through his Spirit (John 16:13), we learn the lesson of grace that enables us to say "No" to overeating, dieting, and making ourselves "fat."

Overeating is not a lifelong "disease." Once you change your mind about dieting and having to be "thin," once you start listening to your body rather than your emotions to tell you when to eat, it usually takes six months to three years to gradually become a "natural eater." Many believe being an overeater is their identity and that it is a condition that must be fought for a lifetime, but what you *really* are is someone designed to eat moderate amounts of the food that appeals to you – in response to physical hunger. We've been brainwashed to believe otherwise and have been bullied into addressing overeating through dieting rather than through returning to who we are quite naturally, especially as born-again Christians, people who are *designed* to live "self-controlled, upright, and godly lives."

It does take time to change attitudes, beliefs, and habits so that you can shed the thinking and behaviors of the "old self" that are related to overeating, but this need not be an area in which you must "always have a struggle." Sanctification, the process of gradually becoming more and more like Jesus as we cooperate with the Holy Spirit's work in us, is indeed a lifelong process, but each specific area of "the flesh" in our lives need not remain an issue for our entire lives. The principles set forth in this book can and do enable women to enter more fully into the process of sanctification, especially pertaining to overeating, resulting in leaving behind those all-consuming obsessions with food, dieting, physical appearance, and weight gain or loss.

Next Step Recommendations

If you have thoroughly read this book and agreed with all or most of it, you have already entered into the process of experiencing the freedom from overeating that God has already given you as his child and regaining the natural eating and physical activity patterns for which you were designed. Yes, the old habits of "the flesh" are often deeply entrenched and the new habits of grace and walking by the Spirit need reinforcement. So, in order to help you stay on the path you've taken by reading this book, you may want to consider *continuing in a small group that studies living in the grace of God by the power of the Spirit and/or non-diet approaches to overcoming overeating.* Those who have gone through Weight of Grace groups and have the most success in becoming "natural eaters" are those who have had a good deal of exposure to "new creation in Christ" and "grace walk" principles or who go on to immerse themselves in those concepts. There are many excellent books and materials available along these lines, all of which could be explored in the context of a small group. Certainly, these could be read on one's own and be of great benefit, but participation in a small group provides many advantages that come from interacting with other believers. (See Ecclesiastes 4:9-12 and Ephesians 4:15-16.)

Those who have gone through Weight of Grace groups and have the most success in becoming "natural eaters" are those who have had a good deal of exposure to "new creation in Christ" and "grace walk" principles or who go on to immerse themselves in those concepts.

The following books emphasize how to go about living in grace and how to "walk by the Spirit." Each of these, except *Be Transformed*, is available through outlets such as amazon.com and Christianbook.com.

- *Be Transformed*, a small group workbook by Scope Ministries International, Inc., available at www.scopeministries.org.
- *Lifetime Guarantee* by Bill Gillham
- *Classic Christianity* by Bob George
- *Grace Walk* by Steve McVey
- *Grace Works* by Dudley Hall
- *Sidetracked in the Wilderness* by Michael A. Wells

I strongly recommend starting with *Be Transformed* because it is formatted for small groups and is based upon the same material that served as the basis for some of the chapters in this book. Continued reinforcement of basic principles regarding grace and its appropriation will not only help you toward freedom from overeating, but also – more importantly – help you find greater intimacy with and dependence upon God, especially if you invite God to communicate with you as you read materials and interact with others over them.

Since we step out in faith to the degree we trust in God, our understanding of and belief in him and his character as a loving and caring heavenly Father is at the root of our ability to appropriate his grace. Resources which will help you deepen your faith and trust in God are:

Since we step out in faith to the degree we trust in God, our understanding of and belief in him and his character as a loving and caring heavenly Father is at the root of our ability to appropriate his grace.

- "FatherCare," the manuscript that is reproduced with permission in Addendum One of this book and available in booklet form from Scope Ministries International, Inc.

- *Our Heavenly Father* by Robert Frost. This book is out of print but still available on ebay® and from various used booksellers online.
- *The Father Heart of God* by Floyd McClung
- *Knowing God* by J. I. Packer
- *Desiring God* and *The Pleasures of God* by John Piper

Below is a list of some of the many books that address how dieting does not work in the long run. These books are secular, but with a biblical mindset it's fairly easy to "eat the meat and spit out the bones." These authors have discovered a truth without knowing it is God's truth – that legalism has with it a curse and that God has already designed us to eat in moderation.

- *Breaking Free From Emotional Eating* by Geneen Roth
- *Diets Don't Work* by Bob Schwartz
- *Inner Eating* by Shirley Billigmeier
- *Intuitive Eating* by Evelyn Tribole and Elyse Resch
- *The Ten Habits of Naturally Slim People* by Jill Podjasek

"Success" and "Failure"

When a friend heard I was writing this book, she called to strongly urge me to make sure I included a section in the book about what to do when one "fails." She said that all I'd known was success in finding freedom from overeating. What about those who, like herself, still had bouts with overeating and weight gain? What I immediately thought when she made these comments was, *This isn't about "success" or "failure,"* and *What is she referring to as "failure"?*

It is not "failure" for someone to overeat, and it is not "failure" for someone to be larger than the cultural ideal. We are all in a process of trusting more and more in Christ and leaning less and less on our "flesh." Labeling a period of time when you eat for reasons other than hunger as a "failure" only adds to the problem because it adds guilt and puts the focus on the "failure" rather than on the *process* of sanctification. Instead, you can see such a period in your life as a signal that there is a need for prayer and to seek God over what the eating indicates is going on "under the hood." Since no one size is good or bad, right or wrong, gaining weight is certainly not a "failure." Focusing on the weight only throws you back into worldly thinking and the greater temptation to get rid of the weight quickly through a means that's not godly (e.g., dieting or overly stringent exercise).

In 2000, I gained eight pounds and have not lost it since. I know this, not because I regularly weigh myself to see if I'm "fat" or "thin," which is a practice I abhor, but because I've had a relatively minor, recurring health problem for several years which requires that I go to the doctor every three to six months, and the nurse weighs me every time. By 2002, I'd given away several articles of clothing that had become too small for me. I purchased some new jeans in a larger size than I'd worn in several years. I may or may not ever lose these eight pounds. I believe that, if they aren't really natural for my body at my age, they'll drop off (possibly when I enter menopause). Just because I gained them, just because I may have

Labeling a period of time when you eat for reasons other than hunger as a "failure" only adds to the problem because it adds guilt and puts the focus on the "failure" rather than on the process of sanctification.

eaten sometimes when I wasn't hungry, I'm not a failure. I didn't "fail." I did have the opportunity to live out what I'm writing about! I was given opportunities to turn to God and to trust him in areas I had not had to consider for a while. I was given the chance to appreciate myself with a little more "meat on my bones," to admire how another shape is as good or better than the way I was before. If there is any success, it is in viewing oneself as being in a process and in a vital relationship with God rather than in a success/fail situation concerning eating or size.

If gaining weight is "failure," should I have viewed my losing weight as a result of going on a special fast with my church family as "success"? Certainly, my co-workers at the time thought I was being quite successful at losing weight (although most of them weren't aware that I was not on a diet). Everyone around me commented constantly about how good I looked. But I was not succeeding or failing at anything. It was the fickle culture giving me gold stars, not God. Unexpectedly, it took over two years before I gained back the weight I'd lost during the fast. Was the maintenance of my weight loss a success? I think it was just a quirk of my metabolism. I certainly didn't work at staying "thin." In fact, I had to work at liking myself even though I'd lost my bust line. If one's goal is losing weight, the likelihood is that she will, at least at some time or other, both "succeed" and "fail." If one's goal is walking in the grace of God, regardless of outward appearances, there is no "succeed" or "fail." There is just a relationship with its ups and downs, although on God's side of the relationship, it's all a steady flow of love, concern, and empowering grace.

If one's goal is losing weight, the likelihood is that she will, at least at some time or other, both "succeed" and "fail." If one's goal is walking in the grace of God, regardless of outward appearances, there is no "succeed" or "fail."

Reflection

1. What have you been postponing until you're "thin"? Are there any of these activities that you absolutely cannot do now?

2. What plans do you have regarding what you'll do after you finish this book?

What Others Have Experienced

- What have you been postponing until you're "thin"? Are there any of these activities that you absolutely cannot do now?

I used to think I'd wear bathing suits if I were thin. By most people's standards, for over 20 years now, I have been "thin" enough to wear a bathing suit, but I've worn one only a couple of times. It turns out I'm too modest to flash that much skin in public. I feel naked or as though I'm in my underwear.

There are two types of activities we postpone until we're "thin" – the ones we wouldn't do anyway and the ones we could be doing right now. It's hard to determine which is which until we try them. I used to wear all muted colors – lots of brown, navy, and black – because my mother told me they were slimming. When I decided to stop waiting until I was "thin" to wear colors I liked, I started to wear red and yellow and, my favorite, teal. I didn't look fatter; I looked prettier. And I felt prettier. It reinforced my belief that I was lovely no matter what size I was.

Very often, postponing certain pleasures has much more to do with self-punishment or people pleasing than with feeling one really cannot do them at a certain size.

Women have reported putting off acting sexy with their husbands, wearing lingerie, playing tennis, having a massage, going on a vacation, or having a baby until they reach a certain level of "thin." But many so-called "large" women do all of these and have a blast doing them. Usually, postponing certain pleasures has much more to do with self-punishment or people pleasing than with feeling one really *cannot* do them at a certain size. The thinking is, *I don't deserve to do this when I'm so fat*, or *Everyone would think I'm a fool if they saw a tub of lard doing this*. Punishing yourself with deprivation or calling yourself names will not motivate you to lose weight. It will make you feel bad about yourself, and you'll probably just console yourself with food. People pleasing is futile because you can never know what every person's standards are, so you'll never live up to them no matter what size you are. Anyway, if someone is so small-minded as to judge you for doing anything that's perfectly moral just because you're larger than the cultural ideal, that's a problem *he* is having.

Putting off activities and experiences may not only be depriving you, but also depriving those around you. They don't get to join you in the fun you aren't having yet.

The challenge to you is to try some of the activities you thought you shouldn't engage in until you're "thin." These are what *you* want to do. You are you *now*, not some time in the future when you might look different. Experiencing who you are now is part of becoming more and more the person you were created to be.

- What plans do you have regarding what you'll do after you finish this book?

When women discuss with each other their ideas about where to go from here, they usually realize how much they need each other.

When women discuss with each other their ideas about where to go from here, they usually realize how much they need each other. It is hard to fight a culture steeped in the diet mentality and the thinness gospel by oneself, especially if some of that culture is living right there at home with you! If you have been reading this book on your own, I hope you make the decision now to seek out a friend or two with whom you can explore further the concepts of grace, being a new creation in Christ, right thinking about God, and how diets don't work.

Homework

1. Read through the following "Identity Beliefs Related to Food and Fat/Thinness" and "Erroneous Beliefs Related to Food and Fat/Thinness" charts.[1] Circle the statements in the "Lies" columns to which you relate and prayerfully consider the statements and Scripture passages given in the corresponding columns.

IDENTITY BELIEFS RELATED TO FOOD AND FAT/THINNESS

Lies about Self	How Lies Affects My Life	Truth	Scripture References
I have no self-control.	Keep constant rein on eating. "I must control or I'll be out of control."	I am a self-controlled person. God has given me a spirit of self-control.	Galatians 5:23 2 Timothy 1:7 Titus 2:11-12
I can never change. (I'll always be fat.)	Live in "give up" mode, avoid risks, appear lazy and unmotivated.	God is always at work in me. He gives me the desire and ability to change.	Philippians 1:6 Philippians 2:13 Philippians 4:13
I am unattractive at this weight. I am ugly.	Live, eat, think, feel like an ugly person (in the way I carry myself and relate to others).	I don't have to buy into the world's fickle ideas of beauty. According to God's values (the true ones), I am beautiful.	Proverbs 31:30 Romans 12:2 1 Peter 3:3-4
I am inferior (based on looks, weight).	Either shy ("no one is interested in me" – uses weight to hide behind) or overly boisterous (to overcompensate, gain attention). Tries to lose weight to gain approval.	Whose values am I living by? If I live by the world's, it is a losing game. God says I am fearfully and wonderfully made. I am made in the image of God.	Psalm 139:13-16 Romans 12:2 1 Cor. 15:10 2 Cor. 10:12
I am limiting myself spiritually. God can't use me because of my weight.	Hold back from ministry opportunities; assume everyone else is thinking what I am thinking about my spiritual inadequacy.	The world says I have to have my act together before I can do anything. God says that in my weakness he is strong. He chooses the foolish things of the world to confound the wise.	Acts 4:13 1 Cor. 1:27 2 Cor. 11:30 2 Cor. 12:9-10
I am a "fat" person (fat identity; fat = bad/ugly).	Live, eat, think, feel like a fat person.	My identity is not based on how my "earthly tent" looks. Identity = who Christ says I am.	1 Samuel 16:7 2 Cor. 5:1-7 2 Cor. 5:16-17 Ephesians 4:24
I am dirty, immoral.	I feel that, if given the chance, I'd have an affair. Therefore, I'll gain weight to protect myself; no one will be attracted, and I won't be tempted.	I am holy and blameless. I can feel sexual temptations, yet not act in a sinful way. The Holy Spirit empowers me to say, "No."	2 Cor. 5:21 Galatians 5:16 Ephesians 1:4 Colossians 1:22 Titus 2:11-12 Jude 24

Lies about Self	How Lies Affects My Life	Truth	Scripture References
I am primarily a sexual being (identity = sex).	Strong driving force to have sex, but feel out of control. Eat to control self/stay fat (less sexy).	I am primarily a spiritual being. My identity is *not* tied to sex.	Romans 8:9, 16 Ephesians 2:1-6 Colossians 3:1-4
I am a guilty (bad) person.	Eat to punish, fat punishes. My outside reflects how I feel on the inside.	I am a forgiven person. The goodness of God is within me.	Micah 7:18-19 Romans 8:1 Colossians 1:13-14; 2:13-14
I am unloved.	Go to food for love. Try to look skinny so someone will love me.	God loves me with an everlasting, unchanging love. I am deeply loved.	Psalm 103:11 Isaiah 54:10 Jeremiah 31:3 1 John 3:1
I am insignificant.	Either "I'm not important so who cares what I look like," or "If I look good, then I will be significant."	I am significant because I am made in the image of God. I am "in Christ" and he lives in me. I am a joint-heir with Christ.	Genesis 1:26-27 Romans 6 Galatians 2:20 1 Peter 1:18-19; 2:9-10
I am a failure.	Food used as a "pacifier" to dull painful emotions. Live in "give up" mode--avoid risks, appear lazy/unmotivated.	I am victorious. The power that resurrected Christ from the dead is inside me.	2 Cor. 2:14-15 Ephesians 1:18-23
I am unfulfilled.	Go to food primarily for fulfillment and pleasure.	I may feel unfulfilled, but God offers maximum fulfillment through an intimate relationship with him that provides fulfillment through him and his provisions.	Psalm 16:11 Matthew 5:6 John 10:10

ERRONEOUS BELIEFS RELATED TO FOOD AND FAT/THINNESS

Lie	Truth	Scripture References
Food soothes or numbs my emotions.	The emotions don't go away. They will find a way to escape, either through physical symptoms or eventually in an emotional blow-up. Going to food rather than to God is "walking in the flesh" (living life in one's own strength). Eventually the consequences will far outweigh the "benefits."	Romans 6, 7, and 8 (especially 8:12-13) Galatians 6:7-8
Food gives me peace.	Jesus is the Prince of Peace. He promises to give me peace.	Psalms 23:1-3, 55:16-18 Isaiah 26:3 John 14:27 Philippians 4:6-7

Lie	Truth	Scripture References
Food gives me pleasure/is my primary way to experience pleasure.	God desires that I find pleasure first and foremost in him. He delights in me, enjoys me. In his presence is fullness of joy. I can trust God to provide pleasure through himself and what he has created.	Psalms 4:7; 16:11; 18:19; 36:8 Jeremiah 31:14 John 10:10
Food gives me a lift. It encourages me, makes me feel better.	God is the "help of my countenance," my encourager. He is beside me, cheering me on. I can trust him to meet my need and desire for encouragement through himself and/or others.	Psalms 30:10-11; 42:11; 43:5 John 14:16, 26 Romans 15:5
Food helps me forget my fears.	God wants to be involved intimately in my life. He wants me to come to him with my fears, and he promises to deliver me from all my fears.	Psalms 34:4; 56:3 Isaiah 41:10; 43:1-2 Philippians 4:6-7 1 Peter 5:7
Food (and making myself fat and bloated) punishes me when I've blown it.	God has already forgiven me. There is no condemnation in Christ Jesus. He wants me to come to him when I blow it so he can remind me of his forgiveness and help me.	Isaiah 43:25 Romans 8:1 Ephesians 1:7-8 Hebrews 4:15-16
Food helps me feel secure and less anxious.	God is my security. He never changes. All things are in his hands. He promises to meet all my needs. I am secure. I can cast my anxieties on him.	Deuteronomy 33:26-28 Isaiah 43:1-2 Philippians 4:6-7, 19 Hebrews 13:5
Food makes me feel loved.	I am already loved. God delights in me and desires that I experience his love when I am feeling unloved.	Deuteronomy 7:7-8 Psalms 36:5, 7-8; 42:8 Jeremiah 31:3 1 John 3:1; 4:19
Food makes me feel satisfied, content.	Food only works for the very short term and the consequences far outweigh the pleasure. Ultimate satisfaction comes from God. He wants to satisfy me when I feel unfulfilled or unsatisfied.	Deuteronomy 8:3 Psalms 36:8; 63:4-5; 81:16; 103:5 Matthew 5:6 John 6:48-51
Fat = bad, shame.	The world's values say a certain size means I should be ashamed. Years ago, "plumpness" was a sign of wealth and beauty. I refuse to measure my worth by the world's gauge. I choose to believe what God says about me rather than what the fickle world system says. I have value and worth no matter what size I am.	Deuteronomy 26:18 Romans 12:2 2 Corinthians 5:7; 10:12 1 Peter 3:3-4
Fat = punishment or vengeance (against my spouse, family member, etc.).	God is the avenger, not me. Bitterness will only hurt me in the long run. I can give up my anger to God and choose to forgive and receive his forgiveness.	Romans 12:19 Ephesians 4:31-32 Hebrews 12:15 James 4:11-12
Fat = protection from rape. (I'm bigger and feel less vulnerable.)	God is better able to protect me than I am. Who is it more important to trust, me or God?	Deuteronomy 32:10 Psalms 20:7; 32:7; 91:1-4

Lie	Truth	Scripture References
Fat = protection from myself because sexual temptations are less.	When I'm "thin," I may *feel* sexual temptation more strongly, but my strength is always the same. The Holy Spirit is my strength, giving me the ability to say, "No."	1 Corinthians 10:13 Galatians 5:16 Titus 2:11-12 2 Peter 2:7-9 Jude 24
Fat = power or Thin = power.	Because I believe I get power through my size, I sometimes feel it's true and, therefore, act more powerful. The truth is that Christ empowers me with his strength. The Holy Spirit is my power source.	2 Chronicles 16:9; 20:3-30 Zechariah 4:6 Acts 1:8 2 Timothy 1:7
Thin = success and/or significance.	The world's definition of success is completely opposite of God's definition. The world says success = performance, looks, others' opinions. God says success = knowing him, living a life of dependence on him. He has declared me significant and valuable already. I don't have to earn it.	*Success*: Jeremiah 9:23-24 John 13:13-16 Galatians 6:14 1 John 2:15-17 *Value*: Deuteronomy 26:18
Thin = happiness.	If I believe this is true, I may feel happier temporarily if I am thin. Yet, eventually other problems in life will surface. The world offers temporal happiness and satisfaction based on externals. Jesus offers deep and long-lasting joy that no one can take away.	John 10:10; 15:11; 17:13 Romans 12:1-2 1 John 2:15-17
Thin = beauty. (Beauty = value.)	The world says beauty is based on externals. The gauge by which it measures beauty constantly changes. God says beauty is based on my inner spirit. Even Jesus did not conform to the world's idea of beauty. Do I really want to strive for something as fleeting and shallow as external beauty or do I want to be a beautiful person in God's eyes? My value is not based on the world's evaluation of my looks. It is based on the unchanging truth of Scripture. I am already of value.	*Beauty*: Proverbs 31:30 Romans 12:1-2 1 Peter 3:3-4 1 John 2:15-17 *Value*: Matthew 10:28-31 1 Peter 1:18-19; 2:4-10
If I look okay on the outside, I'll feel okay on the inside.	That's backwards! Value and worth are inward qualities. Christ has already declared me to be valuable, significant, and worthy. He lives inside me. I am God's child, complete in Christ, holy and blameless, deeply loved. I want my outward appearance to reflect my inward beauty.	Deuteronomy 26:18 Romans 12:2 Colossians 2:10 1 Peter 2:9-10 1 John 2:15-17
If I feel all my emotions, I will be overwhelmed/unable to handle them! (I eat to avoid feeling the emotions.)	God can handle my emotions. He will empower me to express my emotions to him and walk by faith in the midst of them. He will show me the beliefs that are motivating me to feel this way and show me the truth that will result in resolving the emotions.	Psalms 55:16-18; 62:8 Isaiah 43:1-2 Hebrews 4:15-16

Lie	Truth	Scripture References
Life is out of control. I must be in control. I have to control my body, eating, emotions, and environment.	God is in control and is trustworthy. The Holy Spirit will keep me in control. My ways of trying to maintain control only lead to my being more out of control. I can entrust my life to God as I grow in my understanding of who he is.	Psalms 9:10; 103:19; 138:8 Galatians 5:16 Ephesians 5:18 Colossians 1:16-17; 2:20-23
Eating must be controlled by external activities such as dieting, not having sweets around, etc.	God created my body wonderfully and fearfully. As a new creation in Christ, I have the Holy Spirit empowering me from within and a spirit of self-control. It is the Spirit who enables me to remain moderate.	Galatians 5:16; 23 Philippians 2:13 2 Timothy 1:7 Titus 2:11-12
Dieting is the way to lose weight.	Dieting has a huge failure rate. It serves as punishment for being "fat" and is grounded in the idea that something is wrong with me. Rules and regulations increase one's desire to break them. They have no value in controlling sensual desire.	Romans 7:7-8 Colossians 2:20-23
Guidelines set by health organizations must be followed.	God desires to give direction and input in this area. He alone knows my body, how it is made and what works best for it. He has given us bodies which use physical sensations to tell us when we're hungry, thirsty, full enough, too full, not able to digest a particular food, etc.	Psalms 139:14 1 Corinthians 10:23
I absolutely must exercise in order to lose weight.	Pressure and rules only lead to failure. The law arouses sin. The very things we tell ourselves we ought to do are the things we end up least wanting to do. Exercise is of profit, yet needs to be seen in the proper light. God wants to motivate us through His Spirit to activities appropriate for our health and well-being.	Romans 7:7-8 Galatians 3:3,10; 5:18, 24-25 1 Timothy 4:8

2. Read through the following review. Prayerfully think through whether you believe these concepts are true for you. Make notes here of those you find difficult to believe and why it's hard to believe them.

EXPERIENCE THE FREEDOM FROM OVEREATING YOU ALREADY HAVE
REVIEW

1. You can trust God with this area of your life. He is intimately acquainted with and interested in every aspect of your life and wants you to know the truth so that the truth will set you free (John 8:32). You may have confused your impressions of your parents or authority figures with your understanding of the heavenly Father. God is love – 1 Corinthians 13:4-7 describes God's character and his attitude toward you. He is not disgusted with you and impatiently waiting to see when you'll "shape up." See 2 Corinthians 3:17-18 – God is interested in your being free, and that freedom comes from him, his goodness, and his work within your life.

2. When you put your faith in Christ, God transformed you into a "new creation in Christ" (2 Corinthians 5:17). This means that at your very core, where the Holy Spirit indwells your new spirit, you are a person who desires to totally obey and love God (Ephesians 4:24). You are a spiritual being with spiritual gifts and in possession of the fruit of the Spirit. You are, by nature, loving, kind, peaceful, patient, and *self-controlled*. The reason you do not always act in total concert with your new nature is that "sin dwells in your members" (Romans 7:21-24). You have the "sin measles" as a result of having been born dead to God and alive to Satan. However, you are not defined by your sins or behaviors. You are defined by God. He says that, as a new creation in Christ, you are a saint, holy and blameless, with his laws written on your heart, and you are in the process of gradually becoming more like Christ.

3. The process by which you gradually overcome the "sin measles" and by which you are transformed more and more into the image of Christ is through "the renewing of the mind" (Romans 12:2, Ephesians 4:22-24). You have beliefs about everything, but many of your beliefs were formed apart from input from God, so some are erroneous, corrupted, not accurate. As you mature in Christ, the Holy Spirit points out your false beliefs and shows you accurate beliefs through God's Word. These new beliefs motivate your thoughts, actions, and emotions.

4. Overeating can be a symptom of suppressing difficult emotions. Emotions are also symptoms – messengers telling you that there is something going on in your thinking and beliefs. Emotions need to be acknowledged and shared with God. They are not wrong in and of themselves. It is what you do with emotions that is sometimes wrong. Too often emotions can become the authority by which you live, instead of making God's Word your authority, despite what your emotions may be screaming to the contrary. If God says you have self-control, you do, no matter what your emotions or experience tells you. God has given you a way to resolve the negative emotions you feel – by going to him with them, expressing them to him, asking for his viewpoint on the situation at hand, and deciding to accept and act upon his truth. This is the healthy way to express and experience your emotions, whereas "medicating" emotions with food is ultimately ineffective and only a temporary "fix."

5. An emotion many women try to suppress through eating is anger. Anger is the result of having unmet expectations or blocked goals. By acknowledging your goals and expectations and surrendering them to God, you can prevent some anger. However, it is impossible to anticipate your every goal and expectation. When you do feel angry because someone has blocked your goals, sinned against you, or failed to meet your expectations, the "cure" is to forgive. This is for your own sake and God provides the ability to forgive. When you perceive God as the one who is blocking your goals or not meeting your expectations, you need to acknowledge his sovereignty and love, trusting him to work everything out for your ultimate good (Romans 8:28).

6. You are designed in such a way that your body tells you when to eat (physical hunger) and when to stop eating (satiation – being no longer hungry). Our culture has told you that you cannot trust your body to tell you this information, and it is likely that, through dieting and eating for emotional reasons, you have lost touch with these sensations. Because you

are a "new creation in Christ," with a spirit of self-control, you can expect your body to tell you when you are hungry, when you are no longer hungry, and what you are hungry for. A "natural eater" eats when hungry, quits eating when she's had enough, and eats what she really wants to eat.

7. Because there is a tendency to believe that rules are what "keep us in line," you have probably engaged in some form of legalism. In terms of overeating and "fat," this usually means that you have believed that dieting is the solution to your overeating and that certain foods are "right" or "wrong." However, Scripture plainly says that rules not only fail to keep you in line, they arouse and increase your desire to break the rules. The Christian is created to live life *in the Spirit* rather than "by the law." Colossians 2:23 clearly states that rules have no power to restrain "sensual indulgences," and Galatians 5:16-25 (NASB) says that, if we "walk by the Spirit," we "will not carry out the desire of the flesh." Diets don't ultimately work, especially for Christians; life in the Spirit does.

8. Our culture (the "world system") is controlled by Satan. It is corrupt and tries to squeeze you into its mold. The world puts tremendous pressure on you to look a certain way and eat a certain way. In Romans 12:2, you are told to no longer conform to the world system but be transformed by the renewing of your mind. God wants you are to seek heavenly values over earthly values (1 Samuel 16:7b, Colossians 3:2, 1 Peter 3:3-4).

9. There are many conflicting messages in our culture about sex and sexuality. It is common for women to avoid this whole confusing and sometimes painful issue by becoming "fat." As with any other issue in your life, rather than coping through eating, you can turn to God and his truth in order to gain his perspective on sex and the role sex plays in your life. He has seen it all, and he is not too pure or holy to consider, and help you with, your hang-ups and fears regarding sex and what it means to be a woman.

10. Without even realizing it, women sometimes use their "fat" as a way to communicate with or punish their husbands. Instead of coping with marital problems through overeating, you can turn to God to love you, direct you, comfort you, and provide for you in ways your husband never can.

11. Living in the freedom from overeating that you already have includes:
    *   Acknowledging your emotions and going to God with them.
    *   Continuing to be in the process of renewing your mind as empowered by the Spirit.
    *   Not dieting, not weighing yourself.
    *   Eating when you are hungry and stopping when you are no longer hungry.
    *   When hungry, eating what you really are hungry for and not making rules about "good" and "bad" foods.
    *   Staying sensitive to what your body craves and what foods do and do not agree with you, as opposed to eating to satisfy your emotions, eating certain foods because they're on a program or supposed to be "healthy" or "legal," or eating to reward or treat yourself.
    *   Viewing your desire to eat when you are not hungry as a signal that something is going on in your thinking or beliefs or that you want something less tangible than food (such as affection or to avoid angry feelings) and then going to God for his comfort and perspective.
    *   Being willing to feel the feelings you are trying to avoid by eating. God will help you work through whatever you're feeling – anxiety, anger, depression, loneliness, etc. He wants to interact with you about everything you are feeling.
    *   Accepting your appearance as it is, not imposing false or worldly standards on yourself, and letting God determine your ultimate body size.
    *   Dwelling on the "higher" aspects of who you are, seeking character over external beauty and a relationship with God over obtaining temporal goals.

BEFORE YOU FINISH THIS BOOK

Homework Follow-up

1. What Scripture passages do you see as your "friends" in helping you remember the truth when tempted to believe lies about yourself?

2. Which concepts presented in this book do you find hard to believe? What are your reasons for not believing them, and what is it that you believe instead?

Comments on the Homework

- What Scripture passages do you see as your "friends"?

There are certain passages of Scripture that have been very, very helpful for me to have "on hand;" in other words, those I have memorized. Because I often doubt that any progress is being made in my becoming more like Christ, the verse I repeat most often to myself is Philippians 2:13 (GNT): "God is always at work in you to make you willing and able to obey his own purpose." While I was making a habit of accepting myself as beautiful no matter what my size, I not only memorized Romans 12:2, but also sang it with a little tune I made up. I would sing that in the face of commercials for diet programs and photos of models. "Do not conform any longer to the pattern of this world, but be transformed by the renewing of your mind."

Bible passages are not only encouraging words, but also tools for the Holy Spirit to use in renewing our minds.

Because the Scripture is God's Word, Bible passages are not only encouraging words, but also tools for the Holy Spirit to use in renewing our minds. Keeping some key passages stored on your hard drive, so to speak, gives the Spirit an opportunity to pull them up onto your "desktop" and work all that more effectively in lining up your thinking with God's.

- Which concepts presented in this book do you find hard to believe? What are your reasons for not believing them, and what do you believe instead?

There are sometimes theological reasons why women do not agree with the concepts regarding overweight and overeating that I present in Weight of Grace groups. However, this happens rarely. Most women, when they truly explore why they do not agree with Weight of Grace concepts, cannot find any Scripture to contradict them. Instead, what does contradict the concepts is their own deeply felt, long-held inaccurate beliefs about themselves and God. For them, the hardest hurdle is believing in something that doesn't feel right. This is where I suggest just trying new beliefs out for a while, going ahead and behaving as if one is a new creation with a pure heart and as if God really cares about your struggles, but doing it for just a few weeks or months and then evaluating the outcome.

Scripture tells us that our love for God is demonstrated in our obedience to his commandments, and that his commandments are not burdensome because God has equipped us to overcome the world through our faith in Christ (1 John 5:1-5). Our love for God is not just a mushy feeling, but provides the power to act in faith. And, this is almost always apart from our feelings, at first. There are several behaviors and concepts that feel foreign to us, but that is only because they are untried. The ways we have been used to behaving and what we have been used to believing have resulted in emotional pain – frustration, hopelessness, guilt. Though familiar, those behaviors and beliefs are really what's foreign – to the person God created you to be.

Ask God to help you assimilate the concepts presented in this book that he knows will be most transforming for you. Prayerfully explore some of the suggested follow-up materials that present concepts along the same lines. The Spirit is the one who guides us into all truth (John 16:13), as long as we are willing to hear it from him and are not blocking out the truth with our own preconceived notions.

God is extremely interested in leading you into the freedom from overeating that you already have in Christ. I trust that, as you pursue your relationship with him, you will experience his grace and know what it is to "live self-controlled, upright and godly lives in this present age" (Titus 2:12).

Most women, when they truly explore why they do not agree with Weight of Grace concepts, cannot find any Scripture to contradict them. Instead, what does contradict the concepts is their own deeply felt, long-held inaccurate beliefs about themselves and God.

God is extremely interested in leading you into the freedom from overeating that you already have in Christ.

Addendum One

"FatherCare," a manuscript reproduced by permission of
Scope Ministries International, Inc.
700 N.E. 63rd Street
Oklahoma City, OK 73105
405-843-7778
www.scopeministries.org

FatherCare

A Fresh Perspective on the Character of God

INTRODUCTION

Jesus came to reveal the Father! (John 1:18; 10:30; 14:7,9) All that He did, all that He said, all the miracles He performed demonstrated this amazing truth. It was in the humanity of our Lord Jesus that the Father found full and free expression as our Father. The life that Jesus lived and the death that He died was a deliberate act of revealing to humanity God the Father.

In essence, Jesus was the Father here on earth! Time and time again Jesus reiterated this truth—John 5:19-26; 8:18,29,42,54; 10:30; 14:1-13. It is an inescapable fact that Jesus was on earth what the Father is in heaven. **God stepped out of heaven and became a man in the Person of our Lord Jesus Christ so that a Father's love and care could and would be demonstrated in person to heal and comfort those who were so desperately hurting.**

My own personal experience in counseling and ministering to literally thousands of Christians demonstrates that most believers hold an erroneous view of God as Father. What has happened is that they have based their own concept of the Father, not on the inspired Word of God, but on their own past relationship with their earthly fathers, good or bad. It is no small wonder then that the Church is weak and frail – **it knows not the Father!**

You don't trust a stranger, much less love him. To a great host of believers, the Father is some vague, spiritual being or some "cosmic policeman," who is ten million light years away. For all practical purposes He is a stranger to them. **How can we put any confidence in One we hardly know?** (See Psalm 9:10.) The answer is that we don't! Yet, James warns us of the emotional consequences when we lack confidence in God (James 1:6).

How can we break this belief system that has substituted an earthly father for the Heavenly Father? **The answer to this dilemma lies in the Person of our Lord Jesus Christ.** We must learn to see the Father in Him. As we do, the Holy Spirit will begin to change our own erroneous concepts of the Father into the correct one with all of the accompanying benefits.

Within the confines of our evangelical faith we have so sought to identify with Jesus that we have failed to see Him in His primary role, that of revealing the Father. Also, in an emphasis on seeking the Spirit and His gifts, we have also lost sight of the Father. **Jesus is not a substitute for the Father; He is the essence of the Father on earth.**

Paul wrote to the believers at Colosse:

> **For in His physical body every attribute of the Godhead continuously and permanently dwells.** Colossians 2:9, paraphrase

Simply stated, this means that every attribute, every characteristic of the Father exists in the Person of our Lord Jesus Christ. All that the Father is, is in Jesus. **So, we must view Jesus as revealing the Father.** Otherwise, we will miss what he came to do – **UNVEIL THE FATHER.**

FATHERCARE

Life is made up of relationships – some good, some bad – but all necessary. The Bible is God's inspired textbook on relationships. It is important to recognize the basic common denominator inherent in all relationships; that is, the foundational relationship from which all relationships originate, man's relationship to God, the Father/child relationship. It is this Father/child relationship that made Adam's interaction with God so unique, and it was the Father/child relationship that was lost at the Fall, thereby making man's life so desperate.

History shows us that men have always sought after God. Even from the earliest and most primitive of cultures, there has been a pattern of worship – of man's attempt to restore the lost Father/child relationship. However, it does not lie within the capabilities of man to restore this lost relationship. It has to be done by God. From God's perspective, the restoration of the Father/child relationship was so important that He stepped out of heaven in the Person of Jesus Christ to initiate and accomplish the process of restoring the Father/child relationship.

At the same time, the restoration of the Father/child relationship is so frighteningly threatening to Satan that he has made every attempt to hinder and confuse the process of that restoration (2 Corinthians 4:4). For a child of God to know God as Father brings that child into such intimacy with God, producing such worship of God and service for God, that the whole hierarchy of the evil one is threatened.

As we being this study, I want you to do an exercise. Write out a paragraph on who your father was to you as a person. Stop reading here and do that now:

_____

_____

_____

_____

Believe it or not, years of having counselees do this exercise show that you have just described your concept of God as Father! That's right, most people transfer their experiential knowledge of their earthly fathers to the Heavenly Father. This is Satan's masterstroke of confusing the issue, and it is the reason why the vast majority of Christians have either an erroneous or, at the least, a very nebulous concept of God as their Father.

I once asked a missionary, who had come for counseling, to write out who her father was to her as a person. Later, I had her write out who the Father was to her as a Person. It stunned her to realize that she had written out basically the same thing for both. That was not an isolated case. I have found that most Christians have done this. Read a few of the comments that were received from hundreds of surveys taken with teens. The surveys asked them who their fathers were to them and who the Heavenly Father was to them as a Person. The surveys were taken at Christian conferences across the country and those surveyed indicated that they were Christians, active both in their churches and in the organization that sponsored the conferences.

Jennifer, age 15: *My father is a two-faced, irresponsible, mean S.O.B. Always perfect, nobody can ever do anything right. He is selfish and cruel. ... There is no way I can picture God as my Father.*

Lee Ann, age 14: *My dad always seemed sort of far away. It's like he wants to love me, but he doesn't know how to. ... God is sort of distant and hard to reach.*

Kristy, age 17: *Don't have and never knew my real father. ... God is someone who sits on a white throne.*

Tammi, age 15: *My daddy loves me a lot, I think, but I am not sure 'cause my parents are divorced and I haven't seen my father in five years. ... The Father to me is my protector and guide. Sometimes I feel like He doesn't love me as much as other people.*

Chris, age 19: *I hardly know my father. He has always been too busy working to spend time with me and the rest of the family. ... My heavenly Father I think of similarly as my earthly father in that at times I think He's far off and too busy.*

I could multiply what was said by these young people hundreds of times by the adults who have come in for counseling. What I have found is a profound ignorance on the part of Christians about who God is as their Father. The result of this ignorance is far-reaching, affecting the Christian both spiritually and emotionally.

This phenomenon is particularly disturbing when we realize the importance that the Bible puts on knowing God. In fact, for us to know God as our Father is so critically important that God, in the Person of Jesus Christ, stepped out of heaven to reveal Him. The Bible demonstrates that all Jesus did, all that He said, was for this one single purpose of revealing God as our Father. What man had lost at the Fall – the Father/child relationship that existed between Adam and God – God was determined to restore through Jesus Christ!

Studying how Christ revealed the Father is a study that can revolutionize your life, because it brings you into an intimacy with God as your Father that you have not experienced before. The importance of this knowledge is attested to, not only in Scriptures, but by the great authors of Christendom. For example, J. I. Packer, in his book, *Knowing God*, says, "It is the most practical project anyone can engage in. ... Knowing about God is crucially important for the living of our lives."[1]

Kittle's *Theological Dictionary of the New Testament* says this:

> The glorifying of God's name is effected by Christ's work, and to this again it belongs that Jesus should reveal God's name to men as that of the Father. God's name is obscure to men; it is strange and general. But to those whom the Father has given Him, Jesus makes this name manifest, certain, and plain, so that it again acquires specific content: Father.[2]

I have stated over and over again, not only to counselees, but to Christian groups everywhere, that it is imperative for the Christian to know God as Father. A great deal of the Christian's emotional and spiritual problems can be laid at the feet of ignorance, ignorance of God and who He is as Father.

Why Is It Important to Know God as Father?

First, it is important to know God as Father because the Bible commands that we know God.

> ... that the God of our Lord Jesus Christ, the Father of glory, may give to you a spirit of wisdom and of revelation in the knowledge of Him.
>
> Ephesians 1:17, NASB

> But from there you will seek the Lord your God, and you will find Him if you search for Him with all your heart and all your soul.   Deuteronomy 4:29, NASB

> And He said to them, "You shall love the Lord your God with all your heart, and with all your soul, and with all your mind."   Matthew 22:37 NASB

> And those that know Thy name will put their trust in Thee. Psalm 9:10a, NASB

> I have manifested Your name—I have revealed Your very Self, Your real Self— to the people You have given Me out of the world. They were Yours, and You gave them to Me, and they have obeyed and kept your Word.
>
> John 17:6, AMP

To know God intimately, as God desires us to know Him, we need to know Him as Father. It is one thing to know God through His attributes, but it is quite another to know Him as Father. To know God only through His attributes tends toward a sterile, non-intimate relationship, while knowing Him as Father creates an awesome intimacy.

It is an astounding thing to read the Scripture and realize that God, the absolute Sovereign of the universe, desires that we should know Him, and that He should make it possible for us to do so. I repeat, **Christ's primary purpose of coming to this sin-ridden planet was to reveal God as Father, so that we, as his children, might enjoy that Father/child relationship that once existed between God and Adam.**

The very fact that God in the Person of Jesus did come to this earth to reveal the Father shows the importance God attaches to knowing Him. All that Jesus did and all that He said was to make God known as Father. By His life He gave content to the word "Father." It is interesting to note that the word "father" is used 418 times in the New Testament, and over half of the references, some 264, are of God as Father.

Jesus said:

> I and the Father are one.   John 10:30, NASB

> If you had known Me, you would have known My Father also; from now on you know Him, and have seen Him. ... He who has seen Me has seen the Father. ... Do you not believe that I am in the Father, and the Father is in Me? The words that I say to you I do not speak on My own initiative, but the Father abiding in Me does His works.   John 14:7, 9b, 10, NASB

> But He answered them, "My Father is working until now, and I Myself am working. ... Truly, truly, I say to you, the Son can do nothing of Himself, unless it is something He sees the Father doing; for whatever the Father does, these things the Son also does in like manner. For the Father loves the Son,

and shows Him all things that He Himself is doing; and greater works than these will He show Him that you may marvel." John 5:17, 19-20, NASB

Not only are we commanded to know God, but second, knowing God as Father is important for giving meaning to our lives. Packer puts it well:

> Knowing about God is crucially important for the living of our lives. As it would be cruel to an Amazonian tribesman to fly him to London, put him down without an explanation in Trafalgar Square and leave him, as one who knows nothing of English or England, to fend for himself, so we are cruel to ourselves if we try to live in this world without knowing about the God whose world it is and who runs it. The world becomes a strange, mad, painful place, and life in it a disappointing and unpleasant business, for those who do not know about God. Disregard the study of God, and you sentence yourself to stumble and blunder through life blindfolded, as it were, with no sense of direction and no understanding of what surrounds you. This way you can waste your life and lose your soul.[3]

Third, it is important for the Christian to know God as Father for his emotional and spiritual well-being. A person cannot and will not trust a stranger. If God as Father is a stranger to us, for whatever the reason, we cannot and will not trust Him (Psalm 9:10). If we can't trust Him, we will doubt Him. And our doubts about God, while we try to live for God, produce a contradiction in our lives that creates tremendous emotional and spiritual stress (James 1:6). I have yet to have someone come in for counseling who was suffering from emotional stress and turmoil and had a good, Biblical concept of God as Father.

As you progress in this study, you will see how crucial it is to your spiritual development to know God as Father. In fact, as you begin to grasp this great truth of God as your Father, you will realize the tremendous spiritual and emotional benefits that accrue to the Christian who gains this knowledge.

What Are the Benefits that Come from Knowing God as Father?

No relationship is more crucial to children than that of the parent/child relationship. In our culture, we sometimes forget how important the father/child relationship is. I have often stated that every daddy needs a little boy or little girl, and every little boy and little girl needs a daddy. What a loss when we realize that the average father spends approximately six minutes a day with his children. We live in a society that not only condones, but encourages, absentee fatherhood. What a refreshing and astounding difference it makes when we realize that God is our Father and is never absent, but always available to us every moment of every day.

Two passages of Scripture, among many others, confirm this fact of God's fatherhood to us:

A father of the fatherless, and a judge and protector of the widows, is God in His holy habitation. Psalm 68:5, AMP

"And I will be a Father to you, and you shall be sons and daughters to Me," **says the Lord Almighty.** 2 Corinthians 6:18, AMP

Allow me to digress here for a moment to demonstrate how easily we have been deceived into erroneous thinking about God. In this passage from the Psalms, you will note that God selects two segments of society to specifically mention, widows and orphans. It is interesting to note that at the time of this writing, both widows and orphans were considered a detriment to society, a non-productive drain upon the culture.

In this passage, God is called a "judge." Now what image comes to your mind when you think of a judge? Normally, we see in our mind's eye an image of a judge behind his bench, dispensing justice from his perspective – and we feel guilty. Place this mental image of a judge over onto God and we come up with the concept of a "cosmic policeman" just waiting for us to step out of line.

However, God is *not* a judge in that sense. First, all judgment has been placed in Christ (John 5:22). Second, there is no condemnation to those who are in Christ (Romans 8:1). Third, all of our punishment was placed on Christ (Isaiah 53:5). Fourth, God doesn't remember our sins and transgression (Hebrews 10:17). Fifth, our transgression is forgiven and our sins covered (Psalm 32:1). So, if God is not a judge in the way we conceive of a judge, then how are we to define the way "judge" is used in Psalm 68:5?

The way that the word "judge" is used here is "one who evaluates worth"!!! Get this, for it is important – God as Judge is not one who condemns, but one who evaluates what is of worth. In this passage, He is evaluating as worthy the two segments of society which were considered worthless. **Therefore, God doesn't judge you in the sense of passing judgment unto condemnation, but He evaluates your absolute WORTHINESS!!!**

Now, what is a father? William Barclay says this:

> There are two English words which are closely connected, but whose meanings are widely different. There is the word "paternity" and the word "fatherhood." "Paternity" describes a relationship in which a father is responsible for the physical existence of a son; but, as far as paternity goes, it can be, and it not infrequently happens, that the father has never even set eyes on the son, and would not even recognize him if in later years he met him. "Fatherhood" describes an intimate, loving, continuous relationship in which father and son grow closer to each other every day.[4]

It is this "fatherhood" that describes God's relationship to us. Thus, this is the greatest benefit of all in knowing God as Father – a continuing, growing intimacy with the Father.

However, this tends not to be our experience because on what basis do we build our concept of the Father? Humanly speaking, we establish father concepts through experiential relationships with our earthly fathers. Unfortunately, this produces erroneous concepts of a true father, because there is no absolutely perfect human father who can provide a role model for us.

Therefore, it is only through the Bible, our absolute standard of truth, that we can know what a father truly should be. It is the Bible that shows us, in the humanity of Jesus as He lived His life here on earth, the perfect role model as to what a true father is. It is there in the pages of Scripture that we see Jesus as the Father, a real Father in action.

What I am saying is that our normal father concepts tend to be erroneous, and it is only through the love and care of God, as we know Him as Father, that we can establish the proper concept of "father." It is in this Biblical dimension that we discover what a father truly is, that is, by seeing, in the Person of Jesus Christ, the Father at work here in our lives on earth!

A true father, a perfect father, a caring father is one who has the ability and desire to meet his children's deepest needs. And, what are our deepest needs? Let us discuss six of them:

- the need to worship
- the need to be loved and to belong
- the need for well-being
- the need to feel secure
- the need for approval
- the need for acceptance

The Need to Worship

Most people would probably not list worship as one of their deeply felt needs, but it is man's most vital need because man was created for worship and to worship. Worship denied or wrongly expressed can and will cause wrong and/or harmful spiritual and emotional problems, as well as wrong behavior.

The word "worship" comes from the Anglo-Saxon word *weorthscipe*, which evolved into the word *worthship* and then into "worship." Worship is ascribing worth to someone or something. Man was not designed to live independent from God, but to commune intimately with, and totally depend upon, God. In order to live life as it was meant to be lived, to its fullest, man must ascribe to God His ascendant, infinite, absolute worth, His "first-place-ness." Man must worship. Without worship, we do not have God in His rightful place and, therefore, everything else in life is totally out of place. Right worship is ascribing to God His worth and worthiness.

It is through worship, right worship, that we come to know God and experience His love and care. Worship and intimacy are related. The greater the worship, the greater the intensity of intimacy. This is what our Father desires, an intimate relationship with us, His children. When His Spirit indwells us at our rebirth in Christ, He gives us the ability to rightly worship Him, to place Him in His rightful position, to honor Him and, therefore, to return to our deep dependence upon Him in every aspect of our lives – in other words, to be in an intimate, right relationship with our Father.

In a day and age where "self worth" is said to be man's basic need, we need to realize that worth, true worth – a true understanding of who we really are – can only come through worship, right worship – a true understanding of who God really is as the One of ultimate worth. In a sense, that is what this study is all about – to introduce you to who He really is: our loving heavenly Father, the One who meets all our needs out of His love, the One who is worthy of our worship, the only One who can fulfill our need to worship, because of His perfection and greatness and selflessness.

The Need to Be Loved and to Belong

Probably no other words so characterizes Christianity as does the word "love." The profound mystic of the Christian faith is the overwhelming, overpowering, compelling unconditional love that flows from the pages of God's Word. It is a very basic, deeply felt need in all of our lives. We crave love – not a conditional love based on what we have or on what we are able to achieve, but an unconditional love, based upon who we are.

We need to love and be loved. It is the indispensable dynamic of our existence. And, our ability to love and be loved is directly related to our knowledge of God as our Father. The Bible says it best:

> **We love, because He first loved us.** 1 John 4:19, NASB

Two words characterize our Father's love for us and to us. The first word is found in Ephesians 2:4, where the word "great" is associated with God's love for us. The second is found in 1 John 3:1, where the word "manner" (KJV) is associated with God's love.

The word "great" in the Greek is *polus* and signifies "much, many, or abundance." Here I think the word "magnificence" would best describe this love – a superabundance and overflowing of love from our Father to us. The word "manner" in the Greek is *potapos*, and Kenneth S. Wuest says, "The word speaks of something foreign. The translation could read, 'Behold what foreign kind of love the Father has bestowed upon us.'"[5] Actually, our words "exotic" or "incredible" would be suitable translations. What we are being told about our Father's love to us and for us is that it is **INCREDIBLY MAGNIFICENT!!!**

It is said that the love of God must have arms, and we are the arms through which the love of God is demonstrated. Let me share an incident that illustrates God's love for us. My wife, Doris, and I have five children – four boys and a girl. Our daughter is the youngest and the first girl in three generations of Craddocks. You can imagine the fuss made over this little piece of femininity when she pushed her way into this world. But the impact upon Danny, the youngest of the four boys, was something else. What do you do when you have three older brothers and, suddenly out of nowhere, comes a sister who steals the limelight? What you do is break the mold, and that is just what Danny did.

I could write a book about Danny. I will someday when I can safely change the names to protect the guilty. This boy could do more, get into more trouble, find the dirtiest mud hole, create more commotion than all the rest of our kids put together.

When Danny was a preschooler he was always going to marry one of the cute girls on our staff. He invariably had a crush on one or more of them, depending on who was the cutest and most responsive. One Sunday afternoon we had a rather formal tea to introduce new staff members. One young woman, Arlys, was a lovely brunette who came dressed in the prettiest, filmiest, whitest dress you ever saw. She was absolutely breathtaking.

As we adults were chatting, in came Danny, moving along with his dust cloud and looking like he just invented twelve new ways to incorporate dirt and mud into his four-year-old body. Just as he was about to head out the front door, out of the corner of his eye he caught a glimpse of this lovely girl in white and, in a second, he was up in her lap, hugging the life out of her.

I almost fainted. All I could see was a dirty, grimy little guy who was messing up the whitest dress in the room. But all Arlys could see was a little guy who needed loving, and she just loved on and hugged on him as though he were the only little guy in all the world.

God taught me something in that moment. We tend to look at ourselves as though we are the dirty, grimy guys, but God as our Father sees us only as little guys and gals who need lots of loving, and that is why His love is **INCREDIBLY MAGNIFICENT!**

Belonging to God allows us to fulfill the flip side of this need, that of belonging to others. God created us as social beings. He meant for us to relate to one another. In Genesis 2, God said that it wasn't good for man to be alone. The word "alone" in the Hebrew means "to be isolated." No one is an island unto himself. We need to belong.

If we are rightly related to God, enjoying the intimacy of right worship, then He becomes the prime mover in bringing other people into our lives to fulfill the need for belonging. How? He does this through the Church! – a family of like-minded people, born of His Spirit, enjoying oneness in His Spirit, learning to care for one another. Here is where the need to belong can be and should be met.

The Need for Well-Being

Solomon wrote, "All a man's labor is for his mouth and yet the appetite is not satisfied" (Ecclesiastes 6:7, NASB). Man is driven to secure the basics of life – food, clothing and shelter. And once these are secured, man looks for emotional well-being.

However, our Lord made it quite clear in Matthew 6 that a sense of well-being comes, not through what we have or what we can get, but from who our Father is!

> **...do not be anxious for your life, as to what you shall eat, or what you shall drink; nor for your body, as to what you shall put on. Is not life more than food, and the body than clothing? Look at the birds of the air, that they do not sow, neither do they reap, nor gather into barns, and yet your heavenly Father feeds them. Are you not worth much more than they? ... Observe how the lilies of the field grow; they do not toil nor do they spin, yet I say to you that even Solomon in all his glory did not clothe himself like one of these. But if God so arrays the grass of the field, which is alive today and tomorrow is thrown into the furnace, will He not much more do so for you...? Do not be anxious, then, saying, "What shall we eat?" or "What shall we drink?" or "With what shall we clothe ourselves?" For all these things the Gentiles eagerly seek; for your heavenly Father knows that you need all these things. But seek first His kingdom and His righteousness; and all these things shall be added to you.**
> Matthew 6:25-26, 28-33, NASB

We are to seek, first, His kingdom and His righteousness, and then all these things *will* be ours. Our Father promises to meet all of our needs, but only *He* can meet them. Our pursuit of them only leads to failure and frustration. As we relate to our Father, He opens our eyes to see His abundant provision, to see that our well-being is a need He eagerly desires to fulfill.

The Need to Feel Secure

A father is one who provides security. **God our Father guarantees personal security**. This personal sense of security is affirmed and reinforced by the use of the term "Abba Father" in the Bible (Mark 14:36; Romans 8:15; Galatians 4:6). The word *abba* is a transliteration from an Aramaic word that signifies the first words a little baby says of its father. Our modern-day counterpart would be "da da." In other words, the best translation of the word *abba* would be "daddy"!! That is right. God is our "Daddy"! And I am not being disrespectful in the least.

The two words used in unison, "Abba Father," have great significance. The first demonstrates the childlike faith the believer is to have in his heavenly Father, followed by an adult appreciation of that childlike faith.

Let me share a personal chapter out of my own life that will illustrate the security that a daddy brings. When I was quite small, one of the "fun-est" things of all was to get a penny or two and go to Pinelli's corner grocery store and buy some candy. In those days a penny could go a long way toward corrupting a five-year-old addicted to candy. I can remember going to that store and yearningly looking over every piece of candy displayed in the case. I would pick and choose, drooling over what I couldn't afford, changing my mind constantly, asking dozens of questions, taking forever. (Of course, I was driving "old Man Pinelli" crazy in the process.)

However, there was a problem with getting my candy. To get to Pinelli's grocery store, I had to go up a block and over two blocks. This wasn't so bad, but situated at the strategic point midway between my house and Pinelli's was the biggest, ugliest four-foot bully you ever saw. He made the Incredible Hulk look like a ballet dancer. This bully and his buddy had a nasty habit of shaking me down for my pennies. (By the way, when you are three and a half feet tall, a four-foot bully looks immense.) Whenever this happened, I would return home blubbering about the threat to my life and the assault on my funds. I remember my dad telling me to stand up for my rights, but being of sound mind, and not necessarily suicidally depressed, I rejected that advice forthwith.

About the third time this degrading, depriving experience occurred, my dad told me that he would sneak up the alley, and if these two nemeses of my candy run interfered, he would handle them. Well, I can't begin to tell you the difference in my attitude. I was cock-o'-the- walk. I made faces at those two bullies. I flipped my pennies to let them know I was going to get some candy. In short, I was acutely obnoxious. However, I kept looking over my shoulder to make sure that my daddy was there. As long as I knew he was there, I had all the security in the world.

Of course, the moral to the story is that when we know God as our Father, as our *Abba*, our "Daddy," then we have that profound sense of personal security and safety. No matter what we face, the obstacles that lie in our paths, the struggles in our lives, our Father is there!!! He will never leave us nor forsake us! (Hebrews 13:5)

The Need for Approval

Approval comes in many forms, and we all desire it. Everyone desperately seeks parental approval, and when it is not forthcoming, it creates real problems. As Christians we constantly seek God's approval. Jesus said, "Well done thou good and faithful servant" (Matthew 25:22). Proverbs says to give a pat on the back to whom it is due (Proverbs 3:27). Approval is a basic need of life. Through my counseling I have found that men who are younger than forty drive for success, while men over forty seek significance. Both are indicative of a need for approval. Since significance is so closely related to approval, let us look at it for a moment.

Have you ever thought what it is that gives significance? The early Greeks felt that it was determined by parentage. They felt a noble mind and virtue were inherited and could not be acquired.[6] In the rabbinical culture of Paul, his significance was based upon his being Jewish and a Pharisee, on belonging to the tribe of Benjamin and on his learning within the rabbinical schools (Philippians 3:5-6). In our day and age, significance is based upon performance, on what we are able to achieve, on credentials and on what we have. Notice in all these that significance is based on external factors, not internal ones.

Why is significance so important to us? Because it makes us "someone." It allows us to stand apart and above the crowd. It gives us the sense of approval we so deeply desire. But more importantly, in this mixed up, crazy world of ours, it is our way to try to gain a sense of worth. In the world system in which we operate, our approval and, hence, our significance, does not come from our inward sense of worth, but from our accomplishments achieved outwardly. The Biblical pattern is just the reverse.

The drive for approval is so strong that men will neglect their families, their health, all that they have, to gain it. Women will risk their happiness, their children, their futures, everything, to gain it. Why? Because we want so deeply to be somebody, to stand apart from the crowd, to leave an indelible mark on history, to stand approved before men. This drive explains why one survey I saw in a newspaper showed 82 percent of all American men were unhappy with their present employment and were considering changing jobs. A great number of men make a change as they enter their forties because they feel it is their last chance to make an impact upon their world and, thus, their last change for gaining approval.

The Bible tells us that God gives His approval unconditionally in Christ! (Colossians 1:22) But how do we then, as Christians, gain a sense of this approval/significance? Is it through performance or achievement? Is it doing, is it having, or is it through some other means? Obviously, it is through God's means and not through man's efforts. Our Father is far more concerned with who we are than in what we do. In other words, as far as the Bible is concerned, approval and significance is related to **BEING**, not doing. Real, lasting approval comes from a relationship with the Father that insures us that we are His children.

I have mentioned some aspects of what a father is, but there is another factor which would normally go without saying, and that is that a father is one who has children. Really profound, you say! Yes, it is when you consider who the Father is and what that makes us as His children. Under the inspiration of the Holy Spirit, Paul quoted to the Corinthians an astounding truth from 2 Samuel:

> **And I will be a Father to you, and you shall be My sons and daughters, says the Lord Almighty.** 2 Corinthians 6:18, AMP

God, the almighty, majestic God of the universe is our Father!!! This means that we really do have a Father who is **consistent**, who is **kind** and **caring**, **loving** and **thoughtful**. We have a Father who **cherishes** us, who is happy when we are happy, sad when we are sad. He is a Father who brings immeasurable fullness into our lives.

On what basis can I as a Christian really know that I am truly a child of God? How can I have that personal security and knowledge that God accepts me and saves me once for all, for all eternity – that I have the ultimate approval? The assurance that we need can be summed up in one Biblical word, "**ADOPTION**"! However, it is important that you realize that the Biblical concept of adoption is totally different from our idea of adoption today. Our use of the word "adoption" involves children, while the Biblical use of the word involves adults. In other words, we are adopted by God as adult sons and daughters, not just as small children.

The word "adoption" in the Greek is *huiothesias* and is used only five times in the New Testament. This kind of adoption was peculiar to the Romans and was unknown to either the Greek or Jew.[7] It spells out in detail what God has in mind when he uses it in regard to us. William Barclay gives us a most graphic description of Roman adoption in his commentary on Romans 8:12-17.

It is only when we understand how serious and complicated a step Roman adoption was that we really understand the depth of meaning of this passage. Roman adoption was always rendered more serious and more difficult by the Roman *patria potestas*. The *patria potestas* was the father's absolute power over his family; that power was absolute; it was actually the power of absolute disposal and control, and in the early days it was actually the power of life and death. In regard to his father, a Roman son never came of age. No matter how old he was, he was still under the *patria potestas*, in the absolute possession, and under the absolute control, of his father. Obviously this made adoption into another family a very difficult and a very serious step. In adoption a person had to pass from one *patria potestas* to another. He had to pass out of the possession and control of one father into the equally absolute possession and control of another. There were two steps. The first was known as *mancipatio*, and it was carried out by a symbolic sale, in which copper and scales were symbolically used. Three times the symbolism of sale was carried out. Twice the father symbolically sold his son, and twice he bought him back; and the third time he did not buy him back, and thus the *patria potestas* was held to be broken. After the sale there followed a ceremony called *vindicatio*. The adopting father went to the *praetor*, one of the Roman magistrates, and presented a legal case for the transference of the person to be adopted in his *patria potestas*. When all this was completed then the adoption was complete. Clearly this was a serious and impressive step.

But it is the consequences of adoption which are most significant for the picture that is in Paul's mind. There were four main consequences. (i) The adopted person lost all rights in his old family, and gained all the rights of a fully legitimate son in his new family. In the most literal sense, and the most binding legal way, he got a new father. (ii) It followed that he became heir to his new father's estate. Even if other sons were afterwards born, who were real blood relations, it did not affect his rights. He was inalienably co-heir with them. (iii) In law, the old life of the adopted person was completely wiped out. For instance, legally all debts were canceled; they were wiped out as if they had never been. The adopted person was regarded as a new person entering into a new life with which the past had nothing to do. (iv) In the eyes of the law the adopted person was literally and absolutely the son of his new father.

That is what Paul is thinking of. He uses still another picture from Roman adoption. He says that God's Spirit witnesses with our spirit that we really are the children of God. The adoption ceremony was carried out in the presence of seven witnesses. Now, suppose the adopting father died, and then suppose that there was some dispute about the right of the adopted son to inherit, one or more of the seven original witnesses stepped forward and swore that the adoption was genuine and true. Thus the right of the adopted person was guaranteed and he entered into his inheritance. So, Paul is saying, it is the Holy Spirit Himself who is the witness to our adoption into the family of God.

We see then that every step of Roman adoption was meaningful in the mind of Paul when he transferred the picture of adoption into the family of God. Once we were in absolute possession of sin, in absolute control of our own sinful nature; but God, in His mercy, has brought us into absolute possession of Himself. The old life has no more rights over us; God has an absolute right. The past is canceled; the debts of the past are wiped out; we begin again a new life, a life with God. We become heirs of all the riches of God. If that is so, we become joint-heirs with Jesus Christ, God's own Son. That which Christ inherited, and inherits, we also inherit.

It was Paul's picture that when a man became a Christian he entered into the very family of God. He did nothing to earn it; he did nothing to deserve it; God, the great Father in His amazing love and mercy, has taken the lost, helpless, poverty-stricken, debt-laden sinner and adopted him into His own family, so that the debts are canceled and the unearned love and glory inherited.[8]

What Biblical adoption means is that, as a Christian, you are a chosen child of God and God is your Father. He has adopted you as a son or daughter into His family. It means that nothing can ever change that fact – nothing you can do or ever will do changes the fact that you are an adopted child of God. You are indelibly written in the Lamb's book of life forever and ever. And because you are adopted, you are destined to an eternity with the greatest Father in all the universe.

What does this have to do with approval? Medical science tells us that we are the sum total of our parents' genes, a blending of the two. To a large degree, I am what they are. So it is with the new birth. I become one with my Father in heaven. I become in reality an image-bearer, having been created in the image of God. What greater approval and significance can there be than to realize that, as Christians, we are children of the Most High and Holy God? What is so amazing is that God gives so unconditionally – His love, His care and, of course, His approval.

One time, after I led a Bible study, a young mother approached me and requested to see me for counseling. Later, in the privacy of my office, she shared with me about a childhood with a demanding, demeaning father. No matter what she did, it was never good enough. She could never quite measure up to her father's expectations. Even though her father had been dead for a number of years, she was still in a desperate search for his approval.

I wish this were an isolated case, but it isn't. One of the strongest drives of a person's life is for parental approval. And, the higher the expectations of the parent, the harder it is to gain a sense of his or her approval.

What makes it all so hard is that God created man to be loved, accepted, approved, and understood unconditionally. I mean by this that there is innately in us the expectation and need to be received unconditionally. However, we are born into a world system that receives no one unconditionally, but only conditionally based on what a person is able to do, achieve or have. Every person born into this world discovers that there is a direct contradiction between the desire to be received unconditionally and the world's refusal to honor that need. This contradiction produces enormous stress, especially in light of the tremendous drive that we all have for approval.

At the Fall, man's concept of God was shattered and replaced with an erroneous mindset. Man then had no absolute basis of worth, so his own identity was shattered. Because man had no basis of unconditional worth, he had to compensate. He did this by adopting a compensating system of self-imposed standards, which would allow him to gain conditionally what was denied him unconditionally. He tried to gain worth and significance through his performance rather than in his being as was God's original plan before sin entered into the picture.

What happens is that a person is born into a world system with no basis of unconditional worth. This guarantees a poor identity or poor self-image. Therefore, a person doesn't consider himself worthy enough to receive anything unconditionally. Still, those inward drives and needs for approval must be satisfied, so we all opt for a compensating system of self-imposed rules and regulations, standards by which we can measure ourselves and gain the "strokes" we feel we need.

I call this compensating system the "Torah Syndrome." In Hebrew, *torah* means "the embodiment of the law." What we do is impose upon ourselves a standard or "law" to gain "strokes." In other words, if I don't get what I need unconditionally, I impose upon myself a standard which, if I keep it, can give me conditionally what I desire emotionally. For example, I might decide, "If I make straight A's, then I'll know I'm worthy." Usually we have an elaborate set of such rules for ourselves. They enable us to measure our worth through performance.

Reflect back for a moment to your own childhood. Think of the system you adopted to gain approval from your parents. What did you do to be thought of as a good little boy or girl? Every family has their limits and standards. Approval comes, not from who we are, but from our ability to meet these limits and standards. If you do "this and this and this," then you receive the approval you are looking for. This forces you into a performance bias, which sets the stage for the "Torah Syndrome" you create for yourself as an adult.

The moment we impose upon ourselves standards to gain approval, we deny the innate desire for unconditional approval and acceptance. Therefore, we are doomed to failure. We can never do enough, achieve enough, have enough to satisfy that longing. We keep thinking that more standards will provide that sense of approval, but what we really want is *unconditional* approval. Getting caught up in this "Torah Syndrome" causes many Christians to suffer nervous breakdowns.

However, our Father, who created us to be received unconditionally, does receive us unconditionally. His approval is given on the basis of who He has made us to be in Christ, not on the basis of what we do. He loves us, he accepts us, he approves of us as His children.

A story, again involving Danny, my youngest son, demonstrates this unconditional receiving. Danny was accident-prone. Twice, firemen in large ladder trucks had to rescue him from the heights of enormous trees. His body is riddled with the scars from hundreds of stitches. When he was two and a half, it took seven stitches to repair his head when he got too curious about the neighbor digging out a cistern. At three, he cut his finger off in a car door. (Thankfully, a surgeon restored it.) When he was four, it took over a hundred stitches to repair a leg cut open when he fell. What all this did was to build into Danny a healthy fear of anyone in a white smock!

So, when Danny began to complain of a toothache, I took him to a dentist friend of mine; but when Danny saw the white smock, he figured that here was more pain. He fought for his life. In about fifteen minutes, my friend came out and asked me to take Danny somewhere else (like to a home for incorrigible children).

I had another friend named Charley Brown (really), who was a dentist. Charley told me that he could handle Danny. He said he had had twenty hours of child psychology and this was a good opportunity to put into practice what he had learned.

When we arrived at Charley's office, I offered to help out, but it was felt that I would be more of a hindrance than a help. So, I sat in the foyer listening to the shouts, cries, thudding, etc., until finally Charley came out and asked me to come in. It seemed that when he held Danny's arms with one hand and the drill with the other, with the nurse holding Danny's feet, there was no way to get Danny to open his mouth. Here I am afraid that I destroyed in twenty minutes twenty hours of child psychology. I took off my belt (I refer to this as B-therapy) and told Danny if he didn't open his mouth, I would apply B-therapy.

For four sessions, Charley labored with Danny, along with "the belt and I," through all the strugglings, cryings and fightings that only a pain-enlightened four year old can produce. Finally, when it was all through, we were seated in Charley's office when Charley came in, sat down and, without a word, caught Danny up and hugged and loved on him and said, "Danny, I love you!"

Now Danny knew that he had done nothing to deserve this kind of unconditional approval. In fact, if he had gotten what he deserved, he wouldn't nor couldn't sit down for a week. But all the way home, Danny kept saying over and over again to me, "Daddy, that man really loved me!"

The moral of this story is that we have done nothing to deserve God's unconditional love or approval, but He gives it anyway, not on the basis of what we have or haven't done, but on the basis of His Beloved Son. You can't earn God's approval. All of your little systems to gain God's "strokes" won't work with Him. He gives you His approval unconditionally. You simply are to receive it in faith! We could say then with Packer:

> There is tremendous relief in knowing that His love for me is utterly realistic, based at every point on prior knowledge of the worst about me, so that nothing I can do will disillusion Him about me.[9]

The Father knows it all, and He gives you His approval still.

The Need for Acceptance

Approval and acceptance are very closely related. If we feel approved, we will feel accepted. Unfortunately, many Christians do not feel approved or accepted by God. This happened in my case. As a new Christian, I was taught that God didn't love me, but rather he loved the Christ in me. In fact, I was told by many a preacher that there was no good thing in me and that, because of sin, God could only stand to look at me through "rose-colored glasses." The rose-colored glasses represented the blood of the Lord Jesus. All of this really tended to reinforce my own poor self-image.

What a tragedy that a lie of the pit is preached as though it were the truth of heaven. How ridiculous! God doesn't love the Christ in me. **He loves me!** Of course, He loves His Son. That isn't even the issue. The issue is that He loves me, He accepts me unconditionally. It isn't the Christ in me that makes me acceptable to God. It is what Christ did on the cross that makes me acceptable to Him. And God, my Father, accepts me, Jim Craddock, with all my hang-ups, with all my sins, with all my idiosyncrasies, as a person, unconditionally.

For years, as a Christian involved in Christian work, I never believed that God could or would accept me unconditionally. How could He? There was no good thing in me. Well meaning men did me and many, many others a great disservice by telling me this. But, it was through the greatest crisis of my life up to that time that I discovered the truth that was to change my life.

In the ministry I was in, tremendous animosity had arisen between the president and the top directors, of which I was one. On our part, there was an unreasonable reaction to the productivity demands and a frustration over what seemed to us a dictatorial style of leadership. On the president's part, there was a lack of understanding and communication. During those tense, almost unbearable hours, as charge and countercharge were made and many unfortunate statements were said, I was struggling with my own deepened sense of inadequacy and failure. I felt that I couldn't bear what was happening to the ministry I loved and the people I respected.

During one of the breaks in the meetings, when everything seemed so hopeless, one of the directors turned to the president of the organization and said, "You know, I haven't loved you unconditionally as I should, and I just now realized it. Will you forgive me?" This was the breaking point, for from that moment on, God had the victory.

But for me, in that moment, it suddenly dawned on me that God loved me unconditionally – not the Christ in me. It was not what I was able to do for Him, but that He loved me as me. He loved me as a person, not the Christ in me, but Jim Craddock with all of his weaknesses.

It took time, but I came to experience personally His unconditional acceptance. What a relief it was not to have to struggle for his acceptance or His love and approval, but just to receive them by faith. How great it was and is to be unconditionally loved and accepted by the Father in heaven.

Relationship

I mentioned that a father is one who has children and meets the needs of those children, but there is another facet of fatherhood which I want to develop, and it is crucially important to both father and child. It is that of relationship – a relationship involving three factors: a **continuing** relationship, a **growing** relationship and an **intimate** relationship.

A true father/child relationship is always a **continuing** relationship. We see this in the parable of the prodigal son (Luke 15:11-32). Nothing that the son did affected the relationship of the father to the erring son. The father maintained a continuous relationship with the son. What this parable means to us is that our Father maintains a continuous relationship with us. Nothing can affect it. This is important because every child needs a parent that remains unchangeable even in the face of a changeable child. As a father, I am not to respond in kind to my children's outbursts or inconsistent behavior. I am to be unmovable and unchangeable in my love. Unfortunately, I fall short of this, but my Father in heaven does not! (However, it is important to remember that although nothing affects God's relation to us, sin in our lives can and will affect *our* relation with Him.)

If I am faithless, He is faithful (2 Timothy 2:13). If I am impossible, he is kind. If I am angry with Him, He is patient. In other words, what I need desperately is the security of a Father whose attitude of love, kindness, acceptance and approval is not subject to the whims of vacillating emotions. And we do have a Father who is consistent in His relationship with us.

Having had my own teenaged daughter, I have struggled with thoughts and feelings about what I would do if she were immoral and ended up pregnant out of wedlock. Consequently, when the daughter of a friend of mine bore a child out of wedlock, I asked him how he had handled the obviously difficult and painful situation. His reply was, "I loved her as my daughter before this happened, and I love her as my daughter now that it has happened." He had a continuing relationship with his daughter that transcended her behavior.

Don't get me wrong. He didn't condone what she had done. He hated the sin, but he allowed nothing to affect his relationship with his daughter. He deeply loved her and the child she bore. This is illustrative of God's continuing relationship with us. We are his children by His choice, not ours, and having made that choice, He allows nothing to destroy it!

Not only is our relationship with our heavenly Father a continuing one, it must be a **growing** one – one that grows deeper every day. There is one relationship that we have with our children as babies and quite another as they enter into puberty. When my children were small, we packed them everywhere. We couldn't afford babysitters, so we had to. But then, that wasn't really a problem. We loved showing them off. As they grew older, we would take them with us whether they wanted to or not. We would carefully instruct them on what to do, how to act, to be polite, etc. But when the time came for them to be perfect little men and women, they would allow their mother's genetic side to come through and blow the whole thing!

As my children became young adults, it was a different story. By then my relationship with them had taken on new dimensions. When the kids were in junior high and high school, I would have luncheon dates with them. Once a week we would have a date, and off we would go to scarf down a hamburger and a coke. (They referred to this as a "gut-bomb and a belly-wash.") This gave us time to talk, more like adults.

Now that they are adults, my children and I relate as adults. Our relationship has been one that has continued to grow. Unfortunately, this is not true of all father/child relationships. I'll never forget one young lady who approached me after a meeting in a sorority house where I'd spoken. My topic had been on the father/child relationship. She came up afterwards and said, "My father deserted our family when I was two, and I made up my mind that I didn't need a daddy!" Then she dissolved into tears and cried on my shoulder over and over again, "Oh, but I do need a daddy, I do need a daddy!"

Our Father guarantees us a **continuing** relationship with Him, but the growth of that relationship is a great deal dependent upon us. In his book, *Enjoying Intimacy With God*, J. Oswald Sanders graphically describes the various positions of the disciples with Christ:

> Each of the disciples was as close to Jesus as he chose to be, for the Son of God
> had no favorites. ... It is a sobering thought that we too are as close to Christ as
> we really choose to be.[10]

Out of this continuing and growing relationship with our Father, there develops **intimacy**. This intimacy with the Father is not a luxury, but a necessity for our well-being. The whole purpose of this study is to enable you to develop an ever deepening intimacy with the Father as you come to know Him through the Person of His Son, Jesus Christ.

The question is, just how badly do you want this intimacy? Again, quoting from Mr. Sanders, "It would seem that admission to the inner circle of deepening intimacy with God is the outcome of **deep desire**. Only those who count such intimacy a prize worth sacrificing anything else for are likely to attain it."[11] (emphasis mine)

Isn't it astounding that our Father would make such provision for this type of relationship with us, His children? As I said previously concerning His love for us, and I say it again, His love-relationship with us is **<u>INCREDIBLY MAGNIFICENT</u>**!!!

What then is a father? One who begets children, who raises and nourishes them, who meets their needs, and who encourages an ever growing, continuing relationship with them. But, more than all of this, a father is one who loves his children dearly and who tenderly watches over them, cares for them, understands them, talks with them, listens to them, and is vitally concerned for them. This is *our* heavenly Father.

Beginnings

Before we enter into the practical phase of our study, let me share with you how this particular study came about. It all began with a phone call from a tearful young wife and mother (I'll call her Pat), who was requesting an appointment. Because she was so emotionally upset, I set an appointment for the next morning. Pat arrived early, and as we began our discussion, she poured out her feelings. Having grown up in the church, she understood what it meant to be a committed Christian. In the course of our conversation, she related that, although her grandfather had been a pastor and the church an integral part of her family life, her father had divorced her mother when Pat was quite young. This had caused a lot of disillusionment and bitterness on her part.

In the course of our counseling, I had Pat write out who God was to her as a person. She wrote that God was an all powerful, all loving, all knowing being. Later, for some reason, I had her write out who the heavenly Father was to her as a person. I was astounded to see that she had written out that, to her, the Father was a liar, a thief and a sneak.

I pointed out the contradiction to Pat, and we worked through his misconception. But my curiosity was aroused, so I began to ask a number of people the same two questions. Far too often, they did just what this young woman had done, in that they described two different persons! They had one concept of God as God and another of God as Father.

Then I began having counselees write out who their fathers were to them as a person and who the Father was to them as a person. Again, I was astonished to find that almost everyone was saying the same thing about two different persons. It was obvious that they were patterning their concept of God as Father after their experience with their earthly fathers. Two conclusions seemed to emerge: (1) many Christians are "double minded" as it concerns God as God and God as Father, and (2) most Christians pattern their concept of God after their earthly fathers.

The next stage of my own discovery of this great truth of knowing God as Father came as I was speaking to a class of young ladies at Louisiana State University. During some interaction before my evangelistic presentation, I discovered that most of the class was made up of fairly conservative Jewish girls. However, although my message was about Christ, they proved a very attentive and appreciative audience.

Following the class, I was approached by one of the Jewish girls who told me that, if I was willing to listen, she could tell me how I could become world famous. Of course, anytime a cute young lady wants to tell me how to become world famous, I will listen. So, I told her that I would buy her a Coke and off we went to a quiet part of the student union. We had no sooner seated ourselves than she stated, "What you have to say is not only interesting, but imperative for people to hear. However, by mentioning the name of Jesus you cause people to turn off." She then very earnestly begged me to no longer speak of Jesus, but only of God.

This led to a lively discussion – she talking of God and I of Christ. But she had a peculiar habit that was very disturbing to me. Whenever she spoke of God, great tears would come to her eyes. Her sense of the awesomeness of God was amazing. She seemed to have an awareness of God that was missing from my life. Of course, I had Christ, but I came away from that encounter knowing that I did not know God in the way that I ought.

New Dimensions

The more I thought about God as my Father, the more I realized that I really did not know Him as a Father. My intimacy was with the Son. I knew Jesus. I had served Him for years, but I remained ignorant of the Father.

It was during this time of new awareness about God as Father that I received word that my father was dying. I rushed to his bedside, but he had only hours to live. During the confusion of the next few days, I was too busy to think much about this death, but when I caught my plane to go to my next conference speaking engagement, I contemplated my relationship with my father. The thought kept going over and over again in my mind, "I never really knew him!" My father was a good man, a provider. He had his problems, including a bout with alcoholism, but he had "taken the cure" and hadn't had a drink in 25 years. As I thought of the good times and the bad times, I thought over and over, "I never knew the man."

Suddenly, it occurred to me that I had the same feelings about God the Father. I really didn't know Him as Father. It all seemed to come together, for I too had projected the image of my earthly father onto my heavenly Father. When I returned home, I began to search through the Psalms, for the first time seeking out God as my Father. I reveled in the great and graphic descriptions of the majesty of God found in Scripture. I read every book that I could get my hands on concerning God. I studied His attributes, then His names. It was a thrilling experience.

But the greatest thrill of all was when I discovered that Jesus had come to reveal the Father. This was His primary purpose in coming to this sin-ridden planet. By studying the life of Christ, I could see in detail the Father at work here on earth. In Jesus I could see all the characteristics of the perfect Father. It was in Jesus loving that I saw a loving Father. It was in Jesus caring that I saw a caring Father. It was in Jesus approving that I experienced a Father's approval. It was in Jesus' kindness that I saw a kind Father. It was in Jesus' gentleness that I saw a gentle Father. It was in Jesus' acceptance that I knew a Father's understanding. It was in Jesus' security that I knew the security of a Father. It was in a patient Jesus that I saw a patient Father. It was in Jesus that my knowledge of the Father began to become complete.

Let me illustrate this from Scripture. Take the marriage feast at Cana (John 2:1-10). You are familiar with the story. Jesus' mother was in charge of the wedding. She had planned it, executed it, and was obviously anxious over it. Then the unexpected occurred and they were running out of wine. This could have been disastrous. It would have embarrassed the bride and groom and humiliated Mary. But was Jesus going to let this happen? Would he allow the wedding feast to be spoiled and His mother to suffer the indignity of failing in her preparations for the feast? Of course not. He cared! He cared even for the insignificant things in the lives of people. This was the Father at work. The Father cares. Jesus made this very plain in John 5:19-23.

Take the young man born blind (John 9). People were calloused in that culture. To be born blind could only mean that either you or your parents were under God's judgment. This meant a life of total rejection and ridicule, a life of begging, of groveling in the dirt for every measly morsel. Even the disciples were caught up in this mindset.

Why did Jesus heal the young man? To show His own greatness, to give vent to his deity? Of course not! When Jesus looked at that young man, he didn't see a dirty, filthy beggar. He didn't see a man destined to live out his life under the supposed judgment of God. What He saw was a young man who wanted desperately to be able to see. It was the caring Father in the Person of Jesus who cared enough for that young man that He healed him of his affliction. It was the Father at work, a caring, loving Father.

Take the leper in Matthew 8. If you know anything about leprosy, you will know that it is one of the most horrible of diseases known to mankind. Even today, if a person contracts leprosy, he becomes an instant outcast. In the time and culture of Jesus, leprosy was considered a most dreaded disease, one to be greatly feared lest it spread. Being a leper meant a life of living death, outcast from any normal type of life, doomed to eke out an existence with other lepers, fighting desperately for life while scavenging for food among garbage dumps. A leper knew nothing of what it meant just to talk with someone, to be held and touched, to have someone look at him without flinching. A leper could not enter the city nor attend the synagogue. Lepers were ostracized from their own families. For a leper to approach a normal, healthy person meant instant death through stoning.

Yet, here in Scripture we are witness to an incredible event. Driven by desperation, fearing life more than death, a leper walks right up to Jesus. The leper could have been stoned for this. He falls at Jesus' feet and pleads for healing. And what did our Lord do? An incredible thing! He actually reached out and touched that loathsome leper. He put His great arms around the filthy leper and held him and told him, "I will cleanse you! I will heal you!" I wonder, in that pregnant moment, with all the bystanders gaping aghast, what it meant for that man to feel those strong arms of Jesus around him and to hear that soothing, gentle, loving voice say, "I will heal you!"

Why did Jesus do such a thing? Because the Father cared! It was the Father at work in Jesus. When He looked at that leper, He didn't see the loathsome, despicable, dross of human society. He saw a man intensely desperate to be healed, to be normal. Jesus cared – the Father cares!

And what about the little street prostitute who invaded the private garden party of Simon the Pharisee (Luke 7:36-50)? What a potentially embarrassing moment. Here was Jesus, known for His purity and holiness, reclining in the open courtyard of Simon's house. Not only were there guests, but the townspeople were crowded around the courtyard walls waiting to listen to this young teacher who was stirring up all the people. What would they think? I wonder what the reaction would be today if a well-known prostitute ran up to a famous preacher during Sunday services and threw herself at his feet. He would probably be run out of town.

Notice Jesus' amazing reaction. He allows this young woman to wash His feet with her tears and to dry them with her hair. He actually allows her to anoint Him with perfume. Does He leap up in indignation? No. Does He scream at her for her actions? No. Does He cast her out? No. What does He do? He receives her. He doesn't humiliate her or reject her. He is protecting her, a common street prostitute! Why? Because the Father is at work. Now, you can see why I call the love of God the Father **INCREDIBLY MAGNIFICENT**!!!

We know the Father as our own Father through our Lord Jesus! **It is as we see Jesus as a Father that we come to know the Father!**

> **O taste and see that the Lord is good; how blessed is the man who takes refuge in Him!**   Psalm 34:8, NASB

This relationship with God as Father is two-sided. It was initiated by Him, carried on by Him, but it demands a response on our part. As to God's part, Packer puts it well:

> What matters supremely, therefore, is not, in the last analysis, the fact that I know God, but the larger fact which underlies it – the fact that *He knows me*. I am graven on the palms of His hands; I am never out of His mind. All my knowledge of Him depends on His sustained initiative in knowing me. I know Him because He first knew me and continues to know me.[12]

And to man's part, Sanders says:

> Both Scripture and experience teach that it is we, not God, who determine the degree of intimacy with Him that we enjoy. We are at this moment as close to God as we really choose to be.[13]

The Bible calls God's part of the relationship "grace," and the part which is ours is faith." Grace has been called the "divine adequacy." Faith is the human response to our Father's adequacy. As we grow in awareness of His adequacy, we grow in our experience of the love and care and peace of the Father.

Why is it important for us to see the Father in Jesus? Mainly because we are told by Jesus that the Father is spirit (John 4:24), but we can't identify with spirit. Being flesh and blood, we only relate with flesh and blood. How then was the Father to reveal Himself? Obviously, through the Son. Therefore, to know God as Father, you must know Him as such through our Lord Jesus!

Reparenting

There are nine Bible studies in the application section of this booklet. These are to help in a "reprogramming" or a "reparenting" process to replace wrong ideas about God with right ideas about God. These wrong ideas about God have been programmed into us over the years through experiential relationships with our earthly fathers and form a basic part of what we call our "belief system."

Our "belief system" is everything we believe about God, about ourselves, about others and about the world around us. Unfortunately, much of our "belief system" is erroneous; thus, it needs to be changed. God's means of changing our "belief systems" is through the **renewing of the mind** (Romans 12:2). In regard to how we view God as Father, our term "reparenting" is used interchangeable with "renewing of the mind." This process of renewing or reparenting consists of two basic elements: (1) the **putting off** of the wrong ideas about God and (2) the **putting on** of the right ideas about God.

This "putting off" and "putting on" process takes time. This is why the Bible studies at the end of this booklet are designed to be done over a number of weeks. You should schedule your time to spend a minimum of two weeks on each of the studies.

You will note that there are two sections in the back of this booklet: the workbook section and the application section. The workbook section involves a Bible study consisting of questions and answers. Look up the verse related to the question and then write out the answer in the space provided. It would be helpful to also read the passages of scripture both before and after the verse being cited.

The application section is a combination of Scripture memory and prayer. This section has two parts. First, there is a "Relationship Test," which covers ninety characteristics of the Father. Each group of ten characteristics is correlated with a Bible study page in the second part of the application section, which applies the results of the "Relationship Test" to a practical exercise of Scripture memory and prayer.

WORKBOOK SECTION

Jesus came to reveal the heavenly Father, and the purpose of this study is to reinforce this truth in your own mind so that you might enjoy the benefits which are yours as a child of God.

1. In John 10:30, what did Jesus tell the Jews? _____

    _____

2. Read John 14:8. What was it that Phillip wanted to see? _____

    _____

3. Read John 14:9-10. What was Jesus' reply to Phillip? _____

    _____

4. Read John 14:6. How can we come to know the Father? _____

    _____

5. Read John 5:18. Why were the Jews trying to kill Jesus? _____

    _____

6. Read John 5:19. What was Jesus' statement concerning what He said and did? _____

    _____

7. Read John 5:43. In whose name did Jesus come? _____

    _____

8. In John 8:58, Jesus refers to Himself as the "I AM." Read Exodus 3:14 and comment on the

    connection. What was Jesus claiming to be? _____

    _____

9. Read John 17:26. What did Jesus say that He came to do? _____

    _____

10. According to 2 Corinthians 6:18, what are we as Christians and who are we told that God is

    to us? _____

11. Explain Psalms 68:5 in your own words. Before you do, reread "The Need to Feel Secure" section of this booklet (pp. 219-220). _____

    _____

    _____

    _____

12. If God is a Father – a Father to us – we need to know some of the characteristics of God as Father. For example, Paul says in 2 Corinthians 1:3 that God our Father is the God of mercies and comfort. Therefore, two characteristics of our Father are that He is merciful toward us and that He comforts us. From Psalm 3:3-5, list at least four characteristics of what God is to you as a Father.

    _____

    _____

13. According to Zephaniah 3:17, what is your Father's attitude toward you?

    _____

14. In 1 John 4:10, what are you told is God's attitude toward you?

    _____

    In Romans 15:7? _____

15. Do you feel it is important to you to know God as your Father? Why or why not?

    _____

    _____

16. In the following passages, God is described by certain characteristics of a Father. For example, in 2 Corinthians 1:3, God is called the Father of mercies. Look up each passage and fill in the descriptive word or phrase that describes a characteristic of the Father.

    Matthew 5:48: "… as your Heavenly Father is _____."

    Matthew 6:18: "… your Father who sees in secret will _____

    _____."

Luke 11:13:   "... how much more shall your heavenly Father _____

_____?"

John 14:2-3:   "In my Father's house _____."

John 16:23:   "... if you shall ask the Father for anything, He _____

_____."

Romans 1:7b: "_____ from God our Father."

Romans 8:16:   "The Spirit himself bears witness with our spirit that _____

_____."

2 Cor. 1:3b: "... the Father of _____ and God of

_____."

Eph. 1:3:   "Blessed be the God and Father of our Lord Jesus Christ, who has blessed us

with _____

_____."

Eph. 1:17   "that the God of our Lord Jesus Christ, the _____

_____ may give to you _____

_____."

Eph. 3:14-19: "For this reason, I bow my knees before the _____

from whom every family in heaven and on earth derives its name, that He

would grant you, according to _____

to be _____

so that _____

_____

_____

_____

_____

_____."

James 1:17:   "Every _____

is from above, coming down from _____

_____."

1 Peter 1:3:   "Blessed is the _____

who according to His great mercy has _____

_____

_____."

APPLICATION SECTION

RELATIONSHIP TEST INSTRUCTIONS

This test is designed to allow you to rate your relationship with the heavenly Father. Because it is subjective, there are no wrong answers. To insure the test reveals your actual feelings, follow the instructions carefully.

1. To arrive at an accurate relationship rating, it is imperative that you answer openly and honestly. Do not answer the questions from a theological knowledge of God, but from a personal, experiential knowledge. Do not answer from what your relationship ought to be or what you hope it will be, but from what your relationship is with the Father right now. *In other words, if this test is to achieve its purpose, you must be absolutely candid in your answers.*

2. Some people feel that God might be displeased with them if they indicate a negative factor in answering the questions. Nothing could be further from the truth. Ask the Holy Spirit to guide you as you rate your relationship with the Father. He already knows how you feel and accepts you.

3. To guide you as you begin this test, you may find it helpful to phrase questions around each characteristic. For example, "To what degree do I really feel God loves me?" or "To what degree do I really know and experience God's majesty?" Your answers will form the subjective values that you assign each question.

4. It might be helpful to recall times of stress and difficulties as well as normal situations. *Who was God to you during these times?*

5. Moving from left to right, rate your relationship with the Father in terms of the degree to which each characteristic describes your experiential relationship with Him. *Rate yourself according to the following scale, circling the appropriate number that indicates your choice.*

1 - ALWAYS   2 - VERY OFTEN   3 - OFTEN   4 - SOMETIMES
5 - SELDOM   6 - HARDLY EVER   7 - NEVER

AFTER THE TEST:

1. Wherever you have circled a "3" or higher, put an "X" in the column just to the left of the characteristic.

2. Once you have marked all the X's, transfer them to the corresponding columns in the FatherCare Bible study exercises that follow. There are ten characteristics under each FatherCare heading. For each are listed verses and phrases which will help you in the "reparenting" process.

3. Choose a verse from among the key verses listed for each characteristic and begin to memorize the verse you choose. Establish a consistent prayer time when you can begin to pray out loud and choose to "put off" the wrong ideas about God and "put on" the right ideas about God. An example prayer is given at the end of this booklet. It is a good practice to write out your verses several times in longhand as well as to meditate on them.

RELATIONSHIP TEST

FatherCare:

___ Caring	1 2 3 4 5 6 7
___ Loving	1 2 3 4 5 6 7
___ Kind	1 2 3 4 5 6 7
___ Understanding	1 2 3 4 5 6 7
___ Strong	1 2 3 4 5 6 7
___ Calm	1 2 3 4 5 6 7
___ Pleasant	1 2 3 4 5 6 7
___ Approving	1 2 3 4 5 6 7
___ Sensitive	1 2 3 4 5 6 7
___ Listens	1 2 3 4 5 6 7

FatherKing:

___ King	1 2 3 4 5 6 7
___ Majestic	1 2 3 4 5 6 7
___ Awesome	1 2 3 4 5 6 7
___ Great	1 2 3 4 5 6 7
___ Victorious	1 2 3 4 5 6 7
___ Gracious	1 2 3 4 5 6 7
___ Honorable	1 2 3 4 5 6 7
___ Just	1 2 3 4 5 6 7
___ Good	1 2 3 4 5 6 7
___ Righteous	1 2 3 4 5 6 7

FatherSavior:

___ Redeemer	1 2 3 4 5 6 7
___ Merciful	1 2 3 4 5 6 7
___ Forgiving	1 2 3 4 5 6 7
___ Compassionate	1 2 3 4 5 6 7
___ Gentle	1 2 3 4 5 6 7
___ Beautiful	1 2 3 4 5 6 7
___ Cleanses	1 2 3 4 5 6 7
___ Holy	1 2 3 4 5 6 7
___ Pardons	1 2 3 4 5 6 7
___ Reasonable	1 2 3 4 5 6 7

FatherFriend:

___ Friend	1 2 3 4 5 6 7
___ Faithful	1 2 3 4 5 6 7
___ Patient	1 2 3 4 5 6 7
___ Delightful	1 2 3 4 5 6 7
___ Truthful	1 2 3 4 5 6 7
___ Counselor	1 2 3 4 5 6 7
___ Supportive	1 2 3 4 5 6 7
___ Humble	1 2 3 4 5 6 7
___ Joyful	1 2 3 4 5 6 7
___ Discerning	1 2 3 4 5 6 7

FatherProvider:

___ Provider	1 2 3 4 5 6 7
___ Trustworthy	1 2 3 4 5 6 7
___ Adequate	1 2 3 4 5 6 7
___ Generous	1 2 3 4 5 6 7
___ Fair	1 2 3 4 5 6 7
___ Steadfast	1 2 3 4 5 6 7
___ Wealthy	1 2 3 4 5 6 7
___ Concerned	1 2 3 4 5 6 7
___ Satisfies	1 2 3 4 5 6 7
___ Giver	1 2 3 4 5 6 7

FatherProtector:

___ Protective	1 2 3 4 5 6 7
___ Secure	1 2 3 4 5 6 7
___ Preserver	1 2 3 4 5 6 7
___ Alert	1 2 3 4 5 6 7
___ Deliverer	1 2 3 4 5 6 7
___ Defender	1 2 3 4 5 6 7
___ Cherishes	1 2 3 4 5 6 7
___ Advocate	1 2 3 4 5 6 7
___ Forceful	1 2 3 4 5 6 7
___ Courageous	1 2 3 4 5 6 7

FatherLove:

___	Loving	1 2 3 4 5 6 7
___	Considerate	1 2 3 4 5 6 7
___	Comforting	1 2 3 4 5 6 7
___	Encouraging	1 2 3 4 5 6 7
___	Lover	1 2 3 4 5 6 7
___	Accepting	1 2 3 4 5 6 7
___	Intimate	1 2 3 4 5 6 7
___	Pleasing	1 2 3 4 5 6 7
___	Rewarder	1 2 3 4 5 6 7
___	Appreciative	1 2 3 4 5 6 7

FatherTeacher:

___	Instructor	1 2 3 4 5 6 7
___	Wise	1 2 3 4 5 6 7
___	Creative	1 2 3 4 5 6 7
___	Helpful	1 2 3 4 5 6 7
___	Lovingly Kind	1 2 3 4 5 6 7
___	Disciplines	1 2 3 4 5 6 7
___	Hopeful	1 2 3 4 5 6 7
___	Favor	1 2 3 4 5 6 7
___	Light	1 2 3 4 5 6 7
___	Respectful	1 2 3 4 5 6 7

FatherLeader:

___	Guide	1 2 3 4 5 6 7
___	Bold	1 2 3 4 5 6 7
___	Confident	1 2 3 4 5 6 7
___	Perfect	1 2 3 4 5 6 7
___	Devoted	1 2 3 4 5 6 7
___	Commander	1 2 3 4 5 6 7
___	Authoritative	1 2 3 4 5 6 7
___	Loyal	1 2 3 4 5 6 7
___	Sufficient	1 2 3 4 5 6 7
___	Decisive	1 2 3 4 5 6 7

FATHERCARE – THE CHARACTERISTICS OF THE FATHER

As you do each of the following studies, ask yourself these questions:

1.   Does this passage clearly support the point made in the characteristic?
2.   Are there any cross references which might better highlight or emphasize that characteristic?
3.   Have I personally had an experience with God in which this trait was made clear to me? If not, do I have trouble believing God is this way?
4.   As I meditate upon this trait in God's character, what emotions come to the surface and what do they tell me about the condition of my belief system?
5.   How does this characteristic motivate me to greater love for God Himself rather than just to "serve in His name" or to see His gifts?

When you conclude each Bible study, write out a prayer to God, thanking Him for who He is and for how He has shown Himself to you and asking Him to continue to reveal Himself to you as the perfect Father He is. There is a sample prayer on the last page of this section.

NOTE: Unless indicated otherwise, the Scripture references in this study are based on the wording in the New American Standard Version of the Bible. Wording may vary slightly in other translations.

FatherCare:

1. **Caring**: Matthew 6:26; 1 Peter 5:7
   ____ He cares for me as only a loving father can care for his child.
   ____ He not only cares for me, but He cares about me.

2. **Loving**: John 3:16; Romans 5:8; Ephesians 3:14-19
   ____ He loves me for who I am, not for what I do
   ____ His love for me is unconditional and unceasing.

3. **Kind**: Psalm 103:13; Romans 2:4; Ephesians 1:5
   ____ Our Father is a kind and considerate Person to us, His children.
   ____ He always has a kind and encouraging word for me.

4. **Understanding**: Psalm 103:14; 139:1; Hebrews 4:15
   ____ My Father understands me as a person.
   ____ He understands me in my moods, my feelings, my thoughts, my actions.

5. **Strong**: Psalm 93:1; 105:4; 106:8; Ephesians 6:10-13
   ____ My Father is strong and powerful on my behalf.
   ____ His strength becomes my strength. He is the strongest of the strong.

6. **Calm**: Psalm 37:7; Matthew 11:28; John 14:1
   ____ I find my tranquility in my Father's calmness. He is never hurried or harassed.
   ____ He calms the anxious heart and takes senseless activity and turns it into creative productivity.

7. **Pleasant**: Psalm 16:11; 21:6; 147:1
   ____ My Father is absolutely pleasant. What a pleasure it is to be in His presence.
   ____ He is altogether lovely.

8. **Approving**: John 6:27 with Colossians 3:3
   ____ My Father gives me unconditional approval.
   ____ His approval is based on who I am in Him and not on what I do or have.

9. **Sensitive**: Psalm 94:9; 139:1-6, 17-18; Hebrews 4:15
   ____ My Father is sensitive to my every mood and thought.
   ____ He is sensitive to my needs and desires.

10. **Listens**: Psalm 55:17; 102:17; 116:1-2
    ____ My Father listens to me. He takes time to be involved in who I am and what I do.
    ____ He knows what I have to say is important. It is important to me; therefore, it is important to Him.

FatherKing:

1. **King**: Psalm 47:7; 95:3
   ___ My Father is the sovereign king of the whole universe. He is the Kind Most High!
   ___ I am a child of the King (John 1:12). I am a prince/princess. He enables me to think as a child of the King, act as a child of the King, be the child of a King.

2. **Majestic**: 1 Chronicles 29:11-13; Psalm 93:1
   ___ My Father is majestic. He rules and reigns on high. How great He is!
   ___ He desires my participation in His majesty. He freely shares it all with me.

3. **Awesome**: Exodus 15:11; Psalm 99:3
   ___ My Father is awesome in His ability to love and protect me.
   ___ He is awesome in His strength, power and holiness.

4. **Great**: Psalm 86:10; 99:2
   ___ Greatness Becomes my Father. He is before all things, above all things; He presides over all things.
   ___ He makes me an integral part of His greatness. I find my greatness in Him.

5. **Victorious**: Psalm 98:1; Zephaniah 3:17
   ___ My Father is victorious over all things – the world, the flesh and the devil.
   ___ His victory allows me to be victorious.

6. **Gracious**: Psalm 86:15; 111:4; 119:132; Ephesians 1:7-8
   ___ He is gracious to me no matter how I act toward Him.
   ___ He lavishes His grace on me as His precious child.

7. **Honorable**: Philippians 2:9; 1 Timothy 6:15-16
   ___ My Father is distinguished and upright. His name is above every other name.
   ___ I am so very proud of Him. I am proud to call Him Father.

8. **Just**: Deuteronomy 32:4; Psalm 89:14; 99:4
   ___ My Father is absolutely just. I know that He is impartial.
   ___ I know that He will be just with me no matter what.

9. **Good**: Psalm 34:8; 100:5; 106:1
   ___ My Father is good, a good Person in every sense.
   ___ He is so good to me. He insists on giving me everything out of the goodness of His heart.

10. **Righteous**: Deuteronomy 32:4; Psalm 11:7; 111:3; 119:137
    ___ My Father is absolutely righteous, even though He had been tempted in every manner just like me.
    ___ Because He is righteous, He has made me to be righteous, not because of what I do, but because of who I am in Him.

FatherSavior:

1. **Redeemer**: Psalm 19:14; Isaiah 63:16; Jeremiah 50:34
    ___ My Father cared enough to redeem me out of the authority of darkness.
    ___ He redeemed me from the power of sin and from the hold of Satan, and He put me into His kingdom.

2. **Merciful**: 2 Samuel 24:14; Psalm 86:15; Ephesians 2:4
    ___ My Father is always merciful to me, regardless of my circumstances.
    ___ In the dark storms of self-reproach and condemnation, He is always merciful.

3. **Forgiving**: Psalm 86:5; 103:10-12; Hebrews 10:17
    ___ He has forgiven me completely and totally for all my sins and transgressions, past, present and future.
    ___ He forgives, He forgets – He wipes the slate of my heart clean.

4. **Compassionate**: Psalm 103:8,13; 111:4; Matthew 9:36
    ___ My Father's heart is full of compassion for me for He has shared intimately all my pain and hurt and sorrows.
    ___ Through His compassion, He affirms and supports me.

5. **Gentle**: Psalm 18:35; Matthew 11:29; 21:5
    ___ He is a gentle Person. He deals with me so gently.
    ___ My Father's gentleness permeates my being, making me a gentle person.

6. **Beautiful**: Psalm 27:4; 96:6
    ___ He is the lily of the valley, the bright and morning star, the fairest of ten thousand.
    ___ My Father is a beautiful Person, and He believe me to be a beautiful person.

7. **Cleanses**: Isaiah 1:18; Acts 15:9; 1 John 1:9
    ___ The blood of Christ cleanses me from all unrighteousness.
    ___ No matter the defilement, my Father cleanses, moment by moment.

8. **Holy**: Psalm 99:3,5,9; 108:7
    ___ The beauty of holiness shrouds my Father.
    ___ He is absolutely holy, thus He makes me holy.

9. **Pardons**: Psalm 103:3; Romans 8:1; Hebrews 10:17
    ___ He freely pardons me – all my sins, all my transgressions; even the defilement is pardoned. I am free.
    ___ The Father took me as His precious child and sacrificed His Son to pardon me.

10. **Reasonable**: Isaiah 1:18; 1 Corinthians 10:13
    ___ To think that my Father would reason with me. How important that makes me feel.
    ___ He never demands more than I am able to really give. In every way, He is so very reasonable.

FatherFriend:

1. **Friend**: John 15:13-15
   ___ My Father is my friend. He is closer than a brother.
   ___ Since He is my friend, I can call on Him at any time; He is never too busy for me.

2. **Faithful**: Numbers 23:19; Psalm 89:1,2,5,8; 100:5; Lamentations 3:23-24
   ___ My Father is absolutely faithful to me as a person.
   ___ His faithfulness to me never lags and will never end.

3. **Patient**: Psalm 86:15: 103:8; 1 Corinthians 13:4
   ___ My Father is so patient with me. Nothing affects His patience where it concerns me.
   ___ I cannot provoke Him, nor does He ever hold anything against me.

4. **Delightful**: Psalm 18:19; 27:4; Zephaniah 3:17
   ___ My Father delights in me because I am me; that is enough for Him.
   ___ He is a delightful and pleasing Person.

5. **Truthful**: Psalm 86:15; 89:14; 108:4; John 14:6
   ___ My Father is always truthful to me, to everyone. He cannot be untruthful.
   ___ He builds into me truthfulness. I can be truthful because He is truthful.

6. **Counselor**: Job 12:13; Psalm 73:24; Proverbs 19:21; Isaiah 9:6
   ___ There is nothing that I cannot bring before my Father and seek His counsel on.
   ___ He never condemns or belittles what I ask Him. His advice never fails.

7. **Supportive**: Psalm 37:23-24; Isaiah 41:10
   ___ My Father supports and cares for me.
   ___ I know that whatever I attempt, He is there. What He requires of me, He give me the strength and power to do.

8. **Humble**: Matthew 11:29; Philippians 2:6-11
   ___ To think that the King of kings humbled Himself for me.
   ___ Out of my Father's humbleness, I find my humility.

9. **Joyful**: Isaiah 62:5; Zephaniah 3:17; John 15:11
   ___ My Father is always joyful and full of joy. He is a Father of joy.
   ___ His joy for me and in me produces my joy. I can rejoice in Him.

10. **Discerning**: 1 Samuel 16:7; Jeremiah 17:10; Mark 2:8
    ___ My Father is so very discerning. He knows my heart and nothing is hidden from Him.
    ___ I can be myself. I don't have to be a phony since He knows my heart.

FatherProvider:

1. **Provider**: Psalm 23; Isaiah 58:11; Matthew 6:25-34; Philippians 4:19
   ___ My Father provides for my every need – emotional, spiritual and physical.
   ___ I can rest secure knowing that He will provide for me as He has promised.

2. **Trustworthy**: Psalm 9:10; 18:2; 65:5; 2 Corinthians 1:20
   ___ In every way, in every circumstance of life, my Father is trustworthy.
   ___ He is worthy of the trust I place in Him.

3. **Adequate**: 1 Chronicles 29:12; Psalm 73:25-28; 2 Corinthians 3:5
   ___ My Father is totally adequate for all my needs. He is, in and of Himself, totally adequate.
   ___ His adequacy is the basis for my own personal adequacy. My adequacy is in and of Him.

4. **Generous**: Matthew 7:9-11; John 3:34; Romans 8:32; Philippians 4:19
   ___ My Father withholds nothing good from me. He lavishes the riches of His grace upon me.
   ___ He freely and bountifully gives me all good things.

5. **Fair**: Deuteronomy 32:4; Psalm 98:9; 99:4
   ___ How fair in all of His dealings with me is my Father.
   ___ I know that He will never, ever be unfair with me.

6. **Steadfast**: Psalm 31:3; Isaiah 40:8; 2 Thessalonians 3:5; Hebrews 13:8
   ___ What security I can have because my Father is steadfast and unmovable.
   ___ He is like a rock; I can truly trust Him.

7. **Wealthy**: Psalm 50:10; 2 Corinthians 8:9
   ___ My Father owns the cattle on a thousand hills. He is rich beyond comprehension. His wealth is my wealth right now as my present possession.
   ___ My Father's real wealth is me. I am His inheritance.

8. **Concerned**: Matthew 6:28-32; 10:29-31; 1 Peter 5:7
   ___ My Father is deeply concerned with the intimate details of my life.
   ___ I can trust Him because He cares about me.

9. **Satisfies**: Psalm 103:5; 107:9; 128:1-4; 147:14
   ___ In my Father I am fulfilled.
   ___ He satisfies beyond my wildest dreams.

10. **Giver**: Psalm 37:4; John 3:34; Romans 8:32; James 1:17
    ___ No good thing does my Father withhold from me, His child.
    ___ He brings gifts and gives them to me – the gift of the Sprit, spiritual gifts and material blessings.

FatherProtector:

1. **Protective**: Psalm 91; 118:6-9; 2 Thessalonians 3:3
    ___ My Father protects me because He loves me.
    ___ As His precious child, He protects me.

2. **Secure**: Psalm 18:2; Proverbs 3:25-26; 29:25; Hebrews 13:8
    ___ In an insecure world, my Father gives me security.
    ___ The world offers no sanctuary of security; that only comes in Him.

3. **Preserver**: Psalm 97:10; 119:114; Isaiah 54:17: John 10:29
    ___ My Father preserves me and keeps me from all harm.
    ___ He maintains (preserves) His righteousness in me.

4. **Alert**: 2 Chronicles 16:9; Psalm 121:3-4: 139:1-12
    ___ If His eye is on the sparrow, then I know He watches me.
    ___ My Father watches over me even in the night watches. I am never alone.

5. **Deliverer**: Psalm 97:10; 107:6; 1 Corinthians 10:13
    ___ My Father delivers me from the hand of the enemy.
    ___ He delivers me from all temptation.

6. **Defender**: Psalm 10:18; 27:1; 108:13; Zechariah 9:15
    ___ My Father protects and defends me from myself and my enemies.
    ___ He stands up for me and is a shield to me.

7. **Cherishes**: Psalm 18:19; Zephaniah 3:17; Ephesians 5:29
    ___ My Father delights in me.
    ___ He cherishes me as a person dear to His heart.

8. **Advocate**: Hebrews 7:25; 1 John 2:1
    ___ My Father speaks up for me and defends me.
    ___ He proclaims to Satan that I am "not guilty."

9. **Forceful**: Isaiah 40:10-26; Mark 10:27; Luke 1:37
    ___ My Father accomplishes with ease that which man finds impossible.
    ___ He forcefully conquers His enemies and mine.

10. **Courageous**: Psalm 24:8; Acts 14:3; 1 Thessalonians 2:2; 2 Timothy 1:7
    ___ My Father courageously faces the foe on my behalf. I need not fear anything.
    ___ He builds courage in me. In Him I find that courage is not the absence of fear, but the victory over it.

FatherLove:

1. **Loving**: 1 Corinthians 13:4-8; 1 John 4:9-10
   ___ My Father is altogether loving. He is full of love.
   ___ He inspires love and affection in me.

2. **Considerate**: Psalm 139:17-18 (NIV—see marginal note); Isaiah 54:4-7; Jeremiah 29:11
   ___ My Father is so considerate of me. Even when I am wrong, His consideration does not change.
   ___ He never neglects nor ignores me. To Him I am so very important and special.

3. **Comforting**: Psalm 68:5; 94:19; 2 Corinthians 1:3-4
   ___ He comforts me in all the trials and tragedies I face.
   ___ My Father's comfort extends even to the most intimate areas of my life. There is nothing I can't share with Him.

4. **Encouraging**: Isaiah 35:2-4; 40:31; Romans 15:4-5
   ___ My Father encourages me constantly.
   ___ No matter what I face, the pain I feel, the hurt I experience, He is always encouraging me.

5. **Lover**: Romans 5:8; Ephesians 2:4; 3:17-19
   ___ He is the lover of my soul. He tenderly watches over and cares for me.
   ___ I am secure and confident in my Father's aggressive, yet tender, love for me.

6. **Accepting**: Romans 14:3-4; 15:7
   ___ My Father accepts me as a person, with all my hang-ups, all my sins, all my guilt. He accepts me just as I am.
   ___ He accepts me on the basis of who I am, not on the basis of what I do.

7. **Intimate**: Psalm 139; Proverbs 3:32; John 17:23
   ___ My Father is not someone who is ten million light years away; He is with me at all times.
   ___ He is not vague, but real. He is someone who does care and love.

8. **Pleasing**: Psalm 23:6; Matthew 11:28-30; John 1:14; Philippians 2:13
   ___ What a pleasing Person my Father is. His presence is like the radiance of the sun.
   ___ Not only does He try in every way to please me, but He makes me desire to please Him.

9. **Rewarder**: 2 Timothy 4:7-8; Hebrews 11:6; James 1:12
   ___ My Father has promised crowns to me.
   ___ Knowing Him intimately is reward enough in eternity.

10. **Appreciative**: Matthew 24:45-47; Luke 6:38; 2 Corinthians 9:6-11
    ___ My Father always shows His appreciation for my efforts on His behalf.
    ___ He appreciates me as a person.

FatherLeader:

1. **Guide**: Psalm 73:24; 107:30; Isaiah 58:11

    ___ I know, no matter what the call, my Father guides my way step by step.

    ___ His will is not elusive and will-o'-the-wisp, but a definite statement of His desires for me.

2. **Bold**: Psalm 76:3-9; Hebrews 4:16; Revelation 19:11-16

    ___ My Father is bold, bold for me.

    ___ He imparts boldness to me. He makes me to be bold.

3. **Confident**: Isaiah 41:13; 42:8; 45:5; 2 Corinthians 3:5

    ___ My Father is supremely confident. He knows what He is about.

    ___ Out of His confidence, He builds confidence in me.

4. **Perfect**: Deuteronomy 32:4; 2 Samuel 22:31 (NIV); Psalm 18:30 (NIV); Hebrews 7:28

    ___ Can anyone be as perfect as my Father? He is perfect in and of Himself. He is perfect to me.

    ___ He is the perfect Person for me, to make me everything that I could never be in and of myself.

5. **Devoted**: Hebrews 13:5-6; 1 John 3:1-2

    ___ My Father is devoted to me. He pours out His affection and love on me.

    ___ His devotion for me drove Him to the Cross. I am that worthy in His sight.

6. **Commander**: 2 Chronicles 13:12; Psalm 33:9; 47:3,9; Isaiah 55:4

    ___ My Father is the Commander of the host of the Lord.

    ___ He is in charge. Need I fear anything?

7. **Authoritative**: Matthew 7:29; 9:6; 10:1; 28:18

    ___ My Father speaks with authority.

    ___ He commands the attention and obedience of all.

8. **Loyal**: John 10:29; Romans 8:31-39; Hebrews 13:5

    ___ My Father's loyalty to me as His child never ceases.

    ___ He protects loyally. He never embarrasses nor humiliates me. He cares that I remain loyal and obedient to Him.

9. **Sufficient**: 2 Corinthians 9:8; 12:9-10

    ___ My Father is sufficient for every need, for every situation and circumstances of life.

    ___ His sufficiency guarantees that in my weakness His strength will be made perfect.

10. **Decisive**: Psalm 33:9; 2 Corinthians 1:18-20

    ___ My Father is decisive. He speaks and it is done.

    ___ He knows where He is going and how to get there. My indecision is to be swallowed up in His decisiveness.

FatherTeacher:

1. **Instructor**: Psalm 25:8-9; 32:8; John 14:26; 2 Timothy 3:16-17
   ___ My Father carefully, patiently instructs me in everything.
   ___ He prepares me fully to live a life for Him.

2. **Wise**: Job 9:4; 12:13; Psalm 104:24; Romans 16:27; James 1:5
   ___ My Father is wise beyond imagination. I cannot fathom His wisdom, but it is always the best for me.
   ___ He imparts His wisdom to me, so that I might be truly wise.

3. **Creative**: Psalm 102:25; 104:1-24; John 1:3; Ephesians 2:10; 2 Corinthians 5:17
   ___ In His creative genius, He carefully fashions all that is.
   ___ My Father created me twice – once in His image, and again in spirit.

4. **Helpful**: Psalm 10:14; 54:4; 121:1-2; John 14:16; Hebrews 13:6
   ___ My Father is my Helper.
   ___ What I find impossible in my own strength, I find possible in His.

5. **Lovingly Kind**: Psalm 25:6; 86:5; 89:1; 103:10-14
   ___ My Father's loving kindness is constantly extended toward me.
   ___ His loving kindness forms a shield over me, a guard in front of me, a hedge behind me.

6. **Disciplines**: Psalm 94:12; Isaiah 30:20-21; Hebrews 12:5-11; Revelation 3:19
   ___ My Father will not allow me to stray into danger.
   ___ He tenderly corrects me so that I may live life at its best.

7. **Hopeful**: Jeremiah 29:11; 33:3; Romans 15:4
   ___ My Father never gives up on me; He's always optimistic for me.
   ___ He gives me hope out of the great hope within Him.

8. **Favor**: Psalm 30:5; 89:17
   ___ I find my Father's favor in my intimacy with Him.
   ___ His favor suffices. It strengthens and keeps me.

9. **Light**: Psalm 4:6; 27:1; John 1:9; 8:12
   ___ My Father is the light of life, the light of the world.
   ___ In the darkness of my path of life, His light carefully guides my way.

10. **Respectful**: Job 1:8; 2:3; John 15:15; Hebrews 2:9-13
    ___ My Father respects me because He loves me as a person.
    ___ I don't have to earn His respect; He gives it to me freely.

SAMPLE "REPARENTING" PRAYER

A prayer like the one that follows would be appropriate after each of the preceding Bible studies. In your prayer, acknowledge the characteristic of God that you now believe to be true according to His Word. This prayer is an example for the characteristic of "loving."

My Father, I always considered You an unloving God, but now I know that You are a *loving* Father to me. I choose now in faith to put off my false belief and I choose to believe that You are loving to me. I choose to believe what Your Word has to say about You rather than my feelings or reason or past experiences, and I know that Your Word says that You love me as a person and that your love is not based on my performance or on what I have or achieve. Thank You, my Father, for loving me unconditionally.

Addendum Two

"Self-Disciplined Religion," a transcript reproduced by permission of
Unconditional Love Ministries
7986 Mainland Drive
San Antonio, Texas 78250
www.malcolmsmith.org

SELF-DISCIPLINED RELIGION

By Malcolm Smith
Transcribed from an audio tape with permission from
Unconditional Love Ministries
7986 Mainland Drive
San Antonio, Texas 78250

Copies of this and other tapes by Malcolm Smith may be ordered from
Unconditional Love Ministries: 1-800-457-0947
www.malcolmsmith.org

Let's turn to Titus – Paul's letter to Titus – [chapter 2,] verse eleven:

For the grace of God has appeared, bringing salvation to all men, instructing us to deny ungodliness and worldly desires and to live sensibly, righteously and godly in the present age. Titus 2:11-12, NASB

The grace of God has appeared. And if you notice, it tells us that this grace, when it comes, does two things to us. It tells us to renounce – or your word in the Bible I'm reading from is "deny." It's a very strong word, very strong. The word "deny" doesn't really say it unless you get inside the word "deny" and stamp your feet a bit. The word "deny" – it means to renounce, repudiate, reject, absolutely have nothing to do with. The grace of God has appeared, teaching us or instructing us to reject, deny all ungodliness and worldly desires. So that is the first thing, when a person has received the grace of God, they will turn upon sin and have nothing to do with it.

But, secondly, it says, "...and to live sensibly, righteously and godly in this present age." So it isn't only that they have renounced their lifestyle of ungodliness. That's only one side of it. They have embarked upon a new kind of a lifestyle, which is characterized by three words: to live sensibly, righteously, and godly.

Now, I don't have enough time for three words. But I do have time for one word, which I think, actually, could be the most important word in that sentence. I'm not sure about that, but it could be. And the word is "sensibly." If you are born again, you have renounced – done with – ungodliness, and you have taken up a new lifestyle that is called here "being sensible." Now, I know that didn't sound too exciting, and actually I would like to have translated that word by another word. I'm not sure what your version might say. Maybe it says what I would like to have translated it as. That word, in my opinion, should be translated "self-control."

Now, in actual fact it is translated "self-control" elsewhere in the New Testament by this [translation of the] Bible, New American Standard. But here they've chosen "sensibly," and for the life of me, I don't know why. "Self-control" is the word. It's a very important word in the New Testament describing the new-birth kind of life. In fact, right here, in Titus, it keeps on coming up. When he talks about elders, leaders of the church, one of the great characteristics of them, according to verse eight, is that they are self-controlled. You jump down to chapter two, and it says the older men in the church – they should be characterized by being – it says "sensible" in my Bible – self-controlled. It says the older women should be characterized by being self-controlled – in verse five. Then in verse six it says, "…and likewise, the young men should be self-controlled."[1] Then he says here that, in fact, it is the characteristic of everybody. Once the grace of God has come to you – one of the characteristics that stands out – you become self-controlled.

You might remember that when Paul was addressing Felix. (Now this I find fascinating.) When Paul was addressing Felix, a heathen, he's preaching the Gospel to him, and what does he address this man about? Self-control. It would suggest to me that all these people, according to Titus, are to realize that self-control is the center of this Christian life. And when he addressed Felix, self-control was part of the Gospel that he presented.

And then, of course, another one that leaps out is Galatians 5. The fruit of the Spirit is… And down that list is "self-control." This has got to be a very important word – self-control. So, I must ask, "What is this self-control?"

Now, I don't want you to get confused here. It's very easy. In fact, there are some Bible commentators that got terribly confused here. You see, in the days of Paul, there were certain philosophies. There were certain Greek moralists. You know what I mean? You do realize that being moral is not being Christian. You do understand that, don't you? There is no such thing, actually, as Christian morality. We won't get into that. But, morality is not being a Christian. So, the "Moral Majority" can include a lot of human beings. They don't have to be Christians. Because being moral is the cry of what's left after the Fall has blitzed man. Man is not totally lost in terms of not knowing right from wrong, though man is lost unless he comes to Christ. Even in his lost-ness, he does know God is there somewhere, and he does know there's right and he does know there's wrong. In that sense, he's not totally lost. The devil doesn't know right from wrong. Do you understand what I mean by that? The devil thinks right is wrong and wrong is right. He's totally immersed forever into wrong-ness. Man was deceived, so he can tell the difference. He knows there is right. And whenever man moves to that right-ness, we say it's morality.

And the Greeks had perfected that. In fact, there was a group called the Stoics. You might have heard of the Stoics. They were into self-discipline. And many Bible commentators think that Paul took from the Stoics and was talking here about self-discipline. He's not. He's talking about self-control. And there's a *world* of difference between self-discipline and self-control.

What is self-discipline? A self-discipline is an imposition. That is, it comes from the outside. I impose on myself, or I let somebody else impose on me. It's an imposition upon my inner desires, my inner lusts. I allow someone to impose a law on me – that you shall not do that. And so, here this imposition, something from the outside, comes upon me and says you can't do it. And I say, "Okay, okay, I won't do it." But I really would love to do it. I still want to do it. But I'll be *disciplined*. I won't do what I really want to do. I will do what I am *supposed* to do. That's self-discipline. I bring myself under and I grit my teeth and I say I won't do it. And you'd better give me a good reason why I mustn't do it. And so along with morality and along with self-discipline go the reasons, usually high reasons, why I shouldn't do it. And I'll drag myself. I'll whip myself. "You will not do that!" I am self-disciplined.

Now you see that, as far back as the days of Paul, crept into the church. It's in the church today. I've heard it many times. You can read it any time you want. It comes down to something like this: "After all He has done for you..." Now you can hear it's coming now. You can hear it coming. See, now we've given you a reason. We're going to come to you with all your snake pit of lusts and desires and whip you into shape. "And after all He's done for you, the least you can do for Him is..." And then insert in there the latest fad in the Body of Christ. Do you follow what I mean by this? Do you get what self-discipline is? It's something that comes from the outside. You're going to twist your arm and make yourself do what you don't want to do. But you'll do it – for some reason.

I know some people and they are self-disciplined because they feel that's the route to heaven. I tell you this: I heard a man the other day, God bless him. I prayed for that man. I mean that, because he was a preacher, and he was telling the people that when his mummy was dying, he promised her he'd meet her in heaven. And so, since that day, he has tried so hard. He's been disciplined, and he hasn't drunk and he hasn't smoked and he hasn't chewed tobacco, because he wants to see mummy in heaven. That's self-discipline. That's accepted as evangelical preaching, God help us. Do you understand what I'm talking about? Really, I mean!

And then, of course, you go to some churches and they've already got their self-discipline all lined out – that, if you join this church, you can't do this and you can't do this. They've got the list. And you sign at the bottom. Why? To be accepted by the church. So, I'll let someone twist my arm. Self-discipline is saying, "Here is something I shouldn't do, for some reason or other, and so I guess I won't do it." Self discipline is in the world of "you should," "you must," "you ought." You know, those of you that were in the military, you know what it is. You go along with it. I mean, why not? Get off my back, I'll do it. But you forget why, if there ever was a reason. You just do it. Self-discipline.

See, the Pharisees – if any of you are into self-discipline, let me encourage you, the Pharisees were. The Pharisees were *really* into self-discipline. They were very disciplined people. They were disciplined in the way they dressed. They wouldn't dress like heathens. They dressed in a way that they had determined God liked. Poor God, He's brought into all the fashion shows. They decided what God liked and what God didn't like. And so Pharisees dressed very disciplined. And their hours of prayer – you've got to give them A+. I've never yet met anybody that had a disciplined life like the Pharisees. From the minute they got out of bed, almost every hour had some particular expression – a ritual, a prayer, scripture memorization. Who in this audience started at four years old memorizing Leviticus? Every Pharisee did. As soon as you were born into a Pharisee home, four years old and you're memorizing Leviticus. And you move on to Genesis and then Exodus and then Numbers and then Deuteronomy. By the time you're twelve, you can quote the whole jolly lot. That's the beginning of being a Pharisee. By the time you're twenty, you've delved into the Psalms and the Prophets. Man, that's discipline. Strict, rigid discipline. It came into days of prayer, days of fasting, every Wednesday and Friday. Tithing! You didn't only tithe on your money. You tithed on the very leaves on the vegetables in the garden. Did you know that? A Pharisee would go and count the leaves on the herbs that grew in the garden. Every tenth one, he'd pluck it off and put it in the offering plate. You talk about tithing!

But wherever they went, you could feel the results of discipline. It's cold. There is something ice cold about a self-disciplined religion. Highly organized, I'll grant you that. And it looks perfect. It's right – *dead* right. Cold. Distant. And they don't have to say a word. It plays around their mouths – the arrogance, despising. They don't even have to say it: "I thank you, oh God, I'm not as other men." It's coming out of every pore of their skin.

Do you realize they shared that in common with every other religion in the world? And when I see believers today that are self-disciplined, I often have to tell them, "You know, you're not very well disciplined." I mean, if you're going to get into self-discipline, try being a Muslim. I mean go the whole way! Go the whole way! If you want discipline – you say you don't drink alcohol. Well, even the Mormons don't drink coffee. I mean go for it, man. Go for it. Where does this thing end? You'll end up drinking purified water if you're not... If you want discipline, go to the religions of this world, and they have done a perfect job of it.

And it looks so right. Oh, it gets to you. You see a person who's dressed odd and different, and you see a person who, on the hour, every hour, does this, does that; it looks so right. Anyone who's a bit slob-ish, you suddenly feel unspiritual. Paul spoke to this in Colossians 2. He mentions, "Do not handle, do not taste, do not touch..." He says these have "the appearance of wisdom in self-made religion, self-abasement and severe treatment of the body, but are of no value against fleshly indulgence."[2]

"There is a way that seems right to a man, but the end thereof is the way of death."[3] That's the trouble with it. It seems so right. When you look at it, you say it couldn't be wrong. Can a man be wrong because he prays on the hour every hour? Could a man be wrong because he has memorized the Bible? It depends where his heart is at. Yes, he could be wrong. That's why there's a way that seems right. Going off to break the Ten Commandments on the hour every hour does not seem right. There's no doubt where he stands. But, when a person *seems* to be so right, it's hard to say they're wrong.

Jesus went to the Pharisees of His day. In Matthew 23, He says, "You blind Pharisees, first clean the inside of the cup and of the dish, so that the outside of it may become clean also."[4] He has said the cup is not cleaned by scrubbing the outside. And did you notice what He said? Clean the inside *so that* the outside may become clean. That is, you're spending all your time scrubbing the outside. Basically, He said, "Forget the outside. Get to the inside and the outside will take care of itself." So, He is saying that the holiness that He's talking about is not self-discipline. It's something that arises from the inside and moves to the outside.

See, self-discipline, I suppose, in America today, shows up mostly in dieting. I mean that's self-discipline that everybody understands. For some reason – you see, self-discipline always has to have some reason out there. So, for some reason, I guess I'd better diet. The doctor breathing down my neck or a bathing suit hanging in the cupboard that won't fit around my thigh. You know, some reason that I have got to start dieting. So, I impose upon myself these incredible rules. And everything inside me says yes, until the first meal, and then everything says *no*. But I'm disciplined, and I grit my teeth. For a while. Until, apparently, I've got it licked. And then I go and forget the whole thing again. That's always discipline. Because, you see, you don't want to do this. You're accepting the impositions, but you don't *want* to do it. And so, at the first chance, out! You see, you've got all those crazy magazines as you go in the checkout. They're screaming at you. Lose 30 pounds in an hour! New diet! New diet! And people *buy* them! Ah, a new discovery. *I might just do it this time.*

Now I see the church today in America exactly like that. Most believers I know, in the Spirit, are on diets. "I won't do this and I won't do that and I won't do the other. In my heart, I wish I could, but I won't do this. I'm going to be holy. We're going to get this thing on the road." And every passing preacher has got a new fad diet. "Do it my way and you'll be holy in 30 minutes." Come on. "Five steps!" Hey, you do know, don't you, that when you diet and lose weight and gain it right back, you're in a worse state than when you began? And when believers are forever finding new fad ways to try and be holy – try to discipline themselves into holiness – in the long run, you're worse off than when you began. Because, you see, self-discipline is a *sin*. Self-discipline – I mean applied to the things of the Spirit – is a sin. For what is self-discipline? It is but one more action of the flesh.

Now what do I mean by "flesh"? That fills the New Testament. What does it mean? Very quickly, who were you before you came to Christ? I mean, let's take a quick photograph. Who were you? The Bible calls you an "old man." Not old in years. "Old man" means corrupt, decaying, falling apart. So you were old in that sense. What constituted the old man? "*I*, I had determined I would go my own way." "All we like sheep have gone astray. We have turned every one to his own way."[5] That's the essence of it all. I mean forget these big theological words like "original sin." Basically, when all is said and done, it just means man made a choice beyond all choices, a choice out of which every choice would come. "I want it my way," which means I am going to live my life independently of God. I'll acknowledge He's there. I'll tip my cap to Him every Sunday. But I'll do it *my* way. And man died in his spirit. So, the old man, this corrupt man, decaying man, spiritually, is one who is dead in his spirit and has been taken over by his "*I* will do it my way, independently of God." And such a man plays directly into the hands of Satan and is described as being led around by the prince of the power of the air. "The spirit who is now at work in the sons of disobedience"[6] – that's who you were. Do you identify with that? That's who you were. That's the man that is called "dead in sins."

What happened when you were born again? You realized through the preaching of the Gospel that that old man had been taken by Jesus. And when Jesus died, that man died. Everything you were, in rebellion and hostility toward God, was taken to the Cross, and you died. But not only so, Christ came inside of you by His Spirit, and that which was dead in you came alive. You were a new creation. You were born again. And what was not there, is there. Christ now lives inside of you. Your spirit is alive to God, for Christ is in you.

So you still have flesh – this desire to be independent – but it's not you. *You* are Christ in you. *You* are the new creation. That's who *you* are. The Holy Spirit has shed abroad the love of God in your heart.[7] You have eternal life, which is life as God has it. That's who you are. You are a partaker of the new covenant, which says the law of God is written on your heart.[8] That's who you *are*. But I still live in a body of flesh, which means the potential for living independently of God is there. Oh, I'm not the old man. He's gone, he's dead. I, my spirit alive, Christ in me – that's who I am.

But always the pull, always the – what shall I say? – seduction. "Come and do it the old way. Come and be independent. Feel the sweetness of being in control instead of this dependency upon Christ, instead of Christ living in you and Christ living as you." The pull: every temptation you've ever had, really, is a call to live independently of Jesus. I'll get to that again in a moment.

But, you see, now that I've come to Christ, if my flesh has got any sense, it's not going to call me to commit murder. It has half an idea I'll say no to that. So the flesh joins a church. The flesh says, "You do realize that, independent of God, you can be good enough for Him. I mean I know we did all that awful stuff before. We didn't have to, you know. We could have done it this way. We don't need God to be holy. Good grief. All you need to do is try a bit harder. I mean we never used to try, did we? Well, let's start trying now. Now you know the rules; we'll play by them. Come on, you can do it." "Just a little discipline," says the flesh. "Independently of God, you can try a little harder. A little prayer wouldn't hurt. Memorize a few Bible scriptures." "I mean, just get your act together," says the flesh. "I can do it. I can be like Jesus. You see, I can go anywhere you want. If you wanted wild parties, we had a jolly good time there, didn't we? Now then we'll do it this way now. Now we'll have wild meetings if you want. We'll do it any way you want; just do it my way. You see, you must understand, I'm your flesh. I am not as bad as you think. I'm a pretty good chap really. Just give me a chance. I can really achieve being like Jesus if you'll only give me a chance." The flesh – I kid you not – that's the flesh. Anything independent of God – the flesh, that's what it wants to do. Oh, you don't have to be bad, bad, bad. You can be good, good, good. If it's independent of God, it's the flesh.

The flesh has got one phrase. It says, "*I, I* will try to please God." [It says,] "That is God's over there. I'm over here." See what we can do to become acceptable to God, more loveable? Do you see what I'm saying? "I, I, I, I, I will try to be good." And the tragedy is there are millions of believers in America who came to receive the forgiveness of sins, knowing it has got to come from the God side. Only God could achieve my forgiveness. And when we accepted his forgiveness and came in, we said, "Thank you very much. Now, after all you've done for me, you'd better sit back, God. Wait till I show you what I'm going to do for you."

I pastored for a long time in Northern Ireland. I look back sometimes to those days, back in the '60s when it was almost like pastoring a Third World country. I mean we didn't have running water and, for a while, we didn't have electricity. And while I was there, the electricity finally came to where we were pastoring. I mean it was a big deal. When the first person in the congregation got electricity, we all went to the house. We were there for the switching on ceremony. Electricity has come! And then it got kind of ho-hum as, one by one, everybody got it. We'd almost forgotten – you know, it was in the church now. Until the last person, the oldest elder we had, decrepit, poor old chap – and he lived way out in the sticks. In Ireland that's the peat bogs, and he lived way out there. And finally, he was the last one to get electricity. And so the board of elders – we all went out there. The last one and the oldest one was going to get electricity. I'd been to dinner there many times before, and just as it got dusk, he would light the paraffin lamps. Well, tonight we sat around. He let it get a little bit darker than dusk. And then in Irish fashion, he gave that nod to his wife – the patriarchal nod, which meant, "Wife, to your duty." And she got up in that semi-darkness and went to the switch. And you could see the anticipation as she put on the switch. And immediately the room flooded with light. Very slowly, the old man got up, went over to the paraffin lamps and lit them. And he says, "You can put it out now." He said to us, "It's going to be a lot easier to light the lamps after this."

When I saw him do that, I said, "There go so many believers." When Jesus comes and the light is turned on, they say, "Now it's going to be a lot easier to keep the law." No. When Jesus comes, it's no more self-discipline. It's no more struggling to keep the law. Jesus doesn't come to make it easier to keep the law. Jesus comes to give us something entirely beyond the law. Never contradicting it. But far, far beyond it. Far, far beyond it.

This was the trouble with the Galatians. They thought they could begin in the power of the Spirit and come to a holiness by self-discipline. No. You have come into something that is unlike any religion in this world. Every religion has a law. You have a Person, the Person who has come to live within. We have the new heart, the love of God shed abroad, and the essence of that law written within. And what is the essence of law? Love. The Ten Commandments are only love written negatively. Do you understand? If I love you, I won't kill you. If I love you, I won't lie to you. It's love in another way.

So, what's self-control? Self-control is listening to my heart, not a law imposed from the outside. It's listening to who I now am in Christ. And what do I hear when I listen to who I am? I hear that I *want*, I *want* God. I *love* Him now and I want to fulfill the love of God that is in me by loving you. When you're first born again, however weak that may sound down inside of you, that is your new heart. I mean that is the new you. You're not who you were. You are who you are. If you listen – "What do I really want?" You want God. You want to express His love to others.

See, if I don't listen to my heart. If I don't – if I listen to what many other believers are telling me or if I listen to my flesh... I sit down with some believers sometimes. It's like sitting at a fat farm when the ice cream man goes by. I mean I hear, "Oh, I am so weak. You know, I get so tempted and I fail God so much. Pray for me. The devil's always after me." And every Sunday night, "Anybody got a request?" One weak, limp hand goes up. "Pray for me. I'm going to be tempted this week." Haven't you ever heard your hearts? You're talking discipline there, and you're saying when the discipline's on, "I feel so weak." Don't you know who you are? You don't talk like that. *Listen* to your heart.

Tell me this – those of you that feel the biggest failure in this place – when it comes to living the Christian life, I mean, you've blown it. Well, let me counsel you. This is what I do when people come to me in private. Let me do it publicly. Listen to your heart. Listen to your heart. That besetting sin that makes you feel such a failure – let's listen to your heart. Do you *want* that besetting sin? I mean, do you *want* it? Tell me, will you go to that besetting sin and say, "You are my friend. I will protect you. I will justify my right to have you in my life"? Now, some of you are looking at me horrified. Of course, if you listen to your heart, you don't want sin. You'll never protect that besetting sin. You'll never justify its existence. You don't want it. Why? Because the grace of God has appeared, instructing you to deny sin.[9] You don't want it. You've got a new heart. Then give yourself a slap in the face. You're not one of the dieters. You're not sitting there, saying, "I've got to try again, but it's a hopeless job. I'm so weak and the devil's going to get me this week." No, you haven't got to try again. Stand up. Stretch. Throw away the diet sheets. It's over. It's gone. Arise and shine and Christ shall give you light![10] Be who you *are*!

And for some reason, you've never realized who you are. This isn't a second experience. I'm only telling you who you are. This is what happened to you when you came to Christ. And you've had your eyes on the flesh, and you've had your eyes on discipline, and you've tried to turn your flesh into something acceptable to God. Well, you can't. All God ever said about the flesh is crucify it. So forget that. He comes and writes on your heart, not on your flesh. And He says, "What's your heart? What's your heart?" And He says, "I've given you a new heart and Christ lives there. The love of God is there." That's who you are!

Now I'm in a position to handle this nonsense. I'm going to make choices. Can't fool me with the flesh anymore. When the flesh calls me, I say, "I know you. You're not me. Ha, ha, ha. Oh no, you've been crucified with Christ. That's my faith confession right now. I'm not confessing it to make it happen. I'm confessing it because it's happened. You're no longer me. I, I, in my innermost self, I – Christ lives in me; that's who I am. I don't live with you anymore. At this moment I live in harmony with who I am, with Christ in me." This is faith. This is real faith. It is daring to believe the facts of the Gospel – the facts that this "I" was crucified with Christ, but *this* "I" is Christ living in me. That's my faith. I am helpless. I know that I cannot, in my flesh, live the Christian life. It's impossible. The fruit of the *Spirit* is self-control, the fruit of me being joined to the Holy Spirit. And so I choose to live life out of my deepest self. I'm going to choose to be who I want to be.

Am I making sense? I'm living out of who I really am. I'm going to choose to be who I want to be. I'm not going to struggle and try to have my flesh imitate Jesus. I'm going to let Jesus be Himself. And I am going to choose to let Him be Himself. So, it isn't changing my flesh. It's *ex*changing. It's not the flesh; that's crucified. I exchange – let Christ live.

Oh, that involves sacrifice. No doubt about that. There are some things I don't do. I do not do them by choice. And I didn't not do them – that's bad, isn't it – "didn't not" -- you know what I mean, though, don't you? I was not stopping doing those things in response to law. That is self-discipline. I asked in my innermost heart, "What do you really want to do?" And I want to love God, and I want to love you. And anything that stands in the way of that, I want to be rid of it. I do. I want to. And, so, if there is something that I am doing that is going to tear your heart up, I'll stop doing that. And if there is something I am doing that will only fuel my desire to forget God, I'll stop doing that. Oh, there's no law that's saying, "You must, you must, you must." I want, I want, I want to please God. Therefore, if that's the case, I must adjust my life around that. You understand that?

In 1 Corinthians 9, Paul gives the illustration of self-control using an athlete. There's a perfect illustration. If Paul hadn't used it first, I would have thought of it first. It's a perfect illustration. What is an athlete? He gives up a lot of things. Why? Because he wants to. He has his eyes set upon a certain goal. He's looking for a gold medal, a certain kind of accolade, and he wants that more than a lot of things. And so he gives this up and he gives that up. It's no sacrifice. Oh, *you* might look at him and say what a sacrifice, but then you're not running the same as he is. It's no sacrifice to him. The biggest sacrifice to him would be not being allowed to run in the race.

A believer who understands who he is in Christ does not have an imposition from the outside. He has the bursting forth of the life from the inside. And because of that, he *will* make sacrifices as far as the outsiders are concerned. As far as he's concerned, he didn't even notice it.

So I'm going to watch what goes into my head. I'm going to watch what I watch. I'm going to watch what I read. Why? Not because there's a church loading me with rules and regulations. Because Christ lives in me, and I want to know Him more than anything else in life. And I want to be able to love you even as Christ loved you. So, therefore, I'm going to watch my life. Because, you see, I want to bring my life to its total fulfillment that I may be the human being God created me, and Christ redeemed me, to be. I want to fulfill my innermost self, who is Christ living in me. I want to know the meaning to life in this existential moment. I want to *live* this moment.

So, you see, there are some things that I'm not going to get involved in. But, you see, the fun of it is, I'm not obeying the law when I do that – unless you call Christ in me the law; that's okay. Self-control is response to the voice of the Spirit within. So, you see, if it was a law to keep, then I would say, "Well, I've kept all those rules, and you didn't. Hee hee hee." Immediately, despising arrogance flickers around my mouth. But, no, no, see, I'm living from Christ in me. And then, you see, it sets me completely free, because there are some things... He knows me; He knows me better than I know I'll ever know myself. And He says, "Malcolm, you can't do that." And I say, "But he's doing it and you're blessing him." He says, "None of your business. He can; you can't," because He knows *me* – and He knows you, too. So, it's okay for you, but not for me. Do you understand that? You're taken out of law; you're into the Spirit. And the Spirit says, "Don't." The Spirit says, "Do." And I learn to live from within, and He never contradicts the Scripture. Never.

But it's no sacrifice, because I have a new heart. And I make choices. It says, "The grace of God has appeared, instructing us..."[11] The Holy Spirit does not come through us like a tornado, *making* us do something. The Holy Spirit never takes away your free will. He gives it back to you. The devil stole it. Sin stole it. You got so used to being a robot – addict to this, addict to that. When Jesus comes, He sets you *free*. And that takes some getting used to sometimes. That's why new believers get into self-discipline so quickly. Because they're used to that. They're used to someone beating them around the head and saying, "Do this." They can't get used to growing up into real human adults. So that I live – I live? You mean I can do this by myself? Go on, go on. I say, "God, you do it for me. Go on, you do it for me. Send us revival. Go on, you do it." He says, "Get on and you do it. *You* make the choice." I live for the first time. I'm free. *I* make a choice. The grace of God came and instructed *me* to deny ungodliness. I didn't think I could. He says, "Go on. You can. Go on." And when I deny it, and when I say no, and I say yes to Him, I suddenly find that I have been empowered with the Holy Spirit so that I can say no to sin.

Do you get this picture? What about temptation? Guess that's another hour, really. Let me tell you this, that temptation is God's method. That's how He establishes us in the Spirit. Now, you looked at me weird. Temptation is God's method. Look, I'm going to get in a plane on Monday morning, and we're going to take off. Do you know how we take off? It's very simple. You need power, but you have to have opposition. You know that? That's why they have those windsocks on the airport. Tells you which way the wind is blowing. You know you can't take off in a vacuum? You've got to have opposition. Power plus opposition equals flight. This is God's method. He allows flesh to call me, so that I make a choice in the power of the Holy Spirit. And then I am established in the Spirit – to the point where with many temptations, you're not even tempted anymore, because He's done.

See, with the self-disciplined person, they never deal with temptation or sin. Never deal with it. They suppress it. "I mustn't do that." That's not dealing with it. That's just saying you mustn't do it. And as soon as whoever gave you the discipline is out of the way, you'll do it. You say, "You know, my teenage boy – he was such a good boy until he went to school. Then he fell apart." No he didn't. He'd fallen apart the whole time. He was just under discipline. Do you understand that? I mean, I know you thought he was a good boy. He's just like any other boy, right? He turned to his own way. But he liked you so much and he felt so sorry for you, he was going to try and be good. And as soon as you weren't there, he's going to be what he wanted to be all the time. Come on, don't look at me like that. You do the same thing when the pastor isn't watching. Off you go. When the cat's away, the mice play.

Suppress, suppress, suppress. See, good Christians aren't angry. So, I won't be angry. I *won't* be angry! *I won't be angry!* You put anger in the basement. And what does it do? It climbs up the basement window and comes back through the front door under another name. Hey, do you know the people who have the most psychological problems? Evangelicals and charismatics. Absolutely messed up in their heads, because they've suppressed and they've suppressed and they've suppressed. That's not dealing with sin. That's just pretending it isn't there.

What do we do? Temptation comes and I say, "No, no, no. I'm a disciplined man. I'm not going to sin. I'm not going to sin. I'm not going to sin." But the flesh – the flesh is so crazy. The flesh says, "You know, I'm getting tired of this. I know it was my idea, but I'm getting tired of this. I think, under the circumstances, it wouldn't be sin if you did it, you know. I've been looking in the books, and I think, under these circumstances, it's okay to do it." I'll give you about 20 times of saying no and, before you get to 21, you've justified – it's okay this time. Always.

If you say no to temptation out of self-discipline, you will fall into sin. And as soon as you've fallen into sin, flesh condemns you. "How could you have done a thing like that?" And the devil takes it up and hurls accusation against you. And you wallow in guilt and self-loathing. "My flesh isn't as bad as that. I don't know what came over me." And you wallow like that. You love penance, every one of you. You're as Catholic as the next. You love penance. Wallow in it. Wallow in it. Come to church looking miserable because I've sinned and I'm feeling it. And then, finally, when you can take your own whipping no longer, you say, "Well, maybe we could try again." And on Sunday night, "Come and give your life to Jesus." "Well, I know I did it last week, but I'll have another try." Here we go. Dedicate and rededicate and re-rededicate my dedications. "And I promise, and I'm beginning to feel good. That's right. I can do this. I can. I know I'm strong enough. I don't know what came over me last time, but this is it, mates. This is it. We're going to do it." And we feel smug. Oh, do I feel... "I made my dedication. Ha ha. He didn't; I did. I did. I know, yeah. we're going to make it this time. They're going to write a book about me. I mean, I'm going to be such a holy man. This is it." And so it goes on, and so it goes on.

Self-control is nothing like that. Nothing. Self-control begins with God, not outside pressure. Self-control is from within, and when temptation comes, I'm not surprised. If God says that my flesh is only good enough to be crucified, I'm not surprised what it comes up with or what it wants to respond to. I'm not surprised. I just say, "Lord Jesus, I know what I'm feeling right now, and it's real feeling. And there's a part of me that feels it wants to do this thing (whatever it is), but I know who I am. That's not me. That me was crucified with you on the cross. Lord Jesus, you are my life, and I am now surrendering to you that you shall live your life in me and through me at this moment." And when I thus surrender and say, "Lord Jesus, take over and live," I am empowered with all power – and love reigns. Love reigns.

And, let me tell you this. If you fail – let's suppose it. I mean, you might fall into temptation. But if you know what I'm talking about, even when you fail, you're not wiped out. Because you know He still loves you. So, when the devil condemns you, when you've fallen, you won't accept it. You say, "No, He loves me. And the blood of Jesus cleanses me from sin. And I know why I failed, you see. That's the point. I never expected me to be able to overcome this. I know I failed because I forgot to trust Jesus. So I'm back to rest again. It's okay."

You say, "But just a minute. What about... You're saying you don't want to sin. Come on, preacher," says somebody back there. "I want to sin." Yeah, I'm not upset by that either. He isn't; He knows you. Let me tell you two things very quickly. If you look in your heart and, honestly, you want to sin, number one, don't. The grace of God never, ever, ever is easy on sin. The person who says, "I'm under grace. I can sin and get away with it," no, you haven't heard the grace of God yet. Even if you find, when you do what I say – listen to your heart and you don't find there that you want holiness – still don't sin. But I'll tell you what to do. Ask of yourself, in the presence of the Holy Spirit, "How, how do I so misunderstand the meaning of life and so misunderstand what it means for you to live in me, that I should want to do this?" And that's okay. You can do that without condemnation. "'Come, let us reason together,' says the Lord."[12] If there's an area of your life where, honestly, you say, "But I find I do want to do that, and I know it's sin," number one, don't do it. For grace never allows you to do it. Number two, He loves you. He loves you, even admitting that. Acknowledge it fully, and sit down and ask yourself, in His presence, "How on earth could I so misunderstand what life is all about that I should want to do that thing which I know is sin?" And, do you know, He'll tell you? He will. And you will enter into a whole new dimension of Christian living. Instead of saying, "I won't do it. I won't do it. I know I want to. I want to, but I won't." You'll get nowhere with that. But if you say, "Lord Jesus, I really want to do that. What on earth's wrong with me? Please show me," He'll show you – without condemnation. That's exactly – and I don't have time to prove it – but that's exactly what James means when he says, "If any of you lack wisdom..."[13] That's not wisdom in general; that is wisdom in the middle of a problem. "God, I don't know what's going on inside of me." "Well, ask," He says. "Ask." And He won't get mad at you. That's what it says.

This is *living*. *This* is *living*. "He who rules his spirit is better than he who captures a city."[14] But if you don't, "like a city that is broken into and without walls is the man who has no control over his spirit."[15] If you're living by discipline, by law, you are of all believers most miserable. But if you are living by the inner control, basically doing what you want to do, because your wants are one with Christ, you'll end up loving.

What's your response? I would imagine, if your response is my response, it's relief. Because, when you think about it, what I've just said, it fits. It fits. That's how truth should be. It clicks. It fits. And there's a tremendous sense of relief. "That's right. It's right. It feels good. It feels right." It is *good* news.

Of course, I know I've upset some people. And it hurts me that I have. You're the self-disciplined people. You got graduated from West Point. Well, do me one thing – that's all. Do me one thing. Concentrate on the areas in your life that your discipline can't handle. And begin to realize that that's really what it's like all the way through. But you can't live this life, and discipline only makes it look as if you can when you really can't. And then listen to what I've just said again.

And if you're undisciplined, the grace of God does not allow you to meander through life doing your "thing." A person who understands the grace of God is not a religious hippie. If you've been undisciplined, believe me, self-control will bring your whole life into focus, and you will now have the focus to love my God and to love all I know, all he puts in my path. "And I shall do that, whatever it costs. Because that's my goal, that's my desire." And He will begin. Mind you, He will instruct you. See, law dumps the whole lot on you at once. Twenty five rules, sign here, you're in. Grace isn't like that. He comes and He says, "Now, let's begin. Let's show you who you really are." So, to begin with, you're doing things that all the discipline people get all upset about. It's okay; grace is teaching you. And He says, "Let's deal with this. Let's deal with that. Let's deal with this." Gradually, He brings your whole life into focus. That's the grace of God.

Well, there it is. Go and live this life that the grace of God teaches you to live. Can I tell you something? It happened when I was working with some of the "Jesus People." Do you remember the Jesus People? And they came into our church. They had *long* hair. I mean boys, young guys, they had long hair. Some of them didn't wear shoes. None of them wore real shirts. I mean sweatshirts, some with Mickey Mouse on them and others with other things on them. And they came in. They were truly born again. No one really doubted that. But, then, some of the old folk in the church, you know, bless their hearts – I think some of them had seen the grace of God. The trouble is, like so many people, they'd seen the grace of God and then turned their grace into law for their kids. Do you know how that happens? You know God invades me and there's a whole bunch of stuff I don't want anymore, and I turn right around to my kids, who have not been invaded, and I say, "You can't do that." They say, "Why?" I say, "Because I don't do it." Anyway, that's another story.

So, these dear old folk, you know – and they'd seen the grace of God – and they came to me and they said, "These young men – we believe they're born again, but when are they going to get their hair cut? When are they going to start wearing shoes?" I said, "When you give me a scripture and verse for it." They pressured me. They said, "You've gotta go to them and tell them to cut their hair." I said, "No, I won't frustrate the grace of God." I went to them, all right, but not about that. I said to them, "What is the Holy Spirit saying to you about your hair? What's the Holy Spirit saying to you about your feet?" I said, "Just ask the Holy Spirit what's going on." I said, "Check back in a week. We'll talk about it." And, in a week's time, we got together, and we went around the circle. I said, "Well, what's the Holy Spirit saying?" One of the fellas said, "Nothing." The way he put it actually, he said, "I asked the Holy Spirit, 'Do you like my hair?' and the Holy Spirit says, 'Yep.'" And I came to another one. I said, "What's the Holy Spirit saying about your hair?" He said, "I've got to cut it. And I have to put shoes on." We went around – I forget – it was something like 60 to 40 percent. Sixty percent got their hair cut. But then, when they'd said they're going to cut their hair, I said, "Now we're going back around again." I said to the one who said he had to get his hair cut, "Why did you wear long hair in the first place?" He said, "I hated society. I wanted to show society I was nothing to do with them." And he gave me the whole rebel story. Every one of the 60 percent that wanted to get their hair cut now, every one of them had been rebels against society. The 40 percent that the Holy Spirit said they could keep their hair – they wore it long because it was fashion. So, I learned something there. God goes along more or less with the latest fashion in hairstyles. But if you are wearing clothes or wearing hair or not wearing shoes to be a rebel, God is against rebellion, and He said, "Cut your hair. Put shoes on. Put an IBM business suit on, and get in there."

Do you understand why I said that? My dear church members wanted self-discipline. They said, "Everybody cut their hair. Everybody wear shoes. All look the same." The grace of God says, "No. No." God's not against modern hairstyles. God doesn't want you ladies to wear buns just because that was "in" 900 years ago. Nothing special about that. Now, He's not against modern fashions. What He's against is motives, reasons. See how quickly you can teach a new convert, just born again? "Listen to the Holy Spirit; He'll tell you." That was a risk. I had faith in them – I mean faith in the true them. And as I said last night, I have faith in you. Not faith in your flesh. That's crucified. My faith is you were crucified with Christ. But I believe in Christ in you. And I believe in Christ in you, and I *believe* in Christ in you. And I have come here tonight to call forth the true you, to awaken your faith to know who you *are* – that you might arise and shine, for your light is come. You can go out of this place, not bound by a million rules, trying to learn to walk like a centipede. But to be who you *are*, Christ spontaneously living his life in you.

Addendum Three
Facilitator's Guide

FACILITATOR'S GUIDE

First Meeting – Introduction:

- Open the meeting with prayer. (Pray aloud for God's guidance in all that takes place during the meeting.)
- Starting with yourself, have each group member briefly introduce herself by giving the following information:
    - o Name
    - o Occupation
    - o Marital status and number/ages of children
    - o One thing she wishes others knew about her right off the bat rather than finding out by getting to know her over time
- Discuss with the group the format of each meeting and how meetings will flow each week, as follows:
    - o Facilitator opens the meeting with prayer.
    - o Brief discussion of those parts of the assigned chapter that stood out to group members.
    - o Discussion of the assigned chapter's "Reflection" questions.
    - o Discussion of the assigned chapter's "Homework Follow-up" questions.
    - o The assignment for the week is to read from the current chapter's "Comments on the Homework Follow-up" section through the next chapter's "Homework" section and to do the homework.
    - o Close with conversational prayer. (No one has to pray aloud. Eventually the facilitator closes the prayer.)
- Read out loud the "Small Group Guidelines" on page 7.
- Engage in group discussion by having each participant, starting with you, answer the first reflection question on page 12 of Chapter 1: When did you first start thinking of yourself as "fat" and what were some circumstances surrounding your starting to eat more than what seemed appropriate? In other words, when did you start having a "negative relationship" with food?
- After discussing that question, go over with the group what needs to be completed before you meet again:
    - o Read pages 1 through 18.
    - o Do the homework that is given on pages 15 to 18.
- Close with conversational prayer, explaining that no one has to pray aloud and that you will eventually close the prayer.

Second Meeting – Discussion of Chapter 1:

- Open the meeting with prayer.
- Starting with yourself, have each group member briefly state those parts of the reading assignment that stood out to her.

- Starting with yourself, have each group member answer the second and third reflection questions provided in Chapter 1 on page 13. (The first question was discussed during the previous group meeting.) Explain that no one has to answer any given question but everyone is encouraged to do so. Every person who desires to answer reflection question #2 should do so before you move on to discussing reflection question #3.
- Starting with yourself, have each group member answer the "Homework Follow-up" questions provided on pages 18 and 19. (Always have all the participants who want to answer the a question do so before going on to the next question.)
- Go over the assignment for the week, as follows:
  ○ Read from "Comments on the Homework" on page 19 in Chapter 1 through the homework on pages 27 to 30 of Chapter 2.
  ○ Do the homework that is given in Chapter 2. (The homework refers to Addendum One, starting on page 207.)
- End the meeting with conversational prayer.

Third through Fifteenth Meetings – Discussion of Chapters 2 through 14:

- Open the meeting with prayer.
- Starting with yourself, have each group member briefly discuss those parts of the reading assignment that stood out to her.
- Starting with yourself, have each group member answer the reflection questions provided in the chapter that was read during the week.
- Starting with yourself, have each group member answer the "Homework Follow-up" questions provided in the chapter that was read during the week. (Each will have read up to the page on which these questions are listed.)
- Go over the assignment for the week:
  ○ Read from the "Comments on the Homework" section of the chapter that was just read up through the homework of the following chapter.
  ○ Do the homework provided in the new chapter.
- End the meeting with conversational prayer.

NOTES

Will *You* Benefit from Reading this Book?

1. "Do You Know Your ABC's?" is not original to me; however, the authors asked that they not be credited. I have adapted the original slightly in order to fit the context of this book.

Chapter 1

1. *Tufts University Diet & Nutrition Letter*, Vol. 9, No. 6, August 1991, 3-6. Reprinted with permission.

Chapter 2

1. With permission, portions of this chapter are based on information in "FatherCare," an unpublished booklet by Jim Craddock (Oklahoma City: Scope Ministries International, Inc., 1993) and adapted from "Session 9 – Father/God Concept" of Scope Ministries International's *Pneumanetics* (Oklahoma City: Scope Ministries International, Inc., 1992). "Pneumanetics" is a coined word based on two Greek words that together infer "Spirit-led."
2. An excellent book that describes how one's relationship with an earthly father can influence perceptions of the heavenly Father is *Our Heavenly Father* by Robert Frost (Plainfield, NJ: Logos International, 1978).
3. See, for example, *Theological Wordbook of the Old Testament* by R. Laird Harris, Gleason L. Archer Jr., and Bruce K. Waltke (Chicago: The Moody Bible Institute, 1980), Vol. I, 244, under heading 554a.
4. William Barclay, *The Daily Study Bible: The Letters of John and Jude* (Philadelphia: The Westminster Press, 1958), 87.
5. Jim Craddock, "FatherCare" (Oklahoma City: Scope Ministries International, Inc., 1993), 7-8.
6. Ney Bailey wrote a wonderful book titled *Faith Is Not a Feeling*, which is now out of print. However, Amazon.com and other used book outlets can sometimes obtain used copies of this classic.
7. Craddock, "FatherCare," 51.

Chapter 3

1. Bill Gillham, *Lifetime Guarantee* (Eugene, OR: Harvest House Publishers, 1993), 17.
2. "Age Span Sheets" are available from Scope Ministries International, 405-843-7778. Reprinted with permission (Oklahoma City: Scope Ministries International, Inc., 1983).
3. Handout by Jim Craddock and available from Scope Ministries International, Inc. Reprinted with permission (Oklahoma City: Scope Ministries International, Inc., 1994).
4. Bill Bright, "Would You Like to Know God Personally?" (Orlando, FL: NewLife Publications, 1968), 12.

Chapter 4

1. With permission, portions of the information presented in this chapter are adapted from "Session 6 – Belief Systems" of *Pneumanetics*.
2. For a treatment of the word "conformed," see Lawrence O. Richards, *Expository Dictionary of Bible Words* (Grand Rapids, MI: Zondervan Publishing House, 1985), 185.
3. Geneen Roth, *Breaking Free from Compulsive Eating* (New York: NAL Penguin Inc., 1986), 149-150. For more information, see www.geneenroth.com.

Chapter 5

1. Scope Ministries International, Inc., "Sessions 5 – Experiencing My New Identity in Christ," *Pneumanetics* (Oklahoma City: Scope Ministries International, Inc., 1992), 5-6.

Chapter 6

1. With permission, portions of the information presented in this chapter are adapted from "Session 7 – Emotions" of *Pneumanetics*.
2. Colin Brown, Ed. *Dictionary of New Testament Theology*, Vol. I (Grand Rapids, MI: Zondervan Publishing House, 1975), 111.
3. An excellent aid is the poster, "How Are You Feeling Today?" It is available from Creative Therapy Associates, Inc., 800-448-9145 or www.ctherapy.com.
4. "REED" handout is available from Scope Ministries International, Inc., 405-843-7778. Reprinted with permission (Oklahoma City: Scope Ministries International, Inc., 1987).

Chapter 7

1. With permission, portions of the information presented in this chapter's section on anger are adapted from "Appendix B to Session 7" of *Pneumanetics*, 7-17.
2. I have seen versions of this diagram in many settings, such as Christian seminars and classes, and am unsure of its original source. My best guess is that Bill Gothard first popularized some form of this chart in his "Institute in Basic Youth Conflicts" seminars in the early 1970s.
3. With permission, this chapter's homework is adapted from "Appendix B to Session 7" of *Pneumanetics*, 7-17.

Chapter 8

1. Geneen Roth, *Breaking Free From Compulsive Eating* (New York: Bobbs-Merrill Co., 1984), 8. For more information, see www.geneenroth.com.

Chapter 9

1. Nanci Hellmich, "Intuitive eating satisfies body, mind," *USA Today*, April 26, 1995, 5D, reprinted with permission from *USA Today*.
2. Leonard Pearson and Lillian R. Pearson, *The Psychologist's Eat-Anything Diet*. (New York: Peter H. Wyden, Inc.: 1973), 5.

3. Ibid., 6. The authors have "hunger" in quotes to indicate physical hunger that requires psychological, as well as physiological, satisfaction.
4. Hellmich, 5-D.
5. Geneen Roth, *Breaking Free From Compulsive Eating* (New York: Bobbs-Merrill Co., 1984), 31. For more information, see www.geneenroth.com.

Chapter 10

1. With permission, portions of the information presented in this chapter are adapted from "Chapter 10 - Torah Syndrome" of *Pneumanetics*.
2. Bill Gillham, untitled conference, Tahlequah, Oklahoma, June 1990.

Chapter 11

1. For a treatment of the word "conformed," see Lawrence O. Richards, *Expository Dictionary of Bible Words* (Grand Rapids, Michigan: Zondervan, 1985), 185.
2. Susie Orbach, *Fat Is a Feminist Issue* (New York: Berkley Books, 1978), xx-xxi.
3. John Berger, et al., *Ways of Seeing* (London, 1972), p. 47, as cited in Orbach, *Fat Is a Feminist Issue*, 196.
4. Orbach, *Fat is a Feminist Issue*, 7-9.

Chapter 12

1. Bill Gillham, untitled conference, Tahlequah, Oklahoma, June 1990.
2. Geneen Roth, *Breaking Free from Compulsive Eating* (New York: The Bobbs-Merrill Co., Inc., 1994), 164-166. Used with permission. For more information, see www.geneenroth.com.
3. Ibid., 166.

Chapter 13

1. My favorite book on communication skills is *Caring Enough to Confront* by David Augsburger (Scottdale, Pennsylvania: Herald Press, 1981).
2. Regarding the subject of disappointment in marriage, I highly recommend the booklet, "Intimacy in Marriage," by Donna Edwards, Living Well, Inc., P.O. Box 720828, Oklahoma City, OK 73172, 405-924-3574.
3. An excellent book describing how different people express and perceive love in different ways is *The Five Love Languages* by Gary Chapman (Chicago: Northfield Publishing, 1992, 1995).
4. Jimmy Soul, "If You Want to Be Happy."
5. Examples of such Bible studies are the NavPress "Life Changes" series or Tyndale House Publishers' "Life Application® Bible Studies."

Chapter 14

1. Special thanks to Judi Boyer, former Training Director of Scope Ministries International, for creating these useful charts.

Addendum One: FatherCare

1. J. I. Packer, *Knowing God* (Downers Grove, Illinois: InterVarsity Press, 1973), 14.
2. Gerhard Friedrich, ed., *Theological Dictionary of the New Testament*, Vol. 5 (Grand Rapids, Michigan: Wm. B. Eerdmans Publishing Co., 1967), 272.
3. Packer, 14-15.
4. William Barclay, *The Daily Study Bible: The Letters of John and Jude* (Philadelphia: The Westminster Press, 1958), 87.
5. Kenneth S. Wuest, *Word Studies in the Greek New Testament*, Vol. 4 (Grand Rapids, Michigan: Wm. B. Eerdmans Company, 1966), 142.
6. Friedrich, Vol. 8, 2.
7. Wuest, Vol. 1, 134.
8. William Barclay, *The Daily Study Bible: The Letter to the Romans* (Philadelphia: The Westminster Press, 1958), 109-112.
9. Packer, 41.
10. J. Oswald Sanders, *Enjoying Intimacy With God* (Chicago: Moody Press, 1980), 19-20.
11. Ibid., 20.
12. Packer, 41.
13. Sanders, 13-14.

Addendum Two: Self-Disciplined Religion

1. Titus 2:6, personal paraphrase.
2. Colossians 2:23, NASB.
3. Proverbs 14:12, personal paraphrase.
4. Matthew 23:26, NASB.
5. Isaiah 53:6, KJV.
6. Ephesians 2:2b, personal paraphrase.
7. See Romans 5:5b.
8. See Hebrews 10:16.
9. See Titus 2:11-12.
10. See Ephesians 5:14.
11. See Titus 2:11.
12. Isaiah 1:18a, NASB.
13. James 1:5, NASB.
14. Proverbs 16:32b, personal paraphrase.
15. Proverbs 25:28, NASB.

ABOUT WEIGHT OF GRACE MINISTRIES

Our heart and history is in discipleship that points believers to a more personal and dependent relationship with God, to a lifestyle in which God directs and empowers godly living, and to service and witness motivated by God's love and a passion for God's truth.

The mission of Weight of Grace Ministries is to provide Biblical discipleship — through teaching, speaking, small group experiences and personal counsel — that communicates to Christians how God's grace applies to every aspect of their lives.

Our ministries include:

- Short-term, didactic groups of 4 to 12 participants: These small groups combine teaching and interacting with others as group members make practical application to their daily lives.
- Classes on the basics of biblical discipleship counseling.
- Seminars and conferences: From two-hour seminars to two-day conferences, Weight of Grace Ministries can bring to your group or church fresh and inspiring information that teaches believers to find greater intimacy with God, power for godly living in all circumstances, and hope for change no matter what the personal struggle. Topics include:
    - Why diets don't work, especially for Christians
    - What it means to be a new creation in Christ
    - Overcoming anger and bitterness
    - The devastating effects of legalism
    - Emotional healing
    - Overcoming the affects of sexual abuse and molestation

Weight of Grace Ministries, Inc. is a 501(c)(3) organization, funded by the gifts of those who wish to participate in extending God's love and grace to women seeking freedom from debilitating obsessions and emotional difficulties. If you would like to contribute, mail your tax-deductible donation to:

> Weight of Grace Ministries
> 11 N.W. 61st Terrace
> Gladstone, MO 64118

For more information about Weight of Grace Ministries, go to www.weightofgrace.org or email us at info@weightofgrace.org.